MW01113583

Clinical Trials Design in Operative and Non Operative Invasive Procedures

Kamal M.F. Itani · Domenic J. Reda
Editors

Clinical Trials Design in Operative and Non Operative Invasive Procedures

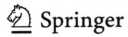 Springer

Editors
Kamal M.F. Itani
Department of Surgery,
  VA Boston Health Care System
Boston University and Harvard Medical
  School
West Roxbury, MA
USA

Domenic J. Reda
Department of Veterans Affairs,
  Cooperative Studies Program
  Coordinating Center
Hines VA Hospital
Hines, IL
USA

ISBN 978-3-319-53876-1   ISBN 978-3-319-53877-8   (eBook)
DOI 10.1007/978-3-319-53877-8

Library of Congress Control Number: 2017932081

Printed on acid-free paper

This Springer imprint is published by Springer Nature
The registered company is Springer International Publishing AG
The registered company address is: Gewerbestrasse 11, 6330 Cham, Switzerland

To Gheed, Fawzi and Karim for their
continuous and unwavering support.
To VA Boston Health Care system, its
patients and staff for being part of my clinical
trials.

Kamal Itani

To the three Mary's in my life.

Domenic Reda

Foreword I

I highly recommend the new text on "Clinical Trials Design in Operative and Non Operative Invasive Procedures" edited by Drs. Itani and Reda. Dr. Itani is a recognized surgical clinical trialist from the Boston VA Medical Center, and Dr. Reda is the Director of the Department of Veterans Affairs Cooperative Studies Program Coordinating Center located in Hines, Illinois. Together they have a wealth of experience in designing, coordinating and conducting clinical trials, which is reflected in the depth and breadth of coverage in this book. The book is an outgrowth of clinical trials courses offered by the American College of Surgeons and the VA Cooperative Studies Program in which they participated and helped to organize. Many of the chapter authors have also participated in these courses, and the book represents a culmination of their considerable expertise in clinical trials.

The text is very encompassing in its coverage, providing a comprehensive resource for any investigator wanting to design, coordinate, execute and analyze a clinical trial. The text is replete with numerous "real world" examples that were carefully chosen to illustrate the concepts being presented. While the text contains material one would normally expect to find about the design, conduct and analysis of clinical trials, it also contains information on unique topics that are often hard to find in the published literature, particularly from one source. For example, the chapter on mistakes in clinical trials "describes some of the mistakes that were made and remedies tried in the design, implementation, conduct, and analysis of over 60 clinical trials and observational studies." The section on "Considerations Specific to Surgical or Procedural Trials" covers a wide array of issues related to studies being conducted in this area, such as surgical training, recruitment and retention, and clinical equipoise, an often overlooked ethical principle in trial design. The chapter on "Publication" highlights issues that investigators need to consider prior to submitting their works for publication, such as having up-to-date protocols and statistical analysis plans (SAP). Many journals now require submitting the study protocol and all protocol amendments, along with the SAP, with the manuscript submission. Reviewers and editors will look at these documents to ensure that the manuscript is consistent with the protocol, particularly the analytic plan. Another relevant chapter involves "Remote Monitoring of Data Quality," which provides a thorough discussion and overview of the U.S. Food and Drug Association's (FDA) guidance on risk-based monitoring (RBM). Because of the increased cost of doing clinical trials and the current capabilities to effectively monitor trial data off-site, RBM is becoming standard practice in many clinical trial settings.

A particularly important topic covered in the book is the chapter on "Trial Registration and Public Access to Data." Trial registration has been mandated by several national and international authorities, including the U.S. FDA (via ClinicalTrials.gov), World Health Organization (WHO), and International Committee of Medical Journal Editors (ICMJE). Registration is also required for publication in many journals, e.g., ICMJE requires trial registration as a condition for publication of research results generated by a clinical trial. Equally important is the reporting of trial results. In the U.S., trial results require posting on ClinicalTrials.gov within one year of ascertaining the primary outcome on the last patient. Thus, investigators need to be mindful of these registration and reporting requirements and plan their trial accordingly.

Another unique feature of the book is the chapter on "Economic Evaluations," which gives a cogent overview of general economic principles relevant to all trials and illustrates them with data from two randomized trials. The chapter concludes with a summary of the lessons learned and recommendations for future research.

So, why this book? While there are many texts on clinical trials, there are none that I know of that target this audience. The book covers many unique issues related to the design, conduct and analysis of clinical trials involving invasive operative and non-operative procedures that would be relevant to surgeons and interventionalists planning trials in this area. Because the book provides comprehensive coverage on many topics not covered elsewhere, it will also be an important resource for those who participate in clinical trials on many different levels, such as investigators, pharmacists, study coordinators, statisticians, health economists, data managers, and regulatory affairs experts.

Peter Peduzzi, Ph.D.
Professor of Biostatistics, Yale School of Public Health;

and

Director, Yale Center for Analytical Sciences
and Yale Data Coordinating Center

Foreword II

I write a Foreword to this book from the perspective of someone who started out like you, as a surgeon and then, later in my career, crossed the line into the very different world of being the clinical editor of JAMA. I went from being worried about anastomotic leaks and wound infections to how to manage hypertension in elderly patients or what medications should be used for diabetes. Transitioning from surgeon to JAMA editor was tough-JAMA is known for its methodological rigor in the review process of research manuscripts-resulting in me being exposed to an intensity of research manuscript reviews like none I experienced in my many years as an academic surgeon. An important misconception was dispelled along the way. I had always assumed that there was a much more substantial body of high quality evidence to support treatment decisions in non-surgical fields such as internal medicine or pediatrics than we had to guide us in surgery. Not true. Certainly, there are many more randomized trials investigating the effects of medications and other sorts of treatments used by non-interventionalists, but even with these trials, considerable uncertainty exists regarding the best treatment approaches for many diseases even when there are numerous RCTs examining various disease entities.

Even though surgeons have done fewer high-quality clinical trials than investigators from other disciplines, some of them have had remarkable effect resulting in substantial improvements in patient care. One breast cancer surgery trial after another showed that less surgery than believed to be necessary resulted in equivalent outcomes. In the span of two generations of surgeons, breast cancer treatment transformed from the disfiguring radical Halstead mastectomy to lumpectomy with radiation to leaving known tumor behind in the axilla of women with sentinel lymph node positive cancers. Surgeons learned via a remarkably well designed trial that accounted for all the pitfalls of clinical trials of interventions that not all laparoscopic approaches are better than their open counterparts-at least for groin hernia operations. Yet, probably the biggest improvement in surgical care in our lifetimes was the introduction of laparoscopic cholecystectomy, which completely replaced the open operation without a single high-quality RCT being necessary.

Not all surgical questions require proof of their utility by performing clinical trials. Yet, when they are necessary they should be performed correctly so that their results are definitive. At JAMA, we review an unfortunately large number of clinical trials that we do not publish because of basic flaws in the design, execution or analysis of clinical trials. Thus, the text "Clinical Trials Design in Operative and Non Operative Invasive Procedures" by Itani, Reda, and colleagues is a welcome addition to the clinical methodology literature. The text is comprehensive covering all aspects of trial design and analysis and the various administrative aspects of trial execution such as IRB considerations, budgeting, funding and getting the trial published. Important emerging concepts such as adaptive trial design and molecular markers and genomic testing are covered.

From a journal editor's perspective, how would I use this book? Of course, all the chapters are useful, but there are certain topics that investigators should pay particular attention to. These are chapters covering material discussing topics where we commonly see mistakes in journal article submitted to JAMA. Trial registration is covered in Chap. 42. Dr. Lucero correctly points out that journals require registration for any study involving an intervention. From our perspective, intervention is not limited to a drug or device. Even quality assurance studies involve an intervention of sorts and requires registration. One of the most common problems we encounter with research manuscripts at JAMA is studies that have incorrect sample size estimation-either because of inadequate consideration of a clinically meaningful difference between groups or inflation of the expected difference in order to keep the number of enrolled subjects small. Investigators trying to sort through these issues will find Chap. 16 particularly helpful.

Missing data either from inadequate follow up of patients or not acquiring all the necessary data when the patients are seen, are common and frequently not adequately considered in clinical research. Chapter 19 with its section on multiple imputation will be helpful in this regard. Many of the common errors we see are summarized in Dr. William Henderson's chapter on mistakes in clinical trials (Chap. 43). Dr. Henderson is a very experienced trialist and his perspective of what can go wrong with a clinical trial deserves serious consideration by young trialists so that they may avoid the pitfalls of their forbearers.

These are just a sampling of chapters in this book and I have highlighted only a few of the problems we see at JAMA that might be rectified had investigators given serious consideration to a book like this one. Clinical research is hard. There are a myriad of pitfalls that any clinical investigator can encounter on the way to answering important clinical questions. Careful consideration of the material presented in this book will help investigators negotiate the complexities of clinical research.

Edward H. Livingston, MD, FACS, AGAF
Deputy Editor for Clinical Reviews and Education
JAMA, Chicago, IL, USA

Preface

Prospective randomized trials evaluating drugs are commonly performed and the results published. Procedures are more likely to be evaluated using small prospective studies without controls usually limited to a few centers or a single investigator expert in the procedure, through a retrospective evaluation of a series of subjects with the intervention or through a retrospective case control study with matching controls. The enthusiasm for new technology, new tools among surgeons and interventionists and the FDA process of allowing them based on patient safety are the major drivers for embracing new technology, procedures and diagnostic tools without proper evaluation for effectiveness, cost and long term results.

Surgeons in particular have been criticized for their lack of scientific approach in evaluating procedures and new technology. Although well designed, properly conducted clinical trials have been published in the last two decades in the surgical and non-operative procedural fields, those specialties are still behind other medical and pharmaceutical specialties in conducting properly constructed clinical trials.

The Department of Veteran Affairs research system was among the first to implement multi-center randomized trials in the various fields of medicine. The Cooperative Studies Program was specifically set up for the purpose of supporting such trials. Some of the largest and most impactful studies have come out of that program. In parallel, the VA Cooperative Studies Program collaborated with the American College of Surgeons to develop a course in the design, conduct and analysis of clinical trials which was sponsored by the American College of Surgeons mostly for surgeons. A similar course was subsequently offered in the VA to VA clinical investigators. Several of the authors of this book have participated in either or both courses and have been encouraged by participants in these courses to come up with this book. This book covers all clinical and statistical aspects for the proper planning, conduct, funding and publication of a clinical trial. It is our hope that this book will be a good reference for any investigator or sponsor planning a clinical trial, especially in the surgical and the non operative invasive fields.

West Roxbury, USA
Hines, USA

Kamal M.F. Itani
Domenic J. Reda

Acknowledgements

We also want to acknowledge the faculty, students and support staff of the best clinical trial courses ever offered at the VA and the American College of Surgeons that both editors had the privilege to lead and participate in.

Kamal M.F. Itani
Domenic J. Reda

Contents

Part XI   Publication

Contributors

Peter Angelos Department of Surgery, The University of Chicago Medicine, Chicago, IL, USA

Ilana Belitskaya-Lévy Cooperative Studies Program Coordinating Center, VA Palo Alto Health Care System, Mountain View, CA, USA

Deepak L. Bhatt Brigham and Women's Hospital Heart & Vascular Center, Harvard Medical School, Boston, MA, USA

Kousick Biswas Cooperative Studies Program Coordinating Center, Office of Research and Development, U.S. Department of Veterans Affairs, VA Medical Center, Perry Point, MD, USA

Judy C. Boughey Division of Subspecialty General Surgery, Mayo Clinic, Rochester, MN, USA

Mary T. Brophy Boston Cooperative Studies Program Coordinating Center, Massachusetts Veterans Epidemiology Research and Information Center, Boston, MA, USA

Marie Campasano Department of Surgical Service, VA Boston Healthcare, West Roxbury, MA, USA

Gregory Campbell GCStat Consulting LLC, Silver Spring, MD, USA

Joseph F. Collins Department of Veteran Affairs, Cooperative Studies Program Coordinating Center, VA Medical Center, Perry Point, MD, USA

Robert George Edson VA Palo Alto Health Care System, Cooperative Studies Program Coordinating Center, Mountain View, CA, USA

Heather L. Evans Department of Surgery, University of Washington, Seattle, WA, USA

Ryan E. Ferguson Boston Cooperative Studies Program Coordinating Center, Massachusetts Veterans Epidemiology Research and Information Center, Boston, MA, USA

Louis Fiore Department of Veterans Affairs Boston Healthcare System, Boston, MA, USA

Jennifer M. Gabany Division of Cardiac Surgery Research (112), VA Boston Healthcare System, West Roxbury, MA, USA

J. Michael Gaziano Medicine, VA Boston Healthcare System, Brigham and Women's Hospital, Harvard Medical School, Boston, MA, USA

William G. Henderson Adult and Child Consortium for Outcomes Research and Delivery Science (ACCORDS) and Department of Biostatistics and Informatics, Colorado School of Public Health, University of Colorado Denver, Aurora, CO, USA

Grant D. Huang U.S. Department of Veterans Affairs, Office of Research and Development, Cooperative Studies Program Central Office, Washington, DC, USA

Denise M. Hynes Health Services Research and Development Service, Edward Hines Jr VA Hospital and Department of Medicine, University of Illinois at Chicago, Hines, IL, USA

Kamal M.F. Itani Department of Surgery, VA Boston Health Care System, Boston University and Harvard Medical School, West Roxbury, MA, USA

Gary R. Johnson VA Cooperative Studies Program, Office of Research and Development, VA Connecticut Healthcare System, Cooperative Studies Program Coordinating Center (151A), West Haven, CT, USA

Ankur Kalra Department of Cardiovascular Medicine, Division of Interventional Cardiology, Harvard Medical School, Beth Israel Deaconess Medical Center, Boston, MA, USA

Tomer Z. Karas Surgical Service, Bruce W. Carter VA Healthcare System, Miami, Miami, FL, USA

Lawrence T. Kim Division of Surgical Oncology, Department of Surgery, University of North Carolina, Chapel Hill, NC, USA

Tassos C. Kyriakides VA Cooperative Studies Program, Office of Research and Development, VA Connecticut Healthcare System, Cooperative Studies Program Coordinating Center (151A), West Haven, CT, USA

Shachar Laks Department of Surgery, University of North Carolina, Chapel Hill, NC, USA

Jennifer E. Layden Public Health Sciences, Loyola University Chicago, Maywood, IL, USA

Eric L. Lazar Department of Surgery, Atlantic Health System, Morristown Medical Center, Morristown, NJ, USA

George Z. Li Department of Surgery, Brigham and Women's Hospital, Boston, MA, USA

Nicole E. Lopez Division of Surgical Oncology, Department of Surgery, University of North Carolina, Chapel Hill, NC, USA

Ying Lu Cooperative Studies Program Coordinating Center, VA Palo Alto Health Care System, Mountain View, CA, USA; Department of Biomedical Data Science, Stanford University School of Medicine, Stanford, CA, USA

Yvonne Lucero Cooperative Studies Program Coordinating Center, Hines Veterans' Affairs Hospital/Loyola University, Hines, IL, USA

Talar W. Markossian Public Health Sciences, Loyola University Chicago, Maywood, IL, USA

Drew Moghanaki Radiation Oncology Service, Hunter Holmes McGuire VA Medical Center, Richmond, VA, USA

Peter R. Nelson Surgical Service, James A. Haley VA Medical Center, Tampa, FL, USA

Leigh Neumayer Department of Surgery, University of Arizona College of Medicine-Tucson, Tucson, AZ, USA

Domenic J. Reda Department of Veterans Affairs, Cooperative Studies Program Coordinating Center (151K), Hines VA Hospital, Hines, IL, USA

Joshua S. Richman Department of Surgery, University of Alabama at Birmingham and the Birmingham VAMC, Birmingham, AL, USA

Mei-Chiung Shih Cooperative Studies Program Coordinating Center, VA Palo Alto Health Care System, Mountain View, CA, USA

Thomas H. Shoultz Department of Surgery, Harborview Medical Center, University of Washington, Seattle, WA, USA

Eileen M. Stock Cooperative Studies Program Coordinating Center, Office of Research and Development, U.S. Department of Veterans Affairs, VA Medical Center, Perry Point, MD, USA

Jennifer Tseng Department of Surgery, The University of Chicago Medicine, Chicago, IL, USA

Hui Wang Cooperative Studies Program Coordinating Center, VA Palo Alto Health Care System, Mountain View, CA, USA

Jiping Wang Department of Surgery, Division of Surgical Oncology, Brigham and Women's Hospital, Dana-Farber Cancer Institute, Boston, MA, USA

Frances M. Weaver Center of Innovation for Complex Chronic Healthcare and Public Health Sciences, Edward Hines Jr. Veterans Administration Hospital and Loyola University Chicago, Hines, IL, USA

Marco A. Zenati Department of Cardiac Surgery, Harvard Medical School, Boston VA Medical Center, Belmont, MA, USA

Part I
Basic Principles

Chapter 1
The Research Question and the Hypothesis

Peter R. Nelson

The Research Question

Getting Started

When first contemplating a clinical trial idea, one should start with a brainstorming session. This is your chance to have fun and simply assemble an inclusive list of ideas that come to mind. These ideas have likely developed from thoughts and experiences over time and may be on note cards or files that have accumulated on your desk or computer in need of some organization. Or, they may be the result of setting aside time dedicated to coming up with an idea either alone or with your research team. For most, it is probably a combination of both. Either way, they may all focus on one disease process with slight variations in concept, or they might cover a wide array of problems within your specialty and likely come from many different sources. Ideas often result from a recent patient, case, or series of cases. They may be the response to a single recent difficult case in which you might have contemplated the need for a new device or a novel application of an existing device. They may arise from hearing a recent presentation at a local grand rounds or at a regional/national scientific meeting or from a recent publication. They may arise from your very own translational research activity. Ideas may also simply arise from idle conversation with a partner or colleague in which you feel there might be a better, safer, or more efficient way to manage a particular clinical problem. And, finally, in this technological and social media age, you might even ask the voice inside your smartphone "What is a good research question?". Try it.

Examples of research ideas that are represented in the referenced clinical trials may have started with simple questions like:

P.R. Nelson (✉)
Surgical Service, James A. Haley VA Medical Center, 13000 Bruce B. Downs Boulevard, Tampa, FL 33612, USA
e-mail: peter.nelson@va.gov

© Springer International Publishing AG 2017
K.M.F. Itani and D.J. Reda (eds.), *Clinical Trials Design in Operative and Non Operative Invasive Procedures*, DOI 10.1007/978-3-319-53877-8_1

- Is total mastectomy necessary? [1]
- Is arthroscopy any good? [2]
- Should we give up on open hernia repair? [3]
- Is surgery necessary for gastroesophageal reflux? [4]
- Can we do endovascular aortic aneurysm repair (EVAR) without incisions? [5]

These ideas start out unrefined, but represent the real thought or feeling you have in reaction to a vexing problem.

Does Your Idea Show Promise?

Before you get too far into thinking about your idea, make an early assessment as to whether or not it is a "good one." This means you need to ask yourself questions like "Is the idea timely and relevant?", "Is the question answerable?", "If so, will the answer change clinical practice?"…meaning "Will it have significant IMPACT?", and "Would it be feasible financially to embark on the study?". These checks and balances begin to address whether or not there is biological rationale for your question if needed; if there is clinical relevance of your question and if so, is there sufficient equipoise within the clinical community surrounding the idea; if the results will be generalizable; and if there is sufficient novelty to the idea to promise the delivery of new knowledge from your efforts? Table 1.1 offers a basic ten-point checklist you can run through to quickly test the merits of your idea.

Refining Your Thoughts

If your idea passes this ten-point evaluation, then it's time to really focus in and start formulating it into a formal "research" question. An essential foundation of clinical trial design is the premise that every clinical trial must center around a

Table 1.1 Ten-point checklist to test a research question	· Do I know the field?
	· Do I know the literature?
	· What areas need further exploration?
	· Has sufficient research already been completed in this area?
	· Could my work fill a gap in the current understanding?
	· If a similar study has been done before, is there room for improvement?
	· Is the timing right for this question to be answered?
	· Would funding sources be interested?
	· Would the target community (i.e., patients, practitioners, health policy makers, etc.) be interested?
	· Will my study have a significant impact on the field?

primary question. The primary question, as well as any related secondary questions of interest (see below), should be carefully vetted, clearly defined, and stated a priori. The primary question should address the key who?, what?, by whom?, when?, how long?, and what result? type questions clearly and succinctly. Therefore, this primary question is the main interest of the trial, whether comparing effectiveness or determining equivalence of two treatments, determining safety and efficacy of a new treatment or procedure, applying existing treatment to a novel cohort of patients or a different disease process, or exploring functional or quality of life impacts of intervention. Logistically this translates into the question being the one that the trial is designed to be capable of answering, the one that the trial is powered to test statistically, and the one that will have the greatest impact following the conduct of a successful trial.

Therefore, the revised versions of the original questions above might start look something like this:

- Can similar results be obtained with breast conservation compared to mastectomy? [1]
- How does arthroscopic surgery impact knee pain and function in patients with osteoarthritis? [2]
- Which is better—open or laparoscopic hernia repair with respect to 2-year recurrence rates? [3]
- How does early laparoscopic anti-reflux surgery compare with optimized medical management for GERD? [4]
- Is percutaneous femoral access comparable to open femoral exposure with respect to overall treatment success following EVAR? [5]

These refined questions now demonstrate clarity in what the researcher is thinking, what will be tested in each of the clinical trials and sheds light on aspects of subject eligibility, what will become the key trial design features, and even what are the critical statistical considerations. Your trial is starting to take shape. Table 1.2 summarizes the key features of the primary research question.

Table 1.2 Primary research question

Key features
· Main interest of trial
· Capable of being answered by trial
· Trial powered to answer this question
· May focus on differences between or equivalence of comparison groups
· States the hypothesis
· Dictates the research design
· Defines the sample
· Identifies the intervention to be studied and the comparison treatment
· Specifies the endpoints/outcomes
· Suggests statistical analytic strategy

Secondary Research Questions

Secondary questions can oftentimes be very important, but at the very least often represent the subtle things that "we really want to know" regarding the treatment of a particular disease process "but were afraid to ask." However, in order to be effective, these questions need to be clearly defined and stated in advance to avoid any question or criticism of post hoc data mining. Secondary questions often dive into more detail within the data generated from a trial and may be aimed at addressing important subgroup analyses, focusing on a single risk factor's association to an outcome, or addressing an alternative, more focused, or less prevalent response variable. However, since these questions are more narrowly focused, the trial is likely not powered to definitively answer them due to the potentially large enrollment that would be required and the statistical challenges that they would present. Therefore, the trialist should avoid the expectation of finding definitive answers to these questions, but should potentially take advantage of the information gained to form the basis for interesting, important future direction for study.

The Hypothesis

The primary research question, once defined, then sets the foundation for subsequent trial design and conduct. First, the primary question must be restated as the primary hypothesis to be tested by the trial. For the researcher, it is more than just simply restating or rewording the question to a statement, but this is where you need to commit to what you think the trial is going to show once it is completed. You need to "pick sides" and define this in advance in a clear statement. The null hypothesis has critical meaning statistically and will be discussed elsewhere, but at this point you need to recognize that it defines that there will be no difference between comparison groups in your trial. Therefore, you need to define whether you agree with this assumption or whether you feel your trial will result in a detectable, meaningful difference for the intervention studied. Importantly, this is another fun part of the process because you eventually get to see if you're "right" once the trial is complete.

For the referenced trial examples, the hypotheses look like this:

- Segmental mastectomy (with or without radiation) provides comparable results to total mastectomy in patients with Stage I and II breast tumors ≤ 4 cm in size [1].
- Arthroscopic knee surgery (i.e., debridement, lavage) will significantly reduce pain and improve functionality in patients with osteoarthritis compared to sham [2].
- Open tension-free hernia repair and laparoscopic tension-free hernia repair are equivalent with respect to 2-year hernia recurrence rates [3].

- Laparoscopic fundoplication can significantly improve outcomes compared to long-term drug treatment for chronic GERD [4].
- Percutaneous femoral arterial access using large bore closure with a preclose technique will provide the same or better results than surgical femoral exposure with respect to vascular complications and overall treatment success following EVAR [5].

Once you've stated your hypothesis, it needs to be testable. This seems implied, but there needs to be clearly defined endpoints and validated measurement tools available to pursue the answer. More on this later.

In addition to the hypothesis, the research question begins to define the other structural components of your trial design. It indicates the type of trial planned whether single- or multi-arm, single- or multicenter, randomized or non-randomized, or explanatory or pragmatic in design, etc. It also begins to define the patient population to be studied and the sample to be enrolled including some direction as to how subjects will be identified, what the control group might look like, and what the initial inclusion/exclusion criteria might look like. It will indicate the intervention to be offered to the subjects and if/how it will be tested for safety, effectiveness, and/or economics. And finally it will define the endpoints and analyses to be used to test the hypothesis and answer the question. These relationships will be developed in the following chapters.

"Practical Exercise"

As a practical exercise, you can use the guidelines put forth in this chapter to identify a research question you are interested in developing. You can then carry this through the entire text and in the end you will have your clinical trial established. One brief example from a vascular surgery perspective could be the treatment of intermittent claudication. Claudication results from the progression of mild to moderate peripheral arterial disease. At this early stage, medical management along with smoking cessation and structured exercise have proved to be effective for upwards of 80% of patients. The Achilles heal of this strategy is the lack of formal programs and the resulting poor compliance with the noninvasive methods in patients without supervision. This unfortunately results in early adoption of invasive intervention with angioplasty/atherectomy/stenting and ultimately the risk of premature acceleration of disease with intervention failure and critical limb ischemia. If one were to develop a research question in this area, he/she might start with:

- Does exercise really help with claudication?

What this question doesn't clearly define are critical concepts like the following. Help? Help how? Help whom? With what degree of claudication? What type of exercise? Within the context of what medical therapy? How frequently?

How intense? How are we going to implement and assess the compliance with exercise? And, how will we determine if exercise actually helps? Therefore, we might refine our question to:

- Do structured walking, stationary bicycle, weight-based resistance, or aquatic exercise offer superior benefit over unsupervised standard care in terms of pain relief, walking distance, and walking duration in patients with peripheral arterial disease compliant with the best medical therapy but suffering from disabling claudication?

Even this question is a little complex since it is potentially asking three questions as to whether the intervention will benefit (1) pain relief, (2) walking distance, and/or (3) walking duration. Therefore, you'd have two options to simplify this issue. First, you could consider a composite endpoint of all three outcome measures together (see Chap. 2). Or, perhaps better, you could determine which of these outcomes you view as having the most critical impact. Let's say you decide that from a patient perspective, pain relief would be considered most important. This would lead to the following primary hypothesis:

- Any structured exercise methodology, when tailored to a specific patient's needs to optimize compliance, will result in overall improvement in pain-free walking ability, when combined with the best medical therapy compared to unsupervised current standard medical practice.

Using this question and hypothesis as a guide, one could begin to envision a randomized prospective clinical trial comparing standard medical treatment consisting of general recommendations for smoking cessation and increased exercise to a structured program with optimized medical therapy, assisted smoking cessation, and structured supervised exercise specifically tailored to an individual patient's comorbidities and physical condition aimed primarily at a pain-free walking goal. Then, the effects of the intervention on walking duration and distance might then be considered the most important secondary questions to ask. Finally, you might then complete the process by considering other secondary questions such as: (1) Will establishment of community-based outreach with long-term monitoring improve compliance and durability of the intervention? and (2) Will patient-specific molecular biomarkers or gene profiles improve traditional clinical prediction models to identify a cohort of subjects in the population that might truly benefit from early intervention? These questions might be more exploratory, but important to pursue as part of this trial at least for proof-of-principle confirmation leading to more detailed subsequent validation trials.

Summary

A clear, thoughtfully designed research question is a critical start to your journey toward a successful clinical trial. You can't answer every question so choose one that can be answered. Once you've defined your primary question, it needs to be relevant, feasible, and generalizable. Your subsequent trial design depends on this primary question as the one you hope to answer, your hypothesis should then translate directly from the question, and your endpoint(s), patient selection, intervention, and analyses will all follow as the process progresses. It is an iterative process, however, and you should continuously reflect back to the original question as the study evolves to maintain focus. Also keep in mind that the results of clinical trials generally have greater relevance when the design is pragmatic, but don't always answer mechanistic questions, and are often a compromise between the ideal and the practical. In any case, dedicated effort spent at this beginning stage often sets your clinical trial up for success.

References

1. Fisher B, Bauer M, Margolese R, et al. Five-year results of a randomized clinical trial comparing total mastectomy and segmental mastectomy with or without radiation in the treatment of breast cancer. N Engl J Med. 1985;31:665–73.
2. Moseley JB, O'Malley K, Peterson N, et al. A controlled trial of arthroscopic surgery for osteoarthritis of the knee. N Engl J Med. 2002;347:81–8.
3. Neumayer L, Gobbie-Hurder A, Jonasson O, et al. Open mesh versus laparoscopic mesh repair of inguinal hernia. N Engl J Med. 2004;350:1819–27.
4. Grant AM, Wileman SM, Ramsay CR, et al. Minimal access surgery compared with medical management for chronic gastrooesophageal reflux disease: UK collaborative randomized trial. Br Med J. 2008;337:a2664.
5. Nelson PR, Kracjer Z, Kansal N, Rao V, Bianchi C, Hashemi H, Jones P, Bacharach JM. Multicenter, randomized, controlled trial outcomes of totally percutaneous aortic aneurysm repair (The PEVAR Trial). J Vasc Surg. 2014;59:1181–94.

Chapter 2
Primary and Secondary Endpoints

Peter R. Nelson

General Concepts

As outlined in the prior chapter, the research questions and resulting hypotheses should lead the investigator directly to the selection of the study endpoints suitable to provide the desired answers. All endpoints, but especially the primary endpoint, need to be clearly defined and redefined at the beginning of the design phase of the trial. Time spent here is critical and should be deliberate. The endpoints chosen must be clinically relevant, focused, discrete, and easily measurable. These endpoints should be equally defined for and applicable to all subjects enrolled, be unbiased, and provide conservative answers to the research questions proposed. Further, these endpoints should ideally be established in and have validity from prior investigation and clinical trials in the field. Avoid relying on a novel, "home grown," untested, non-validated outcome measure, especially as your primary endpoint. You may reserve such novel measurements for secondary endpoints with the hopes of establishing the relevance and validity needed for use in future studies. The importance of this effort is that once a research subject reaches an endpoint, their participation in the study and analyses generally stops, so being confident that the endpoint(s) chosen clearly define the clinical outcome desired is paramount.

Depending on the incidence of the endpoint chosen, a single discrete endpoint may be appropriate for relatively frequent occurrences, or a composite endpoint may be necessary when one of several less frequent events would satisfy censoring a subject to limit the required sample size to power the study. A single endpoint is ideal because it can be well defined, is likely clearly applicable and equally

P.R. Nelson (✉)
Surgical Service, James A. Haley VA Medical Center, 13000 Bruce B. Downs Boulevard, Tampa, FL 33612, USA
e-mail: peter.nelson@va.gov

© Springer International Publishing AG 2017   11
K.M.F. Itani and D.J. Reda (eds.), *Clinical Trials Design in Operative and Non Operative Invasive Procedures*, DOI 10.1007/978-3-319-53877-8_2

measurable for every study participant, and simplifies the analyses required to draw important definitive study conclusions. As indicated, composite endpoints can be useful to create a higher frequency of study events, thus keeping the number of subjects required to power the study manageable. But use caution when deciding on a composite primary study endpoint. The components of a composite endpoint each individually need to be clearly clinically relevant and validated for the disease process and the study being conducted. Ideally, these components should also be interrelated so that, independent of which component triggers an event, it is intuitive to lump them together for the primary analysis. Definition of the composite endpoint is even more important so that throughout the design, implementation, and conduct of the trial it is clear. Finally, in the eventual publication of the trial results, such a composite endpoint needs to be clearly presented. It will be the reader's tendency to split out the components of a composite endpoint and discuss the one most relevant to their practice or most fitting to their bias, and this can undermine the ultimate impact that the study might have.

Whether using a single or composite endpoint, the event and its measure must have established validity and a predetermined hierarchy for event significance should be defined. In some cases, a surrogate endpoint may be considered if necessary to again limit to a manageable sample size, or more importantly to reduce time to an event (and thus overall duration of a trial). A theoretical example would be a biomarker closely correlated with mortality. If the biomarker were to be positive, then the study investigators would not have to wait the months or years for the patient to expire in order to record their event. There may be more practical examples, but in any case, the surrogate endpoint must have an established strong correlation with the true endpoint desired. A list of some commonly used clinical endpoints is shown in Table 2.1, and some pros and cons of their use in your trial are offered below.

Measurement

When defining your trial endpoint(s), you need to consider whether a reliable measurement tool currently exists for accurate assessment of subject outcomes. These measurements should offer sensibility (common sense, clinical relevance), reliability (intra- and inter-observer), validity (true representation of the endpoint, comparison to a gold standard), responsiveness (sensitivity, ability to accurately detect required degree of clinical change), and feasibility (existing technology and expertise, noninvasive, user-friendly, cost-effective). Not every tool will have optimal characteristics in every one of these aspects, but you will need to choose the tool that has the best overall utility for your trial (Fig. 2.1). For example, a relevant, very accurate tool might be available, but it might be invasive and add additional unnecessary risk for the subjects, or it might be prohibitively costly compared to a simpler option. In making these critical decisions, you might opt for a tool that has reasonable sensitivity to detect your endpoint, but is safe, noninvasive, easy to use

Table 2.1 Commonly used trial endpoints

Endpoint	Examples	Pros/cons
Mortality	30-day mortality In-hospital mortality All-cause mortality Disease-specific mortality Long-term mortality Surrogate: event-free survival	Easily defined Multiple sources Generalizable Time to event Missing data points Censored/incomplete data
Morbidity	Short-term complications Longer term sequelae Treatment complications Adverse drug reactions Myocardial infarction Infection Blood transfusion/reaction Length of stay Rehabilitation Return to work/function Overall satisfaction Quality of Life	Commonality and Disease specificity Patient centered Objective auditing Consistent definition Complex measurement Data management Subject variance Blinding
Pain scale	Numerical scale Visual analog scales Surrogate: analgesic usage	Common Generalizable Time course analysis Subjective Subject–subject variance
Procedural	Procedural detail Technical/intraprocedural complications Periprocedural complications Surgical site infection	Procedure specific Translational Short time to event Procedure variability Procedural bias Reporting bias Blinding
Pharmaceutical	Side effects Efficacy Dose response Comparison to standard or placebo	Establish safety and efficacy of novel drug(s) Explore beyond primary indication of a drug Adjunctive use with surgical procedures Side effect profiles Intolerance, compliance Confounding medications Placebo effect
Molecular	Gene expression profiling Single-nucleotide polymorphisms Genome-wide association Protein biomarkers	Adds biological information to clinical data Local and systemic factors Potentially mechanistic Evolving technology Expensive Not real time Limited bioinformatics

(continued)

Table 2.1 (continued)

Endpoint	Examples	Pros/cons
Quality of life (QOL)	Generic health-related QOL Disease-specific QOL	Validated tools Multi-domain constructs Patient centered Expand traditional clinical endpoints Subjective Poor compliance/response rates Multiple tools required Difficult to develop/validate new tools
Economic	Hospital charges Hospital costs (direct, indirect) Quality-adjusted life years (QALYs) Perspective of economic burden Cost-benefit Cost-effectiveness Cost-utility	Aggregate versus itemized costs Health policy comparisons Resource utilization Data availability Data accuracy Generalizability between health-care systems Time/inflation adjustments

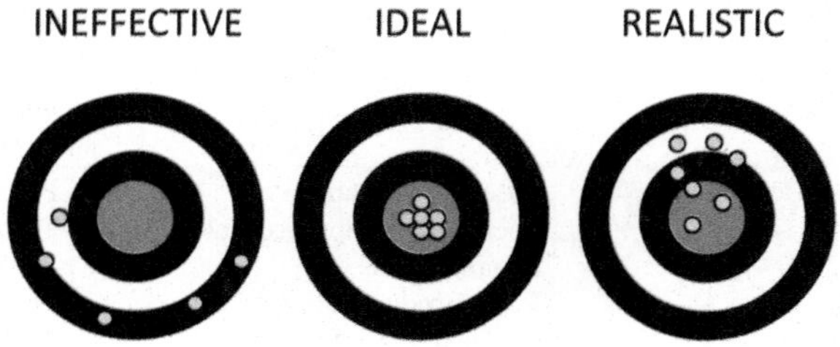

Fig. 2.1 Test characteristics to measure endpoints

INEFFECTIVE   IDEAL   REALISTIC

and interpret, and more affordable. Whatever the situation, once you choose a measurement method, stay with it throughout the entire trial for all subjects, even in cases where new technology might emerge, to ensure consistency and reliability of your data and the ability to comprehensively analyze the full complement of your results.

The Primary Endpoint

The primary endpoint should directly answer the primary research question so is in essence "the answer" to your trial. Like the primary question, defining the primary endpoint requires critical attention at the outset. Selecting the wrong endpoint could prove catastrophic to your trial's success down the road. The primary endpoint has at least three essential features: (1) it needs to be clearly defined a priori and maintained consistent throughout the conduct of the trial; (2) the sample size calculation (discussed elsewhere) will be specifically based on known parameters surrounding this endpoint; and (3) the main conclusions of the trial reported will be focused exclusively on this outcome. Therefore, the primary endpoint absolutely needs to satisfy the features described above as being focused, discrete, easily measurable, applicable equally to all subjects, conservative, and unbiased.

Examples of primary endpoints in representative clinical trials are presented below:

- Composite disease-free survival, distant disease-free survival, and overall survival [1]
- Self-reported pain scoring over two years postintervention [2]
- Hernia recurrence within two years following repair [3]
- REFLUX quality of life score and postoperative complications at one year [4]
- Overall treatment success as defined as successful endovascular aneurysm repair in the absence of major adverse events or vascular access complications [5].

As you can see, these examples include a variety of different endpoints. There are both singular and composite endpoints. There are endpoints that require subject self-reporting, like the pain scale and quality of life assessments, that may require clear instruction and unbiased supervision to be sure the information captured is complete, accurate, and consistent. As the investigator, you should try to stick with discrete, defined objective endpoints whenever available relevant to the subject matter. However, even a seemingly objective endpoint, like hernia recurrence, still requires strict definition depending on who is assigned to determine event occurrence and complete follow-up so that no events are missed in the analyses.

Secondary Endpoints

Secondary endpoints should align with and answer the secondary questions proposed in the study design. They often represent outcomes that are not feasible to assess as an independent primary endpoint, but may well represent "what you really want to study" with the project. They still need to be defined a priori like the primary endpoint, again especially to avoid criticisms of data mining in the post hoc analysis of the study results. They should be limited to a reasonable number that is feasible within the structure and timeframe of the study, but they can be more outreaching, exploratory, and forward thinking. These again may represent endpoints where a definitive answer may not be realized or expected, but that will provide important rationale for future study.

Secondary endpoints can include a wide variety of parameters associated with the trial focus and intervention. They are often designed to provide biological or additional clinical data to support the primary endpoint. In this way, the investigators might start to identify differences in outcomes based on different patient-specific features. These often include patient demographics such as age, gender, race/ethnicity, education, or socioeconomic status. They can also explore specific risk factors or comorbidities that are known or thought to influence the primary endpoint. Finally, they may be aimed to explore specific biological data such as circulating protein biomarkers, molecular genetic differences, or specific pathology findings such as tissue markers that might help to refine the diagnosis and outcomes studied moving toward a truly personalized medicine concept.

Secondary endpoint selection can take on one of the two different general strategies: (1) independent secondary endpoint measurement and (2) subgroup analyses. For the former, the investigators might want to look at the individual components of a composite primary endpoint, for example. The composite endpoint was chosen to allow effective study design and power, but this would allow independent determination of potential differential outcomes for each individual parameter. The result of this type of exploration would presumably lead to assessing the feasibility of powering an additional study specifically to that singular endpoint. Subgroup analyses are common. It is important again to define and limit these up front to avoid the temptation and criticism of post hoc analyses. Things to keep in mind are that the subjects in the trial are likely not randomized based on these subgroup definitions so they may not be equally represented, and by definition, the subgroups will have a smaller sample size and will likely not provide sufficient power for definitive analyses. But again, the focus here is to explore interesting associated outcomes that enhance the primary outcome and fuel further investigation.

For the selected trial examples referred to in the bibliography, the secondary endpoints were as follows:

- Time to treatment failure and recurrence; impact of radiation exposure [1]
- Self-reported assessment of pain and function; objective testing of walking and stair climbing [2]
- Perioperative complications; perioperative mortality; patient-centered outcomes of pain, function, activity [3]
- Health status using a validated questionnaire; serious morbidity; perioperative complications and mortality [4]
- Successful vascular access closure; operation time; ICU requirements; hospital length of stay; blood loss/transfusion; pain scale/analgesia; health-related quality of life; stent graft potency/integrity [5].

As you can see, secondary endpoints can be more numerous. In some cases, they are still fairly well defined and discrete such as time to an event, recorded perioperative parameters, mortality (disease specific or overall), specific objective testing or imaging, or defined validated health questionnaires. Other times, they are more subjective or open-ended such as patient-reported pain and function and complications or impact of a treatment method. In these cases, the endpoints may be reasonable given that they are related to the primary endpoint but not the main focus of the trial.

Pros and Cons of Common Endpoints

The potential strengths and possible pitfalls of commonly used study endpoints are discussed briefly here and summarized in Table 2.1.

Mortality

This is a discrete endpoint that is generally reliable and achievable with direct observation or through established databases such as the Social Security Death Index (SSDI). Disease-specific mortality can sometimes be harder to define or validate. The main downside is time to the event. Mortality may not occur within the timeframe of your study so focusing on a shorter time frame such as peri-operative or 30-day mortality may be feasible, 5-year mortality is often achievable, or identifying a surrogate measure that might provide insight within the desired, feasible timeframe.

Morbidity

These can often be crucial endpoints, but definition is paramount. They may be disease specific which may limit generalizability. They may also vary from subject to subject making data collection/reconciliation critical. They may also be difficult to measure and cause challenges with blinding.

Pain

This is obviously a very subjective endpoint, but is common and often important. Challenges can be partially overcome with validated pain scoring systems incorporating visual and analog scales. Pain can be measured over time. Analgesic use can potentially provide a surrogate measure, but can vary significantly from patient to patient.

Procedural Outcomes

These are often critical procedure-specific outcomes with short timing to an event. Their generalizability can be challenged by uncontrollable regional or practitioner-specific differences in procedural technique. They are susceptible to selection, procedural, and reporting biases, and can pose additional challenges with blinding.

Pharmaceutical

These endpoints are obviously critical for drug studies. An evolving side effects profile, especially for a novel drug, can be the Achilles' heel in these trials creating a lot of regulatory activity and potentially posing safety and ethical concerns for enrollment. Compliance and drug interactions need to be closely monitored. Comparison is typically to an alternative medication or to placebo.

Molecular Information

These endpoints offer promise for a biological or mechanistic rationale to the study intervention and outcomes. Patient to patient variability creates significant variance in the data that often needs to be addressed. The techniques for these analyses are still expensive and do not always offer immediate point-of-care feedback that may impact their utility.

Quality of Life

These patient-centric endpoints are becoming increasingly important to extend beyond typical clinical outcomes in trial design. Validated general health and disease-specific questionnaires are being refined and are increasingly more available making them more generalizable. These resources need to be used as constructed, however, and one needs to avoid the temptation to just use the part of a tool that is of interest or to develop and use an unvalidated survey.

Economics/Costs

The impact of intervention on health-care expenditures is also becoming increasingly important for clinical trial design. The biggest challenge with these endpoints is the availability and accuracy of data and the limited generalizability of the information regionally or between health-care systems. Cost can be studied over time, but adjustments for inflation, etc. need to be anticipated and incorporated.

"Practical Exercise"

To continue our practical exercise, you can use the guidelines put forth in this chapter to identify primary and secondary endpoints for our hypothetical trial. Since we proposed examining various exercise modalities for the non-surgical management of claudication, a reasonable primary endpoint would be reduction in pain induced by walking compared between the two treatment groups—structured exercise versus unsupervised standard care. If not included in the primary endpoint, important secondary endpoints would focus on walking distance, and walking duration compared between the different exercise groups. Standard tools like an ankle brachial index, the 6-min walk test, the Vascular Quality of Life (VascuQol) questionnaire, and the Walking Impairment Questionnaire (WIQ) could be used reliably to measure these endpoints. Another desirable secondary endpoint might be successful avoidance of endovascular or surgical revascularization or amputation over time, but depending on the time to event, this would need definition. Finally, molecular methodologies might be used to add biological rationale to the primary endpoint and/or predictive capability for failure of conservative management and the potential benefit for early revascularization.

Summary

A clearly defined, relevant primary endpoint is critical to successful clinical trial design. Then, selecting appropriate, relevant, reasonably simple, reliable, and valid measurement tools that are sensitive to the disease process and the desired differences examined is essential. If you accomplish this, you are one step closer to empowering your trial to provide a definitive answer to the question being studied. Secondary endpoints, established at the beginning, allow you to explore your data in more depth and to answer related questions that may be (more) interesting, but are not the main focus of the trial, even if the primary endpoint turns out differently than expected. These secondary endpoints establish the premise for future direction of study and the need for additional clinical trials.

References

1. Fisher B, Bauer M, Margolese R, et al. Five-year results of a randomized clinical trial comparing total mastectomy and segmental mastectomy with or without radiation in the treatment of breast cancer. N Engl J Med. 1985;31:665–73.
2. Moseley JB, O'Malley K, Peterson N, et al. A controlled trial of arthroscopic surgery for osteoarthritis of the knee. N Engl J Med. 2002;347:81–8.
3. Neumayer L, Gobbie-Hurder A, Jonasson O, et al. Open mesh versus laparoscopic mesh repair of inguinal hernia. N Engl J Med. 2004;350:1819–27.

4. Grant AM, Wileman SM, Ramsay CR, et al. Minimal Access surgery compared with medical management for chronic gastrooesophageal reflux disease: UK collaborative randomized trial. Br Med J. 2008;337:a2664.
5. Nelson PR, Kracjer Z, Kansal N, Rao V, Bianchi C, Hashemi H, Jones P, Bacharach JM. Multicenter, randomized, controlled trial outcomes of totally percutaneous aortic aneurysm repair (The PEVAR trial). J Vasc Surg. 2014;59:1181–94.

Chapter 3
Intervention and Control Groups

Peter R. Nelson

General Concepts

Like the study endpoints, the interventions and controls of any trial are originally identified in the primary research question, further defining the importance of getting the question right from the outset. Although presented here as the next step in clinical trial design, the establishment of the intervention to be studied occurs concurrently with the conceptualization of the primary research question and is inherently closely linked to the definition of study endpoints since they are likely specific to the intervention. Along with these other critical components of the design phase, the time spent defining the intervention a priori is essential to the eventual success of the trial. In order to move forward, it is critical to establish the intervention as: (1) relevant to advancing the treatment of the disease being studied; (2) having sufficient equipoise in the medical community regarding its potential role in that treatment; and (3) potentially offering something in some way better than the current standard, if one exists, especially if it incurs potential risk to the subjects. Finally, the proper control group needs to be defined for optimal evaluation of the impact of the intervention so that any conclusions drawn are believable, applicable, and generalizable.

There are different approaches to defining the intervention for your trial. It may be that the general nature of an intervention forces the definition because there is only one way to approach it. This would be the case where the intervention has clearly established, specific instructions. However, most interventions are subject to at least a moderate degree of modification based on a specific clinical situation, the preferences/biases of the interventionist involved, learned experiences with the intervention or similar procedures over time, and/or the development of newer

P.R. Nelson (✉)
Surgical Service, James A. Haley VA Medical Center, 13000 Bruce B. Downs Boulevard, Tampa, FL 33612, USA
e-mail: peter.nelson@va.gov

© Springer International Publishing AG 2017
K.M.F. Itani and D.J. Reda (eds.), *Clinical Trials Design in Operative and Non Operative Invasive Procedures*, DOI 10.1007/978-3-319-53877-8_3

technology that may be adopted without significant scrutiny. Therefore, the investigator needs to decide whether he/she wants to be very specific and define every aspect of the intervention, or if they want to leave some decision making to the investigators in the trial.

For the former, your study protocol may mandate the intervention be implemented according to the specific instructions for use (IFU) guidelines defined for that device, procedure, or process. Alternatives, if they exist, in the market or in practice would not be allowed. If this is the case, then you will likely need to anticipate providing specific training for each investigator or selecting only investigators with documented prior experience, or both. You may also want to include a roll-in phase for the trial to be sure each site can demonstrate competency with the intervention. Being this direct as to the details of the intervention has the advantage of knowing that it is being applied uniformly to all study subjects independent of the particular circumstances for any given subject, the study site or particular investigator involved, or what may be done outside the trial parameters. The intervention will not be left up to interpretation, and therefore, the analysis will be cleaner. The potential down side to such fine control over the intervention is that any small departure from the standard could threaten a subject's eligibility to continue in the trial, may present logistic challenges with how to collect and analyze that subject's data, or at the very least will raise concern of the governing institutional review board or data safety monitoring board as to the appropriateness and ethics of the protocol deviation. Finally, this level of micromanagement may negatively impact study enrollment. If a site or an individual investigator feels they offer a "better" approach than what is defined in the protocol, it might lead them to proceed with treatment outside of the trial. In addition to posing unexpected challenges with enrollment targets, this might also have the effect of inappropriately narrowing the subject pool and potentially limiting generalizability.

The alternative is a more pragmatic approach to the intervention. This adopts the concept that there may be more than one way of doing things (within reason) and allows for some investigator discretion as to how to apply the intervention to each individual subject. The advantages of this approach would be better buy-in from the investigators if they are being empowered to manage the intervention and perhaps better enrollment as a result. It also potentially offers the appearance of a "real-world" approach, if it is generally accepted that variations in the technique exist, which may ultimately lead to better generalization of the study results. Your conclusions will reflect "how it's being done in the community." A major limitation of this pragmatic strategy is that the intervention may be applied differently every time for every subject or at least differently in the hands of different investigators. Subtle factors with respect to patient selection and/or variations in procedural technique that may affect the outcomes will not be controlled. For example, if you are studying a certain procedure, but perhaps there are four or five Food and Drug Administration (FDA) approved devices that might be available, you might not mandate a specific device. Alternatively, you might allow the site investigators to choose the device they have the most experience with or think might be best suited for an individual study subject. Although this introduces variation difficult to account for, it may have appeal because it reflects current practice. A potential solution for this, discussed elsewhere in more detail, might be to stratify enrollment and/or structure analyses by the individual investigator or study site, or by the different device(s) in the example above. A secondary endpoint analysis might then explore these variations in the intervention in more detail.

Interventions

The following is a brief discussion of commonly studied categories of intervention. It is obviously not meant to be exhaustive and is intentionally generic in nature, but will provide a decent overview of possible strategies to consider.

Pharmacologic Intervention

Medical or pharmacologic interventions are obviously commonly studied. It may be that you want to study a drug new to the market and compare results to either a prior standard medication or to a placebo control. The trial may focus on testing the drug in healthy subjects to assess dosing (phase I), on initial safety and efficacy of the drug in subjects with the disease of interest (phase II), or most commonly full study of safety, efficacy, and effectiveness in a randomized cohort of subjects with the disease (phase III). These trials might test a novel class of drug where no precedent exists or a novel drug to a previous standard within its same class to establish brand-naming and patent rights. One caution with novel drug studies is to be vigilant keeping up with reported adverse drug events and if they become numerous or raise safety concerns, re-evaluate your willingness to enroll subjects.

Other, sometimes simpler, pharmacologic studies are designed to test existing drugs in novel ways. One such approach may be to explore an off-label indication exploiting known, often unrelated, potentially beneficial, ancillary effects of the drug seen in other studies. This intervention may be studied in isolation or may involve periprocedural use of a medication to improve surgical outcomes in a more complex trial design. Another approach may be focused on optimizing use of existing medical therapy or combination therapies. There may be situations where efficacy has been established in prior studies for individual drugs, but they were not studied in combination. Or, perhaps effectiveness of individual or combination therapy, despite efficacy, has fallen short due to poor implementation into practice, and therefore, structured delivery and follow-up may be the intervention tested. This latter concept may be used to establish "best medical therapy" to which other interventions may then be compared. Finally, the study of individual variable response rates to drugs is becoming more common as advanced molecular tools are becoming available identifying mutations in drug activity and/or metabolism affecting efficacy for both novel and commonly prescribed medications [1].

Procedural Intervention

In the surgical and other interventional fields, procedural or device trials predominate. Like pharmacologic studies, procedural trials may focus on new, conditionally approved/exempted devices or techniques. These, due to their experimental nature and high level of scrutiny, will have more structure and rigid definition to them because FDA approval is likely pending study results. Novel devices or procedures may be studied in a single-arm nature for safety and efficacy, but are more commonly compared to an existing device or procedure, or to best medical management. Beyond these structured device trials, strategies for investigator initiated trials include comparison of a new device to market to the prior standard or market leader, comparison of a minimally invasive approach to a standard open surgical technique, application of an existing device or technique to a new disease of interest, comparison of a novel technique to standard medical therapy, or even comparison of a new or existing procedure to a sham procedural control. The endpoints for these interventions will vary based on the primary question to be answered and need to be carefully defined. However, these investigator-designed protocols present the opportunity to choose between a detailed structured protocol much like investigational device exemption trials versus incorporating a pragmatic strategy with flexibility in the protocol allowing site investigators to adapt where needed.

Regardless of design, many important studies may challenge "gold standard" procedures, supported by years of experience and evidence and the associated dogma, while promising evolution and innovation in the field with the adoption of new technology. For this reason, careful assessment of existing equipoise in the field, selection of investigators who can set aside bias and objectively participate, and in some cases, designing multispecialty studies are critical to trial success. Several of these procedural trial approaches are represented in the selected trial examples referenced [2–6].

Patient Care Intervention

Whether the clinical care focus is medical or surgical, there may be aspects of the inherent patient care that are worth systematically studying. Almost any component of outpatient, inpatient, or periprocedural care is potentially open to investigation. Your interest may be in pre-procedural areas like disease prevention, screening and early detection, strategies to avoid or delay invasive therapies, or preoperative evaluation or optimization. The emphasis may be more periprocedural by examining specific intraprocedural technical steps or adjuncts, adjuvant pharmacologic treatments, anesthetic approaches, or immediate postoperative care. Commonly post-procedural care is the focus of critical study including morbidity prevention, wound care, additional pharmacologic therapy (i.e., antibiotics, analgesia, anticoagulants), nutritional support, physical or occupational therapy, disposition following inpatient treatment, quality of life measures, or short-, medium-, or long-term care for optimal outcomes. There may still be other aspects of care beyond these examples that may be of primary interest and amenable to study.

The interventions in these types of studies may have detailed protocols associated with them, especially if specific devices or applications are being tested, but often they will be more descriptive and broad in nature. Despite this, approach the study design phase with the same level of attention to detail and rigor as seen for more discrete interventions to present a clear strategy, optimize adherence to the protocol, and ensure consistent reliable results. Sometimes identifying new information in these periprocedural components can have as big or bigger impact on clinical practice as developing an entirely new procedural intervention.

In the referenced trials, the interventions studied were as follows:

- Segmental mastectomy with/without irradiation for Stage I and II breast cancer [2].
- Arthroscopic lavage with/without debridement for osteoarthritis [3].
- Laparoscopic mesh inguinal hernia repair [4].
- Laparoscopic fundoplication for gastroesophageal reflux disease (GERD) [5].
- Percutaneous femoral artery access for endovascular aortic repair (EVAR) [6].

Three out of five of these interventions focus on newer, less invasive approaches to existing surgical diseases. The remaining two evaluate surgical intervention in cases where medical management as the standard may be called into question. In all cases, comparative effectiveness of a novel approach to a prior standard is examined.

Control Groups

Once you've determined what makes up your interventional cohort, you need to define the comparator group or the controls. The control group needs to be equally carefully defined as the intervention group so that you don't end up with an ineffective comparison in the end that threatens the validity of your results. Usually, but not always, the control group will be an untreated cohort or a group receiving the "gold standard" accepted treatment. The former might be assessing a new surgical intervention versus standard medical treatment, the latter a new technique being compared to the previously accepted standard procedure. Either way, the focus is on comparative effectiveness of two treatment strategies that have relevance to the disease being studied with promise to change clinical practice if the outcomes are significant. These approaches might require different design components and may pose different challenges with consent and enrollment, but ultimately subjects will be randomized to either the intervention or control arm of the study, so there needs to be support for and established safety with either treatment, and there needs to be sufficient equipoise to warrant the comparison.

In the selected clinical trials, the comparator groups were defined as follows:

- Total mastectomy for Stage I and II breast cancer [2].
- Sham arthroscopic surgery in patients with osteoarthritis [3].
- Open surgical mesh inguinal hernia repair [4].
- Medical management for GERD [5].
- Open surgical femoral exposure for EVAR [6].

Three studies include comparison of a newer, less invasive approach being compared to the prior surgical standard. The other two compare surgical intervention to non-surgical medical controls; both familiar strategies. However, one of the latter groups employs a sham operation in the untreated control group in an effort to control for any placebo effect from the procedure [3]. The use of sham operations in placebo surgery is controversial. It raises significant concerns regarding excessive risk for no expected benefit, but serves as the only way to create true blinding in a procedural intervention trial.

Blinding

To expand upon this, blinding is the process of concealing subject allocation groups from the patients and investigators involved in a clinical trial. Randomization at the outset of a trial minimizes differences between treatment groups, but the best/only way to maintain the rigor of this process throughout the trial is through blinding. Blinding aims to eliminate the introduction of bias with the application of the intervention, in peri-interventional care, or in the assessment of outcomes that might all come from knowing any given subject's treatment assignment [7]. If the investigators or subjects cannot be blinded, blinding data collectors, outcome adjudicators, and/or data analysts can maintain some degree of integrity of the process. In pharmacologic trials, blinding is more easily achieved through the use of placebo controls that can easily mimic the study drug in appearance. In a procedural trial, blinding is more difficult but may be achieved by considering the feasibility and ethics of a placebo/sham surgery that is as close to the intervention surgery as possible but eliminates the therapeutic component. The difficulty is obvious, the control subjects will incur some, even if minimized, risk of an incision, anesthesia, etc., without any expected benefit. Extensive planning and communication with institutional review and ethics boards would be required if a sham procedure is considered. There may be ways to justify placebo surgery through effectively minimizing risk, defending its use based on the potential importance and impact of the interventional procedure being studied, maintaining compulsive compliance with study blinding, and providing detailed informed consent [8]. In patient care trials, subjects in all treatment groups should be treated as equally as possible with respect to all treatments, therapies, assessments, and follow-up. Creative planning such as using identical wound care and surgical dressings, identical blood sampling, identical radiologic imaging, and identical therapy protocols can often achieve effective blinding strategies that are easy to implement and carry no additional risk. Placebo effects resulting in changes in subjects' outcomes unrelated to the therapeutic effect of the intervention, but related solely to their receiving an intervention, participating in a trial, or simply getting the attention of the research team must be considered. However, blinding should be considered integral to trial design, and, if not implemented, justification for not blinding should be explicit and detailed with delineation of the operational safety measures incorporated to otherwise minimize bias and maximize the validity of the findings [9].

"Practical Exercise"

Using these concepts, we can take the next step in the development of our hypothetical trial for the treatment of peripheral arterial disease and intermittent claudication. Our primary research question indicated that we wanted to compare options for structured supervised exercise to standard medical practice as the control. This approach rests on the assumption that standard medical therapy, including counseling on smoking cessation and exercise, but no structured supervision, is ineffective [10]. The intervention here is:

- Supervised exercise along with best medical therapy in patients with disabling claudication.

The control comparator group would then be:

- Standard medical practice with recommendations for best medical therapy and exercise directed through primary care providers.

Subjects will then be randomized to either the supervised exercise protocol or standard medical care. The intervention is then further subdivided to allow the application of various exercise protocols based on some judgment on the part of study investigators as to what might be best suited for each individual subject. Treadmill exercise is the accepted standard, but not everyone can walk on a treadmill. Exercise bicycle sessions, aquatic therapy, and resistance weight-lifting exercises offer alternatives. Incorporating this pragmatic approach will allow more inclusive eligibility and subject enrollment, but will require specific analytic strategies to be defined. The primary endpoint we defined was pain-free walking with secondary endpoints including walking duration and distance and improvements in quality of life. Secondary interventions proposed include structured transition of supervised exercise into community-based programs to optimize long-term compliance and molecular genomic screening to identify subjects that require early endovascular intervention. With these interventions and controls defined, we are ready to identify study subjects and begin recruitment.

Summary

The intervention is the critical focal element of any clinical trial. The control group, when appropriately defined, frames and validates the outcomes of that intervention. The intervention may be a pharmacologic adjunct, a novel or repurposed device or technique, or novel approach to a periprocedural patient care element. Application of the intervention should in most cases be clearly defined following a detailed protocol, but when appropriate, can be pragmatic to allow flexibility for limited adaptation and a "real-world" approach. Comparative effectiveness between two distinct competing interventions, between a novel intervention and a current standard therapy, or an intervention to conservative medical management is common trial design strategies. Comparison to placebo or sham should be considered cautiously and blinding, if appropriate, can eliminate significant bias and provide more objective observations. In every case, there should be sufficient equipoise among experts that the intervention warrants study, is ethical especially when the control group is not offered intervention, and has promise to advance the field with the resulting outcomes.

References

1. Wilson JF, Weale ME, Smith AC, Gratrix F, Fletcher B, Thomas MG, Bradman N, Goldstein DB. Population genetic structure of variable drug response. Nat Genet. 2001;29:265–9.
2. Fisher B, Bauer M, Margolese R, et al. Five-year results of a randomized clinical trial comparing total mastectomy and segmental mastectomy with or without radiation in the treatment of breast cancer. N Engl J Med. 1985;31:665–73.
3. Moseley JB, O'Malley K, Peterson N, et al. A controlled trial of arthroscopic surgery for osteoarthritis of the knee. N Engl J Med. 2002;347:81–8.
4. Neumayer L, Gobbie-Hurder A, Jonasson O, et al. Open mesh versus laparoscopic mesh repair of inguinal hernia. N Engl J Med. 2004;350:1819–27.
5. Grant AM, Wileman SM, Ramsay CR, et al. Minimal access surgery compared with medical management for chronic gastrooesophageal reflux disease: UK collaborative randomized trial. Br Med J. 2008;337:a2664.
6. Nelson PR, Kracjer Z, Kansal N, Rao V, Bianchi C, Hashemi H, Jones P, Bacharach JM. Multicenter, randomized, controlled trial outcomes of totally percutaneous aortic aneurysm repair (The PEVAR trial). J Vasc Surg. 2014;59:1181–94.
7. Karanicolas PJ, Farrokhyar F, Bhandari M. Blinding: who, what, when, why, how? Can J Surg. 2010;53:345–8.
8. Tambone V, Sacchini D, Spagnolo AG, Menga R, Ricci G, Valenti R, et al. A proposed road map for the ethical evaluation of sham (placebo) surgery. Ann Surg. 2016 Sep 14. [Epub ahead of print].
9. Finniss DG, Kaptchuk TJ, Miller F, Benedetti F. Biological, clinical, and ethical advances of placebo effects. Lancet. 2010;375:686–95.
10. Fokkenrood HJP, Bendermacher BLW, Lauret G, Willigendael EM, Prins MH, Teijink JAW. Supervised exercise therapy versus non-supervised exercise therapy for intermittent claudication. Cochrane Database Syst Rev. 2013;(8). Art. No.: CD005263.

Chapter 4
Subject Selection

Peter R. Nelson

General Concepts

Like the endpoints and the interventions in your trial, the subjects targeted for enrollment are initially proposed within your final primary research question. That's why it is critical to get the question right from the outset. Just a word regarding semantics of language. The terms "patient" and "subject" get used interchangeably when it comes to the individuals enrolled in clinical trials. Since we are generally proposing medical trials, all those enrolled will be patients of one sort or another, and it might be they are the very patients that generated the idea for the trial in the first place. However, the term "subject" is generally the preferred nomenclature for a patient who is enrolled into a clinical trial. It is an important distinction because the investigators are often not the medical caregivers for the subjects enrolled in the trial, and so separation is needed between the patient's general medical care and the reporting of a subject's participation in a clinical trial. I will use subject from here forward for consistency.

It is common for all of us to think that once we have a good research idea and have refined it into an actionable research question, finding subjects to enter into the trial will be easy. This can be an "eyes bigger than your stomach" phenomenon, and those more experienced have learned this perhaps the hard way. We all are guilty of thinking and even saying "we see 'a ton' of patients in clinic with disease X that would be amenable to intervention Y." This fuels an initial interest in developing the trial. However, a realistic, detailed appraisal of the actual number of eligible subjects that will be available and then actually entered needs to be conducted. This is obviously critical to powering your study and to its ultimate success.

P.R. Nelson (✉)
Surgical Service, James A. Haley VA Medical Center, 13000 Bruce B. Downs Boulevard, Tampa, FL 33612, USA
e-mail: peter.nelson@va.gov

© Springer International Publishing AG 2017
K.M.F. Itani and D.J. Reda (eds.), *Clinical Trials Design in Operative and Non Operative Invasive Procedures*, DOI 10.1007/978-3-319-53877-8_4

Many important large trials, well designed otherwise, have failed due to poor enrollment often at a huge expense for no definitive results.

Figure 4.1 simply depicts in a Venn diagram the process involved in predicting and then accruing the subjects enrolled in your trial. The outermost circle is the actual or perceived availability of patients in your clinic (or the clinics of multiple proposed sites in a multicenter trial) that might be approachable for screening. You need to base this initial estimate on data from your own practice and/or from national estimates. This number is important because it might speak to the potential impact your trial may ultimately have, but it does not accurately forecast your trial's enrollment. The next circle limits the potential subject pool to those that will meet at least the specific eligibility criteria you define for the trial. More on this below, but suffice to say this circle will be larger if the criteria are loose and will be much smaller if those criteria are more stringent. Moving inward, you then must be able to consent the subject to participate. This might seem like a forgone conclusion once you get this far, but many subjects, perfectly fit for trial inclusion otherwise, will simply not consent just because it is research, or due to other less predictable reasons. This process is well summarized by Lasagna's Law that states "*The incidence of patient availability sharply decreases when a clinical trial begins and returns to its original level as soon as the trial is completed.*" [1]. So, Muench's Third Law provides a ball-park conversion factor by stating "*In order to be realistic, the number of cases promised in any clinical study must be divided by a factor of at least 10.*" [2]. For our diagram, the final circle, colored in red, signifies the number of subjects ultimately consented and successfully enrolled in the study and is exactly 10% the size of the largest outer circle.

Fig. 4.1 Patient selection process

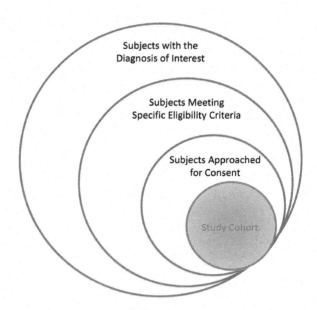

With this basic understanding, you now need to clearly define your target population. This is generally done by first identifying the disease process you are looking to study and then, within this cohort, refining the specific parameters of trial entry eligibility through clear inclusion and exclusion criteria. In general, these criteria will determine just how liberal or stringent enrollment will be for the trial. You'll need to decide how you want to approach this because it can be viewed as a "pay now or pay later" type of strategy. By using a more broad inclusive approach, you will be able to acquire a larger sample size that may generate more variance between subjects and will be more work and cost up front, but will likely offer definitive results at the end. If you opt for more specific, strict entry criteria, then you will end up with a smaller, better defined sample that may offer less "noise" and come with less effort and less cost, but you may then run the risk of not having power to achieve a definitive answer to your research question. This is yet another critical phase of trial planning.

Inclusion Criteria

Start by defining specific inclusion criteria to draw from the larger population of potential subjects with the diagnosis of interest. You can think of this as the "case definition" for the types of patients that are potential candidates for the trial. See Table 4.1 for common categories used for inclusion criteria. This process tends to be a little easier because you tend to know who you want to include, but be specific to be sure you define the target population precisely. The focus may be everyone with a certain disease process or potential eligibility for the intervention of interest, or it may be a specific degree of severity of disease or a specific diagnostic variant. Again, the broader the criteria the larger, but possibly more heterogenous, and the stricter the criteria the cleaner, but smaller, the starting sample.

In the selected clinical trials within the bibliography, the following list depicts the inclusion criteria defined in each trial:

Table 4.1 Inclusion Criteria	• Age range of subjects typical to the diagnosis of interest
	• Gender
	• Race/ethnicity
	• Specific target population/subpopulation
	• Diagnosis of interest
	• Specific target disease stage, class or variant
	• Specific risk factor or exposure of interest
	• Index presentation of disease process (vs. recurrent/secondary treatment)
	• Eligibility for proposed intervention
	• Expected compliance with study protocol and all required follow-up

- Women with operable Stage I or II breast cancer and sufficient breast to allow a cosmetic result following tumor excision [3].
- Subjects under 75 years old with osteoarthritis of the knee and moderate pain despite non-operative treatment for 6 months [4].
- Men 18 years or older with a diagnosis of inguinal hernia [5].
- Subjects diagnosed with gastroesophageal reflux (GERD) by endoscopic or 24 h pH monitoring, or both, 12 months of symptoms requiring maintenance medical treatment, and equipoise regarding management [6].
- Subjects 18 years and older with an abdominal aortic aneurysm measuring ≥ 5 cm and meeting all approved instructions for use criteria for the aortic endograft [7].

In all cases, subjects had to be able to provide informed consent. Note that all these criteria are specific and fairly simple, but in some cases are more broad and inclusive, in other cases more focused and restrictive.

Exclusion Criteria

Setting specific exclusion criteria can prove more challenging. You may have to make some very difficult decisions here that will exclude potential subjects in whom you feel might benefit from the proposed intervention, but they present other confounding medical issues or logistical problems with your overall trial design. One such example might be morbid obesity. Unless this is your primary target population for intervention (i.e., bariatric procedures), then the obese subject, by being at generally higher risk for periprocedural complications compared to non-obese counterparts, may experience endpoints not directly relevant to your intervention. These may, however, be significant enough to create concerns over safety, to produce noise in the data, to present challenges with analyses, and to ultimately threaten definitive conclusions. Therefore, you might administratively choose to exclude morbidly obese subjects and consider a separate trial later in this population if warranted. This is the time to clearly identify known confounding disease processes or risk factors that will interfere with the study design and outcomes and eliminate them.

Consider that in a randomized trial, potential study candidates can be assigned to any of the treatments in the trial, whether it be the experimental treatment being evaluated or the control treatment. Therefore, exclusion criteria must consider the potential safety and contraindications to treatment for all treatments in the trial. For example, a trial might require general anesthesia for one of the surgical arms, but local anesthesia is sufficient for the other arm. However, the exclusion criteria will need to exclude people for whom it is not safe to give general anesthesia. These types of decisions may limit the eventual generalizability of your results. See Table 4.2 for common categories used for exclusion criteria.

Table 4.2 Exclusion criteria

• Age (i.e., often extremes of age)
• Gender
• Race/ethnicity
• Specific disease attributes (i.e., exclusion of advanced or end-stage disease)
• Confounding medical diagnoses
• Prior treatment of target disease process
• Prohibitive anatomic or physical characteristics
• Prohibitive medical risk
• Prohibitive risk for proposed intervention
• Limited life expectancy to achieve outcome or benefit
• Inability to consent
• Vulnerable populations
• Participation in other clinical trials

In the same referenced clinical trials, the following list depicts exclusion criteria defined in each trial:

- Women with Stage advanced III or IV breast cancer; tumor size >4 cm or adherence to the skin; inadequate breast size to allow tumor excision; fixed axillary or chest wall lymphadenopathy [3].
- Subjects with asymptomatic or minimally symptomatic osteoarthritis of the knee; less than 6 months of or inadequate medical therapy; prior arthroscopy within 2 years [4].
- Subjects in American Society of Anesthesiologists (ASA) class IV or class V; subjects with bowel obstruction, bowel strangulation, peritonitis, bowel perforation, local or systemic infection subjects with contraindications to pelvic laparoscopy; a history of previous repair with mesh; a life expectancy of less than two years; or subjects were participating in another trial [5].
- Subjects in ASA class III, IV, or V; morbid obesity (body-mass index (BMI) > 40 kg/m^2); Barrett's esophagus of more than 3 cm or with evidence of dysplasia; paraesophageal hernia; and esophageal stricture [6].
- Subjects with inadequate femoral artery anatomy based on anterior, >50% posterior, or circumferential artery calcification, aneurysm or pseudoaneurysm, or prior femoral artery surgery; prior clip based closure device; existing femoral infection or hematoma; renal insufficiency; life expectancy <1 year; allergy to device components; morbid obesity (BMI > 40 kg/m^2) [7].

As you can see, these are more detailed and cover in some cases a wide range of subject characteristics and risk factors for intervention. Although the inclusion criteria may offer enrollment to a potentially larger cohort of subjects, exclusions will often narrow the focus to those with more straightforward disease and minimal risk to intervention.

Vulnerable Populations

A word about vulnerable populations in clinical research. These represent specific categories of subjects that require additional protections to be in place prior to inclusion for enrollment. These include (1) pregnant women, (2) children, (3) fetuses and neonates, (4) subjects deemed decisionally impaired or mentally ill, (5) prisoners, and (6) students. Pregnant women and their fetuses require special protection because most medications and interventions have not specifically been tested in pregnancy. Also, you must consider the safety, risks, effects for both the mother and the fetus and so consent often requires both parents' agreement. Children require special protection because they are obviously not of legal consenting age. Safeguards should be in place since emotions run high between exposing children to risks versus the availability of what might be their only hope for treatment. Consent is obtained from the parents or legal guardians, but for children over the age of 12, their assent is also required. Prisoners require special precautions to avoid real or perceived advantages like improvements in living conditions or leniency for parole that might serve as enticement. The risks involved in the research must be the same as those for non-prisoner subjects, and selection should be fair for all eligible prisoners. Students require special precautions since they might view involvement as an enticement either for financial gain or for preference in school grading. The investigator(s) may be the students' teacher(s) and therefore in a position of authority which could affect the consent process. This extends to other situations where there is a hierarchical relationship between the investigator and the potential study subject, such as seen with medical residents and fellows. Mentally or decisionally impaired subjects may be the most frequently encountered vulnerable population and one of the more vexing. These individuals may satisfy all inclusion/exclusion criteria, but be unable to comprehend trial involvement let alone the detailed specifics of your trial. Consent must be signed by legal next of kin or guardian, or power of attorney. Again the risks associated must be the same as for those subjects able to consent themselves, and specific precautions need to be in place to address potential enticement, especially in terminal illness. Finally, although these potential subjects may be deemed incompetent to sign consent, they generally still retain the right to decline participation in research, especially if it offers no perceived benefit.

Informed Consent

The concept of informed consent takes on at least two important critical roles. An exhaustive discussion is beyond the scope of this chapter but, briefly, (1) the creation of a detailed informed consent document, and (2) the process of acquiring truly informed consent from the research subject. The required components and guidelines for creating an informed consent document are shown in Table 4.3.

Table 4.3 Informed consent

• Title of trial
• Investigator credentials and contact information
• Detailed description of subject involvement – Written at 8th Grade reading level – Avoid technical or complex terminology – Tailor to subject population
• List any benefits or potential benefits to the subject
• Detail risks and discomforts associated with participation – Define "more than minimal" risk – Statement regarding attempts to minimize risk – Coverage for treatment of study incurred injuries
• Compensation for subjects (if any)
• Confidentiality/data protection plan
• Availability/sharing of protected health information (PHI) – Health Insurance Portability and Accountability ACT (HIPAA) waiver
• Availability of future information, future use of data collected, or future contact for additional trial participation
• Any audio or visual recording of subjects, or use of subject's likeness
• National Institute of Health Certificate of Confidentiality (if applicable)
• Printed names and signatures – Subject – Subject's legal representative – Investigator providing/obtaining informed consent

It is advisable to use a template document that already includes all of these criteria and has been reviewed, vetted, and approved by your Institutional Review Board. This document can be reviewed during the consent process and then is signed by the subject or his/her legal representative if relevant, and by the investigator leading the discussion. A copy is provided to the subject for their records.

This brings us to the second component, acquiring consent. All too often this process is truncated or done at a superficial level, sometimes to avoid scaring the subject away. It is critical to allocate adequate time to spend with eligible research subjects in order to review the trial protocol in detail, explain the associated risks and benefits, and answer any and all questions they may have regarding their participation. This should be conducted objectively, transparently, and without bias. You are not trying to "talk them into" participating in the trial. In spending the necessary time, you are more likely to demonstrate your enthusiasm for the trial, to display confidence and competence to the subjects, and to garner their trust in you as the lead investigator. This is critical to minimize loss of subjects at this very last phase of the enrollment process.

"Practical Exercise"

As the last phase in planning our hypothetical claudication trial, let's see how we might define our study population and address enrollment and informed consent issues. We might start by hoping to enroll every single patent diagnosed with claudication, but given the discussion above we know that won't be feasible. Our inclusion criteria would start with clinically documented reproducible leg pain/fatigue with ambulation supported by noninvasive vascular studies showing a reduced ankle-brachial index (ABI) < 0.85 and/or a stress test demonstrating exercise induced leg ischemia and a further reduction in ABI by >15%. These definitions should adhere to accepted specialty society clinical practice guidelines. Next, we'd want to define exclusion criteria which might eliminate subjects with advanced peripheral arterial disease (PAD) and critical limb ischemia that might require more urgent revascularization, subjects with medical or physical limitations prohibiting their participation in any of the proposed supervised exercise protocols, subjects who have had prior intervention for their claudication, and subjects with alternative causes of their symptoms (i.e., neurogenic, musculoskeletal, etc.). We would limit the age range to the typical presentation of symptomatic PAD, say 50–80 years of age, and would exclude younger subjects whose atypical symptoms would likely be caused by a congenital or musculoskeletal etiology rather than PAD. Men and women would be equally eligible, but this would not be a disease of children or pregnant women. Specific provisions could be made for prisoners to participate if relevant. Finally, subjects would have to have a reasonable life expectancy, should be able to sign informed consent, and should be likely to be compliant with the study protocol. Control patients would meet similar inclusion/exclusion criteria, but would only receive counseling regarding smoking cessation and exercise and would be followed per standard medical practice. This later point might challenge the consent process because eligible subjects might prefer the availability of supervised exercise and not be agreeable to randomization to less supervised standard care. Alternatively, unwillingness to quit smoking or participate in any type of exercise, travel limitations, concerns over the safety and security of remote monitoring, and a bias toward intervention as an immediate definitive treatment over exercise and medical management may all further challenge our ability to gain consent. In the end, using our 10% rule, if we wanted to study 100 subjects as defined, we might need to anticipate screening upwards of 1000 patients who present with claudication—a potentially daunting task.

Summary

To this point, you have clearly and thoughtfully stated your research question and hypothesis, established primary and secondary endpoints for your outcomes, and have defined your intervention and control strategies. Now, you need to identify and enroll the subjects into your trial to put this all to the test. You may feel all the heavy lifting is done in the prior three phases of design, but do not underestimate patient selection and enrollment. Set your inclusion and exclusion criteria so that you get the necessary balance between broad general inclusion and excessively stringent exclusion. This will hopefully provide you with the necessary number of subjects to power your study with reasonable effort and costs associated with the enrollment process, limited heterogeneity in the study groups with manageable variability in the resulting data, and ultimately the definitive answer to your originally proposed question.

References

1. Lasagna L. Problems in publication of clinical trial methodology. Clin Pharmacol Ther. 1979;25:751–3.
2. Bearman JE, Loewenson RB, Gullen WH. Muench's postulates, laws and corollaries, or biometrician's views on clinical studies (Biometric note 4) Bethesda (MD): office of biometry and epidemiology. National Institutes of Health: National Eye Institute; 1974.
3. Fisher B, Bauer M, Margolese R, et al. Five-year results of a randomized clinical trial comparing total mastectomy and segmental mastectomy with or without radiation in the treatment of breast cancer. N Engl J Med. 1985;31:665–73.
4. Moseley JB, O'Malley K, Peterson N, et al. A controlled trial of arthroscopic surgery for osteoarthritis of the knee. N Engl J Med. 2002;347:81–8.
5. Neumayer L, Gobbie-Hurder A, Jonasson O, et al. Open mesh versus laparoscopic mesh repair of inguinal hernia. N Engl J Med. 2004;350:1819–27.
6. Grant AM, Wileman SM, Ramsay CR, et al. Minimal access surgery compared with medical management for chronic gastrooesophageal reflux disease: UK collaborative randomized trial. Br Med J. 2008;337:a2664.
7. Nelson PR, Kracjer Z, Kansal N, Rao V, Bianchi C, Hashemi H, Jones P, Bacharach JM. Multicenter, randomized, controlled trial outcomes of totally percutaneous aortic aneurysm repair (The PEVAR trial). J Vasc Surg. 2014;59:1181–94.

Part II
Study Designs

Chapter 5
Clinical Phases of Device and Drug Evaluation with Emphasis on Early Phase Trials

Domenic J. Reda

Overview of Regulatory Phases for Investigational Agents

The US Food and Drug Administration and regulatory agencies in other parts of the world follow a measured sequential approach to the testing of investigational agents that emphasizes safety. Ultimately an agent must be shown to be both safe and effective before it receives marketing approval. However, at the initial stages of clinical research on the product, studies are generally small with a primary focus on identifying large safety signals. As data are accumulated, later phases of clinical investigation involve larger numbers of study participants where the focus on safety continues through more refined assessments of subtler safety signals with increasing emphasis on establishing efficacy.

The basic regulatory phases (I–IV) for drug development were developed first and are well known. The more recent guidelines for vaccines and biologics use the same structure. Device approval guidelines use a different sequential approach to device evaluation. The following table gives an overview of the regulatory phases for drugs, vaccines, biologics and devices (see Table 5.1).

Regulatory Phases for Device Approval

The Food and Drug Administration Center for Devices and Radiological Health is responsible for the review of marketing applications for devices in the USA. The phases of device evaluation and regulatory approval differ from those for drugs and include feasibility and pivotal trials.

D.J. Reda (✉)
Department of Veterans Affairs, Cooperative Studies Program Coordinating Center (151K),
Hines VA Hospital, Building 1, Room B240, Hines, IL 60141, USA
e-mail: Domenic.Reda@va.gov

© Springer International Publishing AG 2017   41
K.M.F. Itani and D.J. Reda (eds.), *Clinical Trials Design in Operative
and Non Operative Invasive Procedures*, DOI 10.1007/978-3-319-53877-8_5

Table 5.1 Regulatory phases for assessment of investigational agents

	Drugs, vaccines, biologics	Devices
Early	Phase I (includes Phase 0 and proof of concept)	Feasibility (includes proof of concept)
Middle	Phase II (includes Phase IIa and IIb)	Feasibility
Late	Phase III Phase IV	Pivotal

FDA classifies devices based on their level of risk and intended use. Class I devices are deemed to be low risk and are therefore subject to the least regulatory controls. For example, surgical instruments are generally classified as Class I devices. Class II devices are higher-risk devices than Class I and require greater regulatory controls to provide reasonable assurance of the device's safety and effectiveness. For example, contact lenses and ultrasound devices are classified as Class II devices. Class III devices are generally the highest-risk devices and are therefore subject to the highest level of regulatory control. Class III devices must typically be approved by FDA before they are marketed. Class III devices are life-supporting, life-sustaining or important in preventing impairment of human health. For example, replacement heart valves are classified as Class III devices [1].

Class III devices must go through a premarket approval process that involves two stages of clinical studies, feasibility studies and a pivotal trial.

Feasibility Study

A feasibility study may provide support for a future pivotal study or may be used to answer basic research questions about the device. It is often required by FDA prior to the pivotal study to assess basic safety and potential for effectiveness. The sample sizes for these studies are generally between 10 and 40, although they can be larger. Ultimately, the decision to proceed to the next phase of clinical evaluation is based on whether the potential benefit from the device justifies the risk.

Pivotal Study

The pivotal study is the definitive trial assessing the safety and efficacy of the device that will be used to obtain marketing approval. Device trials tend to be smaller than drug trials. Many are difficult to blind, and safety and effectiveness may depend on physician technique. Data from the pivotal study will be used as the primary clinical support for a marketing application. This stage of clinical study must provide a "reasonable assurance of safety and effectiveness" for the marketing application.

Regulatory Phases for Trials of Drugs, Vaccines and Biologics

The International Conference for Harmonization has defined three phases of clinical studies that are required to move a drug out of preclinical testing into clinical testing and ultimately to marketing approval [2]. The FDA Center for Drug Evaluation and Research (CDER) and the FDA Center for Biologics Evaluation and Research (CBER) use the same classification system for drugs, vaccines and biologics.

Phase 0 Trials

In 2007, FDA issued guidance on exploratory INDs [3]. An exploratory IND study is intended to describe a clinical trial that is conducted early in Phase I, involves very limited human exposure, and has no therapeutic or diagnostic intent (e.g., screening studies, microdose studies). Such exploratory IND studies are conducted prior to the traditional Phase I dose escalation, safety and tolerance studies that ordinarily initiate a clinical drug development program. The duration of dosing in an exploratory IND study is expected to be limited. Exploratory IND studies are identified as Phase 0 trials [4].

The FDA Exploratory IND Guidance includes examples of three types of Phase 0 trials: determination of biodistribution, determination of pharmacokinetics and bioavailability, and evaluation of the mechanism(s) of drug action. These trials provide an opportunity to examine a new agent in humans earlier than traditional dose-finding, toxicity-driven Phase I trials. Because a limited number of subtherapeutic doses are administered in the Phase 0 setting, assessment of preclinical toxicology can also be limited before proceeding to Phase I. Thus, Phase 0 trials permit identification of potential therapeutic failures earlier in the drug development process. Only drugs showing sufficient promise are to be evaluated for safety and tolerability in traditional Phase I trials.

For Phase 0 trials, a single dose or a short course (typically fewer than seven days) of low, non-therapeutic, non-toxic doses is administered to a few patients. PK/PD studies are conducted on these patients. It is essential that the drugs being considered for a Phase 0 trial have a high therapeutic ratio in preclinical toxicity models in vivo so that the desired PK or PD effect may be observed without substantial toxicity. Potential cancer chemopreventive agents may be suitable for evaluation in a Phase 0 trial.

Phase I Clinical Studies

Following completion of preclinical testing, trials that involve the initial administration of a drug, vaccine or biologic in humans are identified as Phase I clinical studies. Studies in this phase of development usually have non-therapeutic objectives as their primary intent, although the data from these studies are also used to provide very preliminary data on potential effectiveness. These studies are closely monitored and may be conducted in patients with the medical condition for which the drug may have potential use, e.g., patients with mild hypertension, but are usually conducted in healthy volunteer subjects. Drugs with significant potential toxicity, e.g., cytotoxic drugs, are usually studied in patients with the medical condition of interest.

Phase I trials are often non-randomized and do not employ a control group. However, many designs involve initial assessments of a range of doses for the agent that can include very low subtherapeutic doses. Sample sizes for Phase I are usually between 20 and 100. Studies conducted in Phase I typically involve one or a combination of the following aspects:

Estimation of Initial Safety and Tolerability

The initial evaluation of an investigational new drug in humans is usually intended to determine the tolerability of the dose range expected to be needed for later clinical studies and to determine the nature of adverse reactions that can be expected. Depending on the nature of the investigational agent, these studies typically may include single- or multiple-dose administration. Determination of dose-limiting toxicity, and the maximum tolerated dose are primary goals of Phase I trials.

Although Phase I trials were originally conceived as the first test of safety in humans, Phase I trial designs and objectives evolved over time to maximize information obtained from this early phase of drug development to guide the next phases of clinical research for the drug. Thus, these trials are also used to assess mechanism of action and early evidence of effectiveness.

Pharmacokinetics/Pharmacodynamics (PK/PD)

The preliminary characterization of the pharmacokinetics of a drug is an important goal of Phase I. Pharmacokinetics (PK) is defined as the study of the time course of drug absorption, distribution, metabolism and excretion. PK may be assessed via separate studies or as a part of efficacy, safety and tolerance studies. PK studies are particularly important to assess the clearance of the drug, possible accumulation of parent drug or metabolites and potential drug–drug interactions. Although drug–drug interaction studies are generally performed in phases beyond Phase I, animal and in vitro studies of metabolism and potential interactions may lead to doing drug–drug interaction studies earlier.

Pharmacodynamics (PD) studies assess the mechanisms of action of drugs and other biochemical and physiological effects on tissues and organ systems. PD data can provide early estimates of activity and potential efficacy and may guide the dosage and dose regimen in later studies.

PK/PD studies may be conducted in healthy volunteer subjects or in patients with the target disease. Designs for these studies typically involve taking serial measurements from test subjects after dose administration.

Early Measurement of Drug Activity

Preliminary studies of potential therapeutic benefit may be conducted in Phase I as a secondary objective. Such studies are generally performed in later phases but may be appropriate when drug activity is readily measurable with a short duration of drug exposure in patients at this early stage.

Phase I Trial Designs

There are a wide range of Phase I designs [5]. One of the most frequently used designs is the "3 + 3" design, which is one of the simpler forms of a dose escalation design [6]. A group of three test subjects is treated at a starting dose that is considered to be safe based on extrapolation from animal toxicological data. If none of the three subjects in a cohort experiences a dose-limiting toxicity, another three subjects will be treated at the next higher dose level. However, if one of the first three subjects experiences a dose-limiting toxicity, three more subjects will be treated at the same dose level. If no more than one of the six experiences a dose-limiting toxicity, then the trial proceeds to the next dose level in three new test subjects. The dose escalation continues until at least two subjects tested at a dose level experience dose-limiting toxicities. The recommended dose for Phase II trials is conventionally defined as the dose level just below this toxic dose level.

Not all Phase I designs involve evaluation of various doses of a treatment. Siprashvili et al. conducted a single-center Phase I clinical trial to evaluate the safety and wound outcomes following genetically corrected autologous epidermal grafts in 4 patients with recessive dystrophic epidermolysis bullosa (RDEB), an inherited blistering disorder caused by mutations in the COL7A1 gene encoding type VII collagen. RDEB causes significant disability and is often fatal. Autologous keratinocytes isolated from biopsy samples collected from the patients were transduced with retrovirus carrying full-length human COL7A1 and assembled into epidermal sheet grafts. Type VII collagen gene-corrected grafts were transplanted onto 6 wounds in each of the patients. The primary safety outcomes were recombination competent retrovirus, cancer and autoimmune reaction. Through one year of observation, all grafts were well tolerated without serious adverse events. No clinical signs of malignancy were observed. Recombinant retrovirus and cytotoxic T-cell assays were negative for the majority of time points; a minority was undetermined. Wound healing was assessed using serial photographs taken at 3, 6 and 12 months after grafting. Wound healing was observed in some type VII collagen gene-corrected grafts, but the response was variable among patients and among grafted sites and generally declined over 1 year [7].

Phase II Clinical Studies

Phase II includes the early controlled clinical studies conducted to obtain some preliminary data on the effectiveness of the drug for a particular indication or indications in patients with the disease or condition. This phase of testing also helps determine the common short-term side effects and risks associated with the drug. Phase II studies are typically well controlled, closely monitored and conducted in a relatively small number of patients, usually involving several hundred people.

A series of Phase II trials may be conducted before a decision to proceed to a Phase III clinical study is made. Phase II is usually considered to start with the initiation of studies in which the primary objective is to explore therapeutic efficacy in patients.

Phase IIa Studies

Early Phase II clinical studies are identified as Phase IIa studies. These are generally exploratory with a primary objective of evaluating clinical efficacy, pharmacodynamics or biological activity. These may be conducted in healthy volunteers or in patients with the target medical condition. Phase IIa trials may be non-randomized, using historic or concurrent controls or a pre-post design where test subjects serve as their own control.

Late Phase II clinical studies, known as Phase IIb, are dose range finding studies in patients with efficacy as the primary endpoint. Phase IIb trials are usually randomized and concurrently controlled to evaluate the efficacy of the drug and its safety for a particular therapeutic indication. Studies in Phase IIb are typically conducted in a group of patients who are selected by relatively narrow criteria, leading to a relatively homogeneous population and are closely monitored.

An important goal for this phase is to determine the dose regimen for Phase III trials, including dose range and frequency and timing of administration. Early studies in this phase often utilize dose escalation designs to give an early estimate of dose–response, and later studies may confirm the dose–response relationship for the indication in question by using parallel dose–response designs. Confirmatory dose–response studies may be conducted in Phase II or left for Phase III. Doses used in Phase II are usually but not always less than the highest doses used in Phase I.

Proof of Concept Studies

Proof of Concept (Proof of Principle) studies are an early stage of clinical drug development when a compound has shown potential in animal models and early safety testing. This step of proof of principle or proof of concept often links between Phase I and dose ranging Phase II studies. Thus, a Proof of Concept (POC) study can be thought of as a type of Phase IIa trial. Cartwright et al. describe a proof of concept study as "the earliest point in the drug development process at which the weight of evidence suggests that it is 'reasonably likely' that the key attributes for success are present and the key causes of failure are absent… Tools for POC include biomarkers, targeted populations, pharmacokinetic (PK)/pharmaco-dynamic (PD) modeling, simulation, and adaptive study designs" [8].

These small-scale studies are designed to detect a signal that the drug is active on a pathophysiologically relevant mechanism, as well as preliminary evidence of efficacy in a clinically relevant endpoint. Sponsors use these studies to estimate whether their compound might have clinically significant efficacy in other diseases states as well. For example, a drug with potential therapeutic efficacy for treatment of epilepsy may also be evaluated for its ability to treat other conditions (e.g., migraine, neuropathic pain, anxiety, depression) [9].

Example

Cartright et al. [8] provide an example of a proof of concept trial which was conducted by Lachmann et al. [10]. ACZ885, a monoclonal antibody against interleukin 1β, was administered to four patients with Muckle–Wells syndrome, an autoimmune disease in which interleukin-1 has a central role. In these four patients, a single-intravenous injection resulted in complete clinical remission within 8 days, with biomarkers of inflammation returning to normal ranges over the same time period. Because the antibody performed as designed, the proof of concept was demonstrated.

Phase IIb Studies

Phase IIb studies can be used as pivotal trials, if the drug is intended to treat life-threatening or severely debilitating illnesses as in oncology indications [11].

Additional objectives of clinical trials conducted in Phase II may include evaluation of potential study endpoints, concomitant medications and target populations (e.g., mild versus severe disease) for further study in Phase II or III. These objectives may be accomplished employing exploratory analyses, examining subsets of data and by including multiple endpoints in trials.

Phase II Trial Designs

Although many Phase II designs are non-randomized, many efficient randomized clinical trial designs have emerged and randomized Phase II designs are becoming more common [12]. There are three categories of randomized Phase II designs: (1) randomization to parallel non-comparative single-arm experimental regimens where the decision whether a single-arm shows evidence of efficacy is independent of the data from the other arms; (2) randomized selection (or pick the winner) designs for selecting the most promising experimental regimen among several similar experimental regimens [13, 14]; and (3) randomized screening design for comparing an experimental regimen to standard of care [15].

Phase III Clinical Studies

Phase III studies are larger trials that usually include a control group and random treatment assignment to the investigational agent or control. They are intended to gather the additional information about effectiveness and safety that is needed to evaluate the overall benefit–risk relationship of the drug. Phase III studies also provide a basis for extrapolating the results to the general population. Phase III studies usually include several hundred to several thousand participants.

Phase III begins with the initiation of studies in which the primary objective is to demonstrate, or confirm therapeutic benefit. Studies in Phase III are designed to confirm the preliminary evidence from Phase II that a drug is safe and effective for use in the intended indication and target population. These studies are intended to provide the basis for marketing approval. Studies in Phase III may also further explore the dose–response relationship or explore the drug's use in wider populations, in different stages of disease, or in combination with another drug. For drugs intended to be administered for long periods, trials involving extended exposure to the drug are ordinarily conducted in Phase III.

A trial designed and executed to obtain statistically significant evidence of efficacy and safety as required for marketing approval by regulatory agencies such as FDA is identified as a Phase IIIa trial. A Phase IIIB is a study started prior to approval and whose primary intention is support of publications rather than registration or label changes. The results are not intended to be included in the submission dossier.

Procedural Trials

Trials of a procedural technique do not fall under the purview of regulatory agency review before the technique can be used in general surgical practice. Thus, a new surgical technique or refinement of an existing technique can move from use by a few expert surgical practices that were instrumental in developing the technique to more widespread use without class I evidence to assess the benefit:risk ratio of the new technique.

For example, laparoscopic cholecystectomy moved into widespread use in the early 1990s without rigorous evidence from a randomized clinical trial comparing it to open cholecystectomy. Rather, its widespread adoption was driven by observational data indicating its safety and effectiveness and patient preference for a less invasive procedure, which quickly moved use of the technique from a few specialty centers to widespread use in general surgical practice [16–18].

References

1. Faris O. Clinical trials for medical devices: FDA and the IDE process. http://www.fda.gov/downloads/Training/ClinicalInvestigatorTrainingCourse/UCM378265.pdf.
2. International Conference on Harmonisation of Technical Requirements for Registration of Pharmaceuticals for Human Use. General considerations for clinical trials E8. Current Step 4 Version, 17 July 1997. http://www.ich.org/fileadmin/Public_Web_Site/ICH_Products/Guidelines/Efficacy/E8/Step4/E8_Guideline.pdf.
3. U.S. Department of Health and Human Services Food and Drug Administration Center for Drug Evaluation and Research (CDER). Exploratory IND studies, Jan 2006.
4. Kummar S, Doroshow JH. Phase 0 trials: expediting the development of chemoprevention agents. Cancer Prev Res (Phila). 2011;4(3):288–92.
5. Ivy SP, Siu LL, Garrett-Mayer E, Rubinstein L. Approaches to phase 1 clinical trial design focused on safety, efficiency, and selected patient populations: a report from the clinical trial design task force of the National Cancer Institute Investigational Drug Steering Committee. Clin Cancer Res. 2010;16(6):1726–36.
6. Le Tourneau C, Lee JJ, Siu LL. Dose escalation methods in phase I cancer clinical trials. J Natl Cancer Inst. 2009 20;101(10):708–20.
7. Siprashvili Z, et al. Safety and wound outcomes following genetically corrected autologous epidermal grafts in patients with recessive dystrophic epidermolysis bullosa. JAMA. 2016;316(17):1808–17.

8. Cartwright ME, Cohen S, Fleishaker JC, Madani S, McLeod JF, Musser B, Williams SA. Proof of concept: a PhRMA position paper with recommendations for best practice. Clin Pharmacol Ther. 2010;87(3):278–85.

9. Schmidt B. Proof of principle studies. Epilepsy Res. 2006;68(1):48–52.

10. Lachmann HJ et al. Treatment of Muckle Wells syndrome with a fully human anti-IL-1β monoclonal antibody (ACZ885)—initial results from a proof of concept study. Ann Rheum Dis 2006;65(suppl II):76.

11. Bahadur N. Overview of drug development. Novartis; 2008. http://www.ich.org/fileadmin/Public_Web_Site/Training/GCG_-_Endorsed_Training_Events/APEC_LSIF_FDA_prelim_workshop_Bangkok__Thailand_Mar_08/Day_1/Clinical_Dev_Plans_-_Namrata_Bahadur.pdf.

12. Simon R, Wittes RE, Ellenberg SE. Randomized phase II clinical trials. Cancer Treat Rep. 1985;69:1375–81.

13. Mandrekar SJ, Sargent DJ. Randomized phase II trials. Time for a new era in clinical trial design. J Thorac Oncol. 2010;5(7):932–4.

14. Simon R. Optimal two-stage designs for phase II clinical trials. Control Clin Trials. 1989;10:1–10.

15. Sargent DJ, Goldberg RM. A flexible design for multiple armed screening trials. Stat Med. 2001;20:1051–60.

16. Cuschieri A, Dubois F, Mouiel J et al. The European experience with laparoscopic cholecystectomy. Am J Surg. 1991;161385–388.

17. Dubois F, Berthelot G, Levard H. Laparoscopic cholecystectomy: historic perspective and personal experience. Surg Laparosc Endosc. 1991;152–57.

18. Spaw AT, Reddick EJ, Olsen DO. Laparoscopic laser cholecystectomy: analysis of 500 procedures. Surg Laparosc Endosc. 1991;12–7.

Chapter 6
Overview of the Randomized Clinical Trial and the Parallel Group Design

Domenic J. Reda

Clinical Research Milestones Before the Advent of the Modern Randomized Clinical Trial

We highlight here some of the key advances in history that eventually came together as the randomized clinical trial. In fact, many point to a passage in the book of David around 600 BCE as the earliest recorded description of a "trial." In this passage, the servants of King Nebuchadnezzar II ask whether they can undergo a 10-day trial during which they are given only legumes, vegetables and water to drink. They went on to suggest that the King can then compare their looks to those who ate the King's food. So we appear to have a small comparative nutritional trial described here.

In fact, this passage not only contains the trial protocol as described above, but also gives the results of the trial. After 10 days, the boys who ate the "experimental" diet looked healthier than those who ate the King's food. In essence, this passage describes a two-parallel-group trial. However, it would be another 2500 years before randomization, blinding and informed consent would be incorporated into clinical research.

Avicenna, the Persian physician, published the Book of the Canon of Medicine around 1030 CE, in which he proposed seven rules for the systematic evaluation of drugs on diseases. In 1747, James Lind conducted a non-randomized intervention trial assessing the role of citrus fruits for the treatment of scurvy. In 1836, French physician Pierre-Charles-Alexandre Louis conducted what is now considered the forerunner of the modern quantitative epidemiologic study on the treatment of

D.J. Reda (✉)
Department of Veterans Affairs, Cooperative Studies Program Coordinating Center (151K), Hines VA Hospital, Building 1, Room B240, Hines, IL 60141, USA
e-mail: Domenic.Reda@va.gov

© Springer International Publishing AG 2017
K.M.F. Itani and D.J. Reda (eds.), *Clinical Trials Design in Operative and Non Operative Invasive Procedures*, DOI 10.1007/978-3-319-53877-8_6

pneumonia with blood letting. His key methodologic contributions include exact observation of patient outcome, assessment of the natural progress of untreated controls, precise definition of the disease prior to treatment and careful observation of deviations from the intended treatment [1].

Between 1915 and 1931, the concepts of randomization and blinding emerged. Greenwood and Yule (1915) were the first to suggest random allocation to generate truly comparable treatment groups. R.A. Fisher and Mackenzie (1923) first applied the principle of randomization for agricultural experiments. Amberson et al. [2] published in 1931 the results of a trial for the treatment of pulmonary tuberculosis with a gold compound. This trial used a double-blind placebo-controlled design, created matched pairs of participants and then randomized within each matched pair. In 1944, the British Medical Research Council published the results of a placebo-controlled trial of the antibiotic patulin to treat the common cold [3].

Streptomycin for the Treatment of Tuberculosis

The breakthrough trial that signaled the emergence of the randomized clinical trial as the gold standard for clinical research was the British Medical Research Council multicenter trial on streptomycin of the treatment of pulmonary tuberculosis [4]. Sir Austin Bradford Hill, considered one of the fathers of modern clinical research, was the lead author. Key advances in methodology introduced in this trial included a statistically justified sample size and the use of random number sampling to enable the random assignment of participants to treatment.

Fifty-five participants were randomly assigned to 2 g daily of streptomycin divided into four doses taken every 6 h and 52 received placebo. Treatment duration was four months. The outcomes were assessed by changes in the radiographic appearances using a panel of three who were blinded to treatment assignment. Mortality and radiologic improvement showed statistically significant benefit to streptomycin. Of 55 patients assigned to streptomycin, four (7%) died within 6 months, while 14 of 52 patients on placebo (27%) died within the six months. Considerable radiologic improvement was observed in 27 (51%) of the streptomycin patients and four (8%) of the placebo patients.

Because the results were so striking, the trial received much attention. In addition, the rigorous methodology was noted and the era of the randomized clinical trial had begun.

The Benefits of Randomization

A RCT is an intervention study in which the treatment assignment is random rather than systematic. Randomization confers several benefits.

- It removes the potential for bias in the allocation of participants to the intervention or the control group. Note that for treatment assignment bias to be minimized, random assignment is necessary but not sufficient. Equally important is concealing the randomization code list from the investigator who is entering the patient into the trial until after the person has provided informed consent and is determined to be eligible for randomization.
- It tends to produce comparable groups on measured as well as unmeasured prognostic factors and other participant characteristics. This is a key difference from observational studies, where comparability of groups cannot be assumed, often necessitating covariate adjusted analyses to control for inherent differences between the groups. Even so, in an observational study, there could be unmeasured covariates that differ between groups.
- It gives validity to statistical tests of significance. In other words, incorporating an element of randomness in the trial forms the basis for using statistical methods to draw inferences from the data.

Sir Austin Bradford Hill developed a list of conditions that should be evaluated to determine whether there is a causal link between exposure (or treatment) and a change in a medical condition [5]. These criteria for causality include:

1. Strength of statistical association
2. Consistency of findings
3. Specificity of association
4. Temporal sequence
5. Biological gradient (dose–response)
6. (Biological or theoretical) plausibility
7. Coherence (with established knowledge)
8. Experimental evidence
9. Analogy (based on similar phenomena)

The randomized clinical trial is uniquely qualified to provide the necessary experimental evidence and is also optimized to assess the temporal link between treatment and medical condition. Thus, it has the potential to satisfy more elements on this list than other types of clinical research.

Trial Timing

When is the optimal time to conduct a randomized trial to evaluate a new medical treatment? When a procedure is new, it may be undergoing a rapid phase of refinement in technique, and data are limited regarding benefit and risk. Thus, there is not enough justification at that phase to conduct a definitive RCT.

Once a procedure is in widespread use, even without benefit of evidence from a RCT, it is probably too late to do the definitive trial. The procedure may have already become an accepted standard of care. In addition, it would be difficult to get clinicians to participate in such a trial, and potential study participants may be unwilling to accept randomization.

Somewhere between these two extremes is when the timing to conduct a RCT is optimal. There should be enough evidence of benefit and risk to justify further investigation, the procedure is probably stable enough to allow a trial with the procedure well defined and unlikely to change during the trial, but the evidence for benefit, especially in comparison with the current standard of care, is not so compelling that the trial is not needed.

We refer to this as the experimental and control treatments being in a state of equipoise, or uncertainty, regarding the comparative benefits and risks of the two. Equipoise must exist in order to conduct a trial. In fact, equipoise justifies randomization between the experimental and control treatments.

Ethics

Clearly a trial must be ethical in order for it to proceed. There are certain questions that are not suited to be answered in a randomized clinical trial. For example, the link between smoking and lung cancer was first discovered in a case–control study and the association was quite strong. A randomized clinical trial to assess the link between the two would have been considered unethical.

Feasibility

Finally, a trial must be feasible. The trial may be so expensive that funding cannot be obtained. The study exclusion criteria may be so restrictive that it is difficult to recruit. The proposed outcome measures may be too difficult to measure reliably. The length of the trial, frequency of visits or data collection burden may be so high that participants tend to leave the study early. The available treatment options may not be desirable.

Let us go back to the smoking and lung cancer relationship and imagine that we are able to get a RCT funded (despite the ethical issues). Let us assume we want to select a group of non-smokers to eliminate any contamination from prior exposure. There will be several feasibility issues that will arise. First, you would have to get a group of non-smokers to agree to randomization, knowing they have a 50% chance of being assigned to the smoking group. Next, you would need them to remain compliant with the assigned treatment regimen, i.e., continue to smoke for the duration of the trial if allocated to smoking. Finally, because of the long latency period, you would need to follow participants for a long time. Thus, even if we could get beyond the ethics, the ability to successfully complete the trial is unlikely.

Randomization Is Not Enough, What Happens After Randomization Is Just as Important

As the hypothetical smoking example illustrates, things can go wrong after randomization. Thus, one needs to consider the potential for bias to be introduced into the trial after randomization and how that can be minimized in the design and also the conduct of the trial.

Bias can be introduced in several ways, including:

1. Biased assessment of outcomes
2. Decisions by the clinical investigator to alter the treatment
3. Failure of the study participant to remain compliant with the assigned treatment
4. Deviations from the study protocol
5. Poor quality or missing data
6. Participant withdrawing from the study early

Blinding of the study treatment can help minimize the likelihood of many of these. However, even in a double-blind trial, differences in tolerability and effectiveness of the treatment regimens can cause differences in treatment adherence and follow-up rates between the randomized groups. The preferred strategy is to keep the participant in the trial regardless of their compliance with the treatment regimen, of course, if they agree to continue follow-up. This would allow continued collection of data on the participant and assessing the impact of these individuals on the trial results.

The Two-Parallel-Group Trial

The most frequently used clinical trial design is the two-parallel-group design. The MRC trial on streptomycin for pulmonary tuberculosis used this design as well as multitudes of trials since. In this basic design, participants are randomized to one of two treatment groups and then followed over time for assessment of outcomes.

The null hypothesis is that there is no difference between the two treatment groups in the outcome of interest. The two-sided alternative hypothesis is that there is a difference between the groups. Figure 6.1 shows the hypothesis for both a two-sided and a one-sided trial.

If the outcome measure is continuous, then the mean changes from baseline to a specific time point after randomization can be compared using a t-test for two independent groups. If the outcome measure is a proportion, the two proportions can be compared using the Chi-square test of homogeneity or the normal approximation to the binomial or Fisher's exact test. If the outcome measure is a time to event endpoint, such as survival, the two survival distributions can be compared using the log-rank test.

Fig. 6.1 Null and alternative hypotheses, two-parallel-group trial

Two parallel group trial (two - sided hypothesis)
Null hypothesis $\rightarrow H_o : \Theta_A = \Theta_B$
Alternative Hypothesis $\rightarrow H_A : \Theta_A \neq \Theta_B$

Two parallel group trial (one - sided hypothesis)
Null hypothesis $\rightarrow H_o : \Theta_A \geq \Theta_B$
Alternative Hypothesis $\rightarrow H_A : \Theta_A < \Theta_B$

where Θ_A and Θ_B are the population parameters for groups A and B, such as the mean, proportion or hazard rate for each group

The Multiple-Parallel-Group Trial

There are situations when evaluation of multiple experimental treatments in comparison with a control is desired. One approach would be to do a series of two parallel group trials, each one comparing one experimental treatment to the control. However, efficiencies can be gained by evaluating the multiple treatments in one trial.

In the multiple-parallel-group design, participants are randomized to one of several experimental treatments or control. In such a design, the null and alternative hypotheses are more complicated and there are a number of possibilities. For example, the investigator may be interested in comparing each experimental treatment with control, but there is no interest in how the experimental treatments compares to each other. Another investigator may be interested in how all the possible treatments compare to each other.

This needs to be determined when the study is designed as the number of possible comparisons has an impact on the type I error of the trial and the sample size. Let us say you have a three-group trial and you are interested in making comparisons with all three groups. Then, the null and alternative hypotheses are shown in Fig. 6.2.

Note we now have three different ways we can reject the null hypothesis. If each of these comparisons was made using alpha = 0.05, then the probability of type I error for the study or the probability of erroneously rejecting the null hypothesis is approximately 0.13, rather than 0.05. One simple and frequently used solution is to use a Bonferroni adjustment of the alpha level for each comparison. For Bonferroni adjustment, the number of desired comparisons is determined (here it is 3) and then

Fig. 6.2 Null and alternative hypotheses, three-parallel-group trial

Null hypothesis $\rightarrow H_o : \Theta_A = \Theta_B = \Theta_C$
Alternative Hypothesis $\rightarrow H_A : \Theta_A \neq \Theta_B$ or $\Theta_A \neq \Theta_C$ or $\Theta_B \neq \Theta_C$
or at least two groups differ

where Θ_A, Θ_B and Θ_C are the population parameters for groups A, B and C, such as the mean, proportion or hazard rate for each group the overall alpha for the trial is divided by the number of comparisons, which provides the alpha level to be used for each comparison. In this example, with three possible comparisons and the overall alpha level set at 0.05, then each pairwise comparison would use an alpha of 0.05/3 = 0.0167.

If you were only interested in comparing each of the experimental treatments (A and B) to control (C), then there would be only two pairwise comparisons and the alpha for each comparison would be 0.025.

While Bonferroni adjustment is frequently used because of its simplicity, it is not as accurate as newer methods and tends to be conservative, that is, it fails to statistically detect differences that other methods show to be statistically significant. Some of these methods are covered in the chapter on Advanced Statistical Methods.

Example

The monotherapy of hypertension trial was a seven-parallel-group trial that included six different antihypertensive agents and placebo [6]. A total of 1292 men with diastolic blood pressures of 95–109 mm Hg, after a placebo washout period, were randomly assigned to receive placebo or one of six drugs: hydrochlorothiazide (12.5–50 mg per day), atenolol (25–100 mg per day), captopril (25–100 mg per day), clonidine (0.2–0.6 mg per day), a sustained-release preparation of diltiazem (120–360 mg per day), or prazosin (4–20 mg per day). The drug doses were titrated to a goal of less than 90 mm Hg for maximal diastolic pressure, and the patients continued to receive therapy for at least one year.

Participants who did not achieve goal blood pressure in the initial phase stopped the initially assigned treatment and proceeded to phase B where they were randomized to one of five treatments. In phase B, participants could not be randomized to placebo or to an active treatment they had already received in the initial phase.

This trial also demonstrated that the structure of the treatment algorithm within each group can be pragmatic and attempt to replicate clinical practice. The drugs and their doses (listed from low to medium to high) were hydrochlorothiazide (12.5, 25, and 50 mg daily), atenolol (25, 50, and 100 mg daily), clonidine (0.2, 0.4, and 0.6 mg in divided doses given twice daily), captopril (25, 50, and 100 mg in divided doses given twice daily), prazosin (4, 10, and 20 mg in divided doses given twice daily), a sustained-release preparation of diltiazem (120, 240, and 360 mg in divided doses given twice daily), and placebo. Prazosin was started at 1 mg given twice daily for two days to minimize the risk of hypotension with the first dose. All medications were started at the lowest dose, and the dose was increased every two weeks, as required, until a diastolic blood pressure of less than 90 mm Hg was reached without intolerance to the drug on two consecutive visits or until the maximal drug dose was reached. This phase lasted four to eight weeks.

This study was conducted double-blind, a feat in itself given the differences in the treatment regimens.

Conclusion

Equipoise, ethics and feasibility are key factors in the design of a trial. While randomization confers several benefits that make the randomized clinical trial the gold standard for assessing the effects of treatments, good trial conduct is also needed so that bias is not introduced after randomization.

The two-parallel-group trial, in which participants are randomly assigned to either an experimental treatment or control and then followed to assess response to treatment, was the earliest of the trial designs used in large-scale randomized clinical trials. The design can be extended to the multiple-parallel-group design, where multiple treatments are evaluated simultaneously in one trial.

References

1. First Clinical Research. First clinical research milestones. http://www.firstclinical.com/milestones/. Accessed on 3rd Jan 2017.
2. Amberson JB, McMahon BT, Pinner M. A clinical trial of sanocrysin in pulmonary tuberculosis. Am Rev Tuberc. 1931;24:401–35.
3. Medical Research Council. Clinical trial of patulin in the common cold. Lancet. 1944;2:373–5.
4. Medical Research Council. Streptomycin treatment of pulmonary tuberculosis. Br Med J. 1948;2(4582):769–82.
5. Bill AB. The environment and disease: association or causation? Proc R Soc Med. 1965;58:295–300.
6. Materson BJ, Reda DC, Cushman WC, et al. Single-drug therapy for hypertension in men—a comparison of six antihypertensive agents with placebo. N Engl J Med. 1993;328:914–21.

Chapter 7
Non-inferiority and Equivalence Trials

Domenic J. Reda

Overview

In the "early" era of randomized clinical trials, which spans from 1946 to the late 1970s, many, if not most trials, sought to establish whether a new treatment has greater efficacy than the existing standard of care. For medical conditions where there was no known treatment to be effective, the natural comparator was no treatment or placebo. For medical conditions where there was an accepted treatment, the comparator was an "active control." With rapid development of new treatment modalities in many medical conditions, new treatments showed preliminary evidence that they could be superior to the existing standard of care, and thus, the traditional parallel group approach was appropriate.

As more effective treatments became available, the likelihood that a new treatment was more effective decreased. However, the new treatment might have other benefits compared with the standard of care, such as greater tolerability or improved side effect profile, or a more convenient treatment regimen, such as once daily dosing versus twice a day.

Thus increasingly, the intent of these trials shifted toward establishing that the effectiveness or efficacy of the new treatment was as good as, or similar to, that of an existing treatment. The earliest trials seeking to establish similarity used the traditional parallel group approach where if the null hypothesis were not rejected, then similarity was established.

However, this approach was inconsistent with the theoretical underpinnings of hypothesis testing and the role of the null and alternative hypotheses. The classical approach is to assume the null hypothesis unless the data collected in the trial indicate strong support for the alternative hypothesis. Thus, the null hypothesis can

D.J. Reda (✉)
Department of Veterans Affairs, Cooperative Studies Program Coordinating Center (151K),
Hines VA Hospital, Building 1, Room B240, Hines, IL 60141, USA
e-mail: Domenic.Reda@va.gov

© Springer International Publishing AG 2017
K.M.F. Itani and D.J. Reda (eds.), *Clinical Trials Design in Operative
and Non Operative Invasive Procedures*, DOI 10.1007/978-3-319-53877-8_7

be rejected in favor of the alternative. However, when the null hypothesis is not rejected, this does not establish that the data prove the null hypothesis, rather the data are insufficient to reject the null [1]. Thus, the traditional parallel group approach cannot be used to show that an experimental treatment is similar to a control treatment.

Hypothesis Testing

For a traditional 2 parallel group trial, the null and alternative hypotheses for a two-sided and a one-sided null hypothesis are shown in Fig. 7.1.

The corresponding hypothesis testing framework for non-inferiority and equivalence trials is shown in Fig. 7.2.

For an equivalence trial where the primary outcome measure is the 30-day hospitalization rate, let us assume that the equivalence margin is 8%, group A receives the treatment and group B the control. The null hypothesis states that the 30-day hospitalization rate differs by at least 8% in the two groups, in either

Fig. 7.1 Null and alternative hypotheses for traditional parallel group trials

Traditional parallel group trial (two-sided hypothesis)
Null hypothesis $\rightarrow H_o : \Theta_A = \Theta_B$
Alternative Hypothesis $\rightarrow H_A : \Theta_A \neq \Theta_B$

Traditional (2) parallel group trial (one-sided hypothesis)
Null hypothesis $\rightarrow H_o : \Theta_A \geq \Theta_B$
Alternative Hypothesis $\rightarrow H_A : \Theta_A < \Theta_B$

where Θ_A and Θ_B are the population parameters for groups A and B, such as the mean, proportion or hazard rate for each group

Fig. 7.2 Null and alternative hypotheses for equivalence and non-inferiority trials

Equivalence trial (two-sided)
Null Hypothesis $\rightarrow H_o : |\Theta_A - \Theta_B| > \delta$
Alternative Hypothesis $\rightarrow H_A : |\Theta_A - \Theta_B| \leq \delta$
δ is the equivalence margin

Non-inferiority trial (one-sided)
Null Hypothesis $\rightarrow H_o : \Theta_A < \Theta_B - \delta$
Alternative Hypothesis $\rightarrow H_A : \Theta_A \geq \Theta_B - \delta$
δ is the non-inferiority margin

Fig. 7.3 Reject and do not reject regions for traditional two-sided hypothesis test

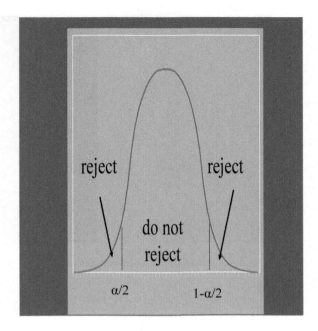

direction. The null hypothesis is rejected in favor of the alternative hypothesis if the data indicate a high likelihood that the 30-day hospitalization rates are within 8% of each other.

If we decided to conduct a non-inferiority trial with a non-inferiority margin of 8%, then the null hypothesis states that the 30-day complication rate for the experimental treatment is more than 8% worse than that for the control treatment. The null hypothesis is rejected in favor of the alternative hypothesis if the data indicate a high likelihood that the 30-day hospitalization rate for the experimental treatment is no more than 8% worse than that for the control treatment.

This reversal of the intent of the alternative hypothesis from establishing a difference in traditional parallel group trials to establishing similarity (either equivalence or non-inferiority depending on the structure of the alternative hypothesis) impacts how statistical tests are done.

Figure 7.3 shows the null hypothesis rejection region for a traditional two-sided null hypothesis.

This contrasts with an equivalence trial design where the reversal of the rejection region results in two one-sided tests, both of which require rejection in order to reject the equivalence null hypothesis [2]. This is shown in Fig. 7.4.

For a non-inferiority trial, a standard one-sided hypothesis test can be done. The need for two one-sided tests for an equivalence trial is specific to the two-sided hypothesis test situation. However, for a non-inferiority trial, one must still appropriately choose the (one-sided) rejection region so that it is consistent with the alternative hypothesis.

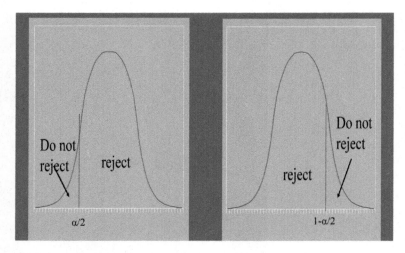

Fig. 7.4 Two one-sided tests for an equivalence trial

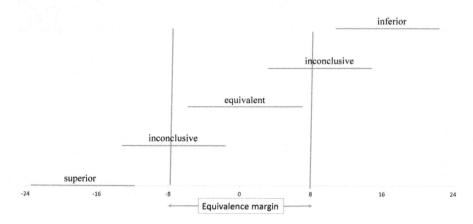

Fig. 7.5 Possible equivalence trial results

Confidence Interval Approach for Equivalence and Non-inferiority Trials

The results of equivalence and non-inferiority trials are more typically shown in a figure that displays the equivalence (or non-inferiority) margin and the confidence interval for the test statistic comparing the results for the two groups [3]. Figures 7.5 and 7.6 show possible trial outcomes for an equivalence trial with an equivalence margin of 8% and a non-inferiority trial with a non-inferiority margin of 8%.

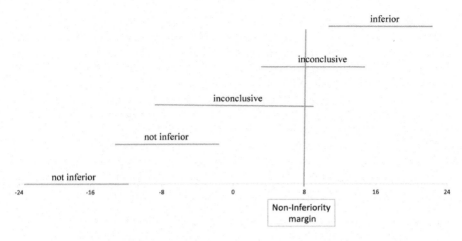

Fig. 7.6 Possible non-inferiority trial results

Example: Oral Versus Intratympanic Steroids for Treatment of Idiopathic Sudden Sensorineural Hearing Loss

Rauch et al. [4] conducted a multicenter unblinded randomized clinical trial to compare the efficacy of intratympanic steroid administration to oral steroids for treatment of idiopathic sudden sensorineural hearing loss (SSNHL). At the time the trial was initiated, standard therapy for SSNHL was a 14-day course of oral prednisolone. More recently, otolaryngologic surgeons had begun administering methylprednisolone as a series of injections into the ear canal, which was expected to produce results at least as good as oral steroid therapy, if not better, due to local concentration of the steroid into the affected area. In addition, the investigators thought intratympanic administration may have some inherent advantages because the likelihood of systemic effects would be much lower. Preliminary data from two very small studies indicated that intratympanic injection was likely as effective as oral steroid but did not appear to be more effective.

Thus, the investigators designed the trial using a non-inferiority design. Eligibility criteria included unilateral sensorineural hearing loss that developed within 72 h and was present for 14 days or less. The pure tone average (PTA), which is calculated as the arithmetic mean of the hearing thresholds at 500, 1000, 2000, and 4000 Hz in the affected ear, must have been 50 dB or higher, and the affected ear must have been at least 30 dB worse than the contralateral ear in at least 1 of the 4 PTA frequencies. Hearing must have been symmetric prior to onset of sensorineural hearing loss based on participant recall, and the hearing loss must have been deemed idiopathic following a suitable otolaryngologic evaluation.

Because oral steroid treatment has long been the standard of care for sudden hearing loss, many patients screened for enrollment in the study had referring physicians that already had initiated this treatment. Therefore, pre-enrollment steroid usage of less than 10 days was acceptable as long as audiometric criteria were met on the day of enrollment.

One hundred twenty-one patients received 60 mg/d of oral prednisone for 14 days with a 5-day taper and 129 patients received 4 doses over 14 days of 40 mg/mL of methylprednisolone injected into the middle ear.

The primary end point was the change in hearing at 2 months after treatment. Non-inferiority was defined as less than a 10 dB difference in hearing outcome between treatments. In the oral prednisone group, PTA improved by 30.7 dB compared with a 28.7 dB improvement in the intratympanic treatment group. Recovery of hearing on oral treatment at 2 months by intention-to-treat analysis was 2.0 dB greater than on intratympanic treatment (95.21% upper confidence interval, 6.6 dB). Thus, the null hypothesis of inferiority of intratympanic methylprednisolone to oral prednisone for primary treatment of sudden sensorineural hearing loss was rejected.

Example: ACOSOG Z6051—Laparoscopic-Assisted Resection Versus Open Resection of Stage II or III Rectal Cancer

The Alliance for Clinical Trials in Oncology published the results of a trial in 2015 comparing laparoscopic-assisted resection to open resection in participants with stage II or III rectal cancer [5]. This was designed as a non-inferiority trial. A total of 486 patients with clinical stage II or III rectal cancer within 12 cm of the anal verge were randomized after completion of neoadjuvant therapy to laparoscopic or open resection. The primary efficacy outcome measure was a composite of circumferential radial margin greater than 1 mm, distal margin without tumor, and completeness of total mesorectal excision.

Assuming a baseline rate of 90% oncologic success (circumferential radial margin results negative, distal margin results negative, and total mesorectal excision complete or nearly complete) for the open resection arm, the sample size of 480 patients (240 per arm) provided 80% power to declare noninferiority if oncologic success rates were truly identical, using a 1-sided z score with $\alpha = 0.10$ for falsely declaring noninferiority when the true oncologic success rate for laparoscopic resection was 84%.

Two hundred forty patients with laparoscopic resection and 222 with open resection were evaluable for analysis. Successful resection occurred in 81.7% of laparoscopic resection cases and 86.9% of open resection cases and did not support non-inferiority (difference, -5.3%; 1-sided 95% CI, -10.8% to ∞; P for non-inferiority = 0.41). The investigators concluded that the findings do not support the use of laparoscopic resection in these patients.

Choosing a Non-inferiority Design Versus a Traditional Parallel Group Design

As noted earlier, the intent of a traditional parallel group design is to determine whether there is a difference between treatment and control while for a non-inferiority (or an equivalence) design, the intent is to establish similarity. When deciding between these two approaches, the following questions should be considered: (1) If a traditional design is considered, does the experimental treatment show preliminary evidence of superiority or is there a theoretical basis that supports an expectation of superiority? (2) If a non-inferiority design is considered, does the experimental treatment offer other possible advantages if its efficacy is shown to be similar to that of the control. If so, then these should be considered as possible secondary questions in the trial, e.g., safety and tolerability, quality of life, treatment compliance. (3) Even if superiority of the experimental treatment is possible, is it sufficient to establish similarity?

Choice of the Non-inferiority (or Equivalence) Margin

In a traditional parallel group design, before the required sample size can be calculated, the investigators must decide how large a difference between experimental and control groups would warrant a conclusion that the experimental treatment is more effective. Thus, choice of δ for a parallel group trial is often thought of as the minimum difference necessary to establish superiority.

In trials that are intended to establish similarity, δ is considered to be the maximum difference allowed to establish similarity. Originally, it was thought that establishment of similarity would warrant a smaller δ than would be used for establishment of superiority. Thus, sample size requirements were often larger for these trials than for traditional trials. However, this thinking has evolved over time and sample size requirements for the two types of designs tend to be the same. Mulla et al. [6] provide good insights on how to consider the non-inferiority margin.

In addition, equivalence designs are in the minority and many trials intending to establish similarity use non-inferiority designs. Note that because non-inferiority trials use a one-sided hypothesis test, the overall alpha for such a trial is generally 0.025, rather than 0.05. This avoids the problem of using less conservative criteria to establish similarity than would be used to establish superiority.

Non-inferiority Is Not Transitive

As long as the result for the experimental treatment is no more than δ worse than that for the control treatment, the former will be shown not inferior to the latter even if it is a little less effective. One could imagine doing a series of trials, each with a new experimental treatment in comparison with the experimental treatment from the previous trial, with a little slippage in efficacy each time. Table 7.1 summarizes this series of studies.

As a result of this potential problem, regulatory agencies additionally require that an experimental treatment be shown to be more effective than placebo when non-inferiority is demonstrated with an existing treatment known to be effective.

Poor Study Conduct Makes Establishing Non-inferiority Easier

In a traditional trial, the primary foci of study conduct include recruitment, study dropouts, completeness of data, adherence to protocol, and precision of data. All of these have a negative impact on study power, either by reducing the actual sample size achieved or by increasing the variability of the measurements. Since power is the likelihood of rejecting the null hypothesis if the null is false, then reduced power makes it more difficult to reject the null and increases the likelihood of missing an important difference in outcomes between the experimental and control treatments.

In non-inferiority trials, the effect of poor study conduct is the same insofar as it reduces effective sample size, increases variability and makes the experimental and control treatments appear to be more similar. Thus, problems with study conduct **increase** the likelihood of establishing non-inferiority (or equivalence) erroneously, i.e., make it more likely to reject the null in favor of the alternative hypothesis. As a result, greater attention needs to be paid to these study conduct issues in non-inferiority trials than in parallel group trials. Regulatory agencies may not

Table 7.1 Non-inferiority is not transitive

Response rate		Conclusion
Drug A: 50%	Placebo: 30%	Drug A superior to placebo
Drug B: 45%	Drug A: 50%	Drug B equivalent to Drug A
Drug C: 40%	Drug B: 45%	Drug C equivalent to Drug B
Drug D: 35%	Drug C: 40%	Drug D equivalent to Drug C
		Is Drug D superior to placebo if it has been shown to be equivalent to Drug C (and therefore Drugs A and B)?

accept the results of a non-inferiority trial if the completeness and precision of the collected data differ substantially from that assumed for the power and sample size calculation.

Guidance on Non-inferiority Trials

In November, 2016, the US Food and Drug Administration released its **Guidance for Industry on Non-Inferiority Clinical Trials to Establish Effectiveness** [7]. Many of the concepts in this chapter have been included in this guidance. Of particular interest is the following:

Reasons for Using a Non-Inferiority Design

The usual reason for using an NI active control study design instead of a superiority design is an ethical one. Specifically, this design is chosen when it would not be ethical to use a placebo, or a no-treatment control, or a very low dose of an active drug, because there is an effective treatment that provides an important benefit (e.g., life-saving or preventing irreversible injury) available to patients for the condition to be studied in the trial. Whether a placebo control can be used depends on the nature of the benefits provided by available therapy. The International Conference on Harmonisation guidance E10: Choice of Control Group and Related Issues in Clinical Trials (ICH E10) states:

In cases where an available treatment is known to prevent serious harm, such as death or irreversible morbidity in the study population, it is generally inappropriate to use a placebo control. There are occasional exemptions, however, such as cases in which standard therapy has toxicity so severe that many patients have refused to receive it.

In other situations, where there is no serious harm, it is generally considered ethical to ask patients to participate in a placebo-controlled trial, even if they may experience discomfort as a result, provided the setting is non-coercive and patients are fully informed about available therapies and the consequences of delaying treatment [ICH E10; pps.1314].

Aside from this ethical reason, there may be other reasons to include an active control, possibly in conjunction with a placebo control, either to compare treatments or to assess assay sensitivity (see section III.D). Caregivers, third party payers, and some regulatory authorities have increasingly placed an emphasis on the comparative effectiveness of treatments, leading to more studies that compare two treatments. Such studies can provide information about the clinical basis for comparative effectiveness claims, which may be helpful in assessing cost effectiveness of treatments. If a placebo group is included in addition to the active comparator, it becomes possible to judge whether the study could have distinguished treatments that differed substantially, e.g., active drug versus placebo. Such comparative effectiveness studies must be distinguished from NI studies, which are the main focus of this document. The word noninferior is used here in a special sense. The methods described in this document are intended to show that a new treatment that demonstrates non-inferiority is effective, not that it is as effective as the active comparator. A new treatment may meet the standard of effectiveness (that it is superior to placebo) without justifying a conclusion that it is as effective or even nearly as effective as the active comparator.

Summary

With the availability of effective treatments for many medical conditions, the use of placebo-controlled traditional parallel group trials intended to show superiority of the experimental treatment has decreased. Non-inferiority (and equivalence) trial designs were developed to demonstrate similarity between an experimental treatment and an active control. While the outward structure of such trials seems identical to those of traditional parallel group trials, there are important differences in the underlying null and alternative hypothesis, approaches to sample size calculation and analysis of data. In addition, greater attention needs to be paid to good study conduct in these trials to reduce the likelihood of erroneously establishing non-inferiority.

References

1. Blackwelder WC. Proving the null hypothesis in clinical trials. Control Clin Trials. 1982;3 (4):345–53.
2. Schuirmann DJ. A comparison of the two one-sided tests procedure and the power approach for assessing the equivalence of average bioavailability. J Pharmacokinet Biopharm. 1987;15 (6):657–80.
3. Jones B, Jarvis P, Lewis JA, Ebbutt AF. Trials to assess equivalence: the importance of rigorous methods. BMJ. 1996;313:36–9.
4. Rauch SD, Halpin CF, Antonelli PJ, et al. Oral versus intratympanic corticosteroid therapy for idiopathic sudden sensorineural hearing loss: a randomized trial. JAMA. 2011;305(20):2071–9.
5. Fleshman J, Branda M, Sargent DJ, et al. Effect of laparoscopic-assisted resection versus open resection of stage II or III rectal cancer on pathologic outcomes: the ACOSOG Z6051 randomized clinical trial. JAMA. 2015;314(13):1346–55.
6. Mulla SM, Scott IA, Jackevicius CA, et al. How to use a noninferiority trial. JAMA. 2012;308 (24):2605–11.
7. U.S. Department of Health and Human Services Food and Drug Administration Center for Drug Evaluation and Research (CDER) and Center for Biologics Evaluation and Research (CBER). Nov 2016. http://www.fda.gov/downloads/Drugs/GuidanceComplianceRegulatory Information/Guidances/UCM202140.pdf.

Chapter 8
Factorial Designs

Domenic J. Reda

Definitions and Examples of Factorial Designs

At its most basic level, a factorial trial tests the effects of two treatments in one trial in a way that examines the treatments alone or in combination with each other. In this instance, we can design a 2 by 2 factorial trial. Let us say we have two treatments, A and B, and we would like to evaluate them in a factorial design. We can randomly assign study participants as follows:

Randomization 1: treatment A or no treatment A (perhaps a placebo version of A)
Randomization 2: treatment B or no treatment B (perhaps a placebo version of B)

Here, each patient will undergo randomization 1 and randomization 2 simultaneously. Table 8.1 shows the formation of four groups by this factorial randomization.

However, the design is more often represented as follows (Table 8.2):

For factor 1, treatment A and placebo A are identified as the levels of factor 1. Correspondingly, treatment B and placebo B are the levels of factor 2.

Within a factor, the levels are not constrained to have one be a placebo (or perhaps no treatment). They could be differently intensities or different types of treatment within a similar class. Tables 8.3 and 8.4 show two other possible 2 by 2 designs as examples.

As mentioned earlier, a 2 by 2 factorial design is the most basic of these designs. The number of factors can increase, and the number of levels within a factor can increase. For the example in Table 8.4, if aspirin alone was incorporated into the trial as another choice for post-stent antithrombosis therapy, then the trial would have a 2 by 3 factorial design. If it were desired also to assess the effect of two types

D.J. Reda (✉)
Department of Veterans Affairs, Cooperative Studies Program Coordinating Center (151K),
Hines VA Hospital, Building 1, Room B240, Hines, IL 60141, USA
e-mail: Domenic.Reda@va.gov

© Springer International Publishing AG 2017
K.M.F. Itani and D.J. Reda (eds.), *Clinical Trials Design in Operative
and Non Operative Invasive Procedures*, DOI 10.1007/978-3-319-53877-8_8

Table 8.1 Four groups formed by a factorial randomization

Group 1	Group 2	Group 3	Group 4
Treatment A + treatment B	Placebo A + treatment B	Treatment A + placebo B	Placebo A + placebo B

Table 8.2 Representation of a 2 by 2 factorial design

Factor 1	Factor 2	
	Treatment B	**Placebo B**
Treatment A	Treatment A + treatment B	Treatment A + placebo B
Placebo A	Placebo A + treatment B	Placebo A + placebo B

Table 8.3 Representation of a 2 by 2 factorial design where levels of a factor are different intensities of a treatment

Factor 1	Factor 2	
	Low-dose B	**High-dose B**
Low-dose A	Low-dose A + low-dose B	Low-dose A + high-dose B
High-dose A	High-dose A + low-dose B	High-dose A + high-dose B

Table 8.4 Representation of a 2 by 2 factorial design where levels of a factor are different types of treatment within a class

Stent type	Post-stent antithrombosis therapy	
	Clopidogrel	**DAPT**
BMS	BMS + clopidogrel	BMS + DAPT
DES	DES + clopidogrel	DES + DAPT

Note: *BMS* bare metal stent, *DES* drug-eluting stent, *DAPT* dual antiplatelet therapy (clopidogrel + aspirin)

Table 8.5 Representation of a 2 by 3 by 2 factorial design

Stent type	Rosuvastatin		
	Post-stent antithrombosis therapy		
	Clopidogrel	**Aspirin**	**DAPT**
BMS	BMS + clopidogrel	BMS + aspirin	BMS + DAPT
DES	DES + clopidogrel	DES + aspirin	DES + DAPT
Stent type	**Atorvastatin**		
	Post-stent antithrombosis therapy		
	Clopidogrel	**Aspirin**	**DAPT**
BMS	BMS + clopidogrel	BMS + aspirin	BMS + DAPT
DES	DES + clopidogrel	DES + aspirin	DES + DAPT

Note: *BMS* bare metal stent, *DES* drug-eluting stent, *DAPT* dual antiplatelet therapy (clopidogrel + aspirin)

of statin drug as part of the trial, then the trial would have a 2 by 3 by 2 factorial design (Table 8.5).

Advantages and Disadvantages of a Factorial Trial

The main advantage of a factorial design is that it provides the ability to answer multiple questions about treatment effects within one trial. For example, the following questions could be asked in a factorial design as shown in Table 8.4 where post-stent thrombosis is the primary outcome measure.

Is there a difference in post-stent thrombosis:

1. between bare metal and drug-eluting stents?
2. between clopidogrel given alone or with dual antiplatelet therapy (DAPT)?
3. between bare metal stents and drug-eluting stents for those given clopidogrel alone?
4. between bare metal stents and drug-eluting stents for those given DAPT?
5. between clopidogrel and DAPT for those given bare metal stents?
6. between clopidogrel and DAPT for those given drug-eluting stents?

This does not exhaust all the possible questions that can be asked regarding post-stent thrombosis with this design. The reader may wish to examine the structure of the trial and identify other possible questions that could be answered. Thus, by overlaying two different treatment modalities in one trial, a factorial design provides the opportunity to examine treatment effects of a therapy alone and in combination with other therapies.

Another advantage is that in placebo-controlled factorial designs, recruitment into the trial may be easier. Referring to the design shown in Table 8.2, let us assume that a factorial design was not considered and the investigator decided to conduct two different trials. The first would compare treatment A to placebo, and the second would compare treatment B to placebo. In each of these trials, a participant would have a 50% chance of receiving placebo. However, in the trial represented in Table 8.2, the participant would have a 25% chance of receiving (double) placebo.

There are three main disadvantages to a factorial design. The first is that the complexity of the trial is considerably increased, which can impede the investigator's ability to successfully complete the trial.

The second disadvantage is that the interpretation of the results can be more complicated if it turns out that a treatment level in factor A modifies the effect of a treatment level in factor B.

The third is that the sample size requirement will increase considerably if it is possible that the effect of one factor will modify the effect of the other factor. For example, in the list of questions above, questions 3–4 imply that the difference between bare metal and drug-eluting stents may depend on whether clopidogrel is given alone or in combination with aspirin, while questions 5–6 imply that the difference between clopidogrel alone and clopidogrel combined with aspirin depends on the type of stent. All four of these questions reflect subgroups in the overall study. Only questions 1 and 2 are based on the entire sample size. We go a bit deeper into this issue in the next several sections of this chapter.

Main Effects

Let us return to the example in Table 8.3. If the effect of low-dose treatment *A* is the same regardless of the dose for treatment *B* and the effect of high-dose treatment *A* is the same regardless of the dose for treatment B, then we can draw a conclusion about whether the effect of low-dose treatment *A* differs from the effect of high-dose treatment *A* without needing to consider what dose of treatment *B* the participants received. It turns out we can also ask whether low-dose treatment *B* differs from high-dose treatment *B* without needing to consider the dose of treatment *A*. We refer to these as the factor 1 main effect (low-dose *A* and high-dose *A* differ) and the factor 2 main effect (low-dose *B* and high-dose *B* differ). Main effects are also described as marginal effects. The factor 1 effect can be assessed by ignoring (or combining) the low-dose *B* and high-dose *B* columns. Similarly, the factor 2 effect can be assessed by ignoring (or combining) the low-dose *A* and high-dose *A* (Table 8.6).

Interactions

When the factor 1 effect depends on the level of factor 2, or vice versa, then there is effect modification between the two factors, also known as an interaction effect. When interaction is present, we can no longer make a statement about the main effect of factor 1 or 2. Rather, in order to determine whether the effect of low-dose *A* differs

Table 8.6 Representation of a 2 by 2 factorial design and the main effect for the two factors

Factor 1	Factor 2		
	Low-dose *B*	High-dose *B*	Main effect of factor 1
Low-dose *A*	Low-dose *A* + low-dose *B*	Low-dose *A* + high-dose *B*	Low-dose *A*
High-dose *A*	High-dose *A* + low-dose *B*	High-dose *A* + high-dose *B*	High-dose *A*
Main effect of factor 2	Low-dose *B*	High-dose *B*	

Types of Interactions

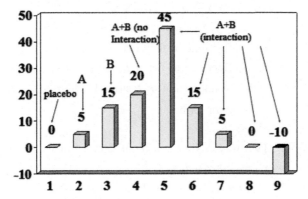

Fig. 8.1 Figure types of interactions. Column 1—there is no placebo effect. Column 2—the effect of A is 5. Column 3—the effect of B is 15. Column 4—the combined effect of A and B is additive and =20 (no interaction). Column 5—the combined effect of A and B is larger than either alone (interaction). Column 6—the combined effect of A and B is the same as B alone, i.e. there is no added benefit to A in the presence of B (interaction). Column 7—the combined effect of A and B is the same as AB alone, i.e. there is no added benefit to B in the presence of A (interaction). Column 8—the combined effect of A and B is the same as placebo, i.e. A and B each cancel the effect of the other (interaction). Column 9—the combined effect of A and B is worse than either alone and worse than placebo (interaction)

from that of high-dose A, we need to consider the dose level of B. Essentially, an interaction effect means that the comparison of low- and high-dose A for those who received low-dose B is different from the comparison of low- and high-dose A for those who received high-dose B. The reverse also holds when interaction is present. In other words, the margins of the table are ignored and the appropriate comparisons are within the 2 by 2 table, i.e. the four cells.

Another way of considering interaction is the following. When no interaction is present, the effects of factor 1 and factor 2 are additive. Any departure from an additive relationship between factor 1 and factor 2 is an interaction. Interaction effects can take many forms. Figure 8.1 shows several scenarios indicating the presence of interaction.

Statistical Analysis

When the outcome measure is continuous, analysis of variance is used to examine main and interaction effects. The statistical models for a 2 by 2 factorial design with a continuous outcome measure are:

Two-way ANOVA with interaction $\rightarrow$

$$x_{ijk} = \mu + \alpha_i + \beta_j + (\alpha\beta)_{ij} + \varepsilon_{ijk};$$
$$i = 1, 2; \quad j = 1, 2; \quad k = 1, 2, \ldots, n$$

$\alpha_i \rightarrow$ effect due to factor A

$\beta_j \rightarrow$ effect due to factor B

$(\alpha\beta)_{ij} \rightarrow$ interaction of factors A and B

$\varepsilon_{ijk} \rightarrow$ error term

Two-way ANOVA without interaction $\rightarrow$

$$x_{ijk} = \mu + \alpha_i + \beta_j + \varepsilon_{ijk};$$
$$i = 1, 2; \quad j = 1, 2; \quad k = 1, 2, \ldots, n$$

$\alpha_i \rightarrow$ effect due to factor A

$\beta_j \rightarrow$ effect due to factor B

$\varepsilon_{ijk} \rightarrow$ error term

The analytic steps are:

- Perform two-way ANOVA with interaction
- If the interaction is not statistically significant

    - Perform two-way ANOVA again but with no interaction term
    - Examine the significance level of factor A and factor B

- If interaction is statistically significant

    - Transform the problem into a one-way ANOVA with each group defined by the levels of factors A and B
    - For example, a 2×4 factorial becomes a one-way ANOVA with 8 groups
    - Then proceed as if you have an 8 parallel group trial. Use a multiple comparison procedure to determine which pairs of groups are different

If the outcome measure is binary, then a similar approach can be followed using logistic regression. If the outcome is a time-to-event outcome (survival analysis), then Cox regression can be used. Note that for binary and time-to-event outcomes, the multiple comparisons step will use a more sophisticated process to perform multiple comparisons.

Effect of Interaction on Sample Size

During the design of a factorial trial, the investigator will need to determine whether it can be assumed there is no interaction. Here, the nature of the medical condition being considered, and the known effects of the treatments may help inform that decision. However, absent good evidence that interaction is unlikely, the study should be designed assuming interaction is possible. Unfortunately, this will have the effect of increasing the sample size for the study, often substantially. A fourfold increase in sample size would not be unusual.

Let us assume we have designed a 2 by 2 factorial trial that will have 1000 participants in total, equally divided among the four groups. If no interaction can be assumed, then the comparison of the two levels of factor A (the factor A main effect) will involve 500 participants assigned to one level of factor A and 500 assigned to the other level. However, if interaction is present, then the analysis will involve a comparison of the four groups constructed by the 2 by 2 design and each pairwise comparison of any of the four groups will involve 500 total (250 per group), or half the sample size available for a test of a main effect. However, the relationship between power and sample size is quadratic rather than linear.

BARI 2D—A 2 by 2 Trial

The Bypass Angioplasty Revascularization Investigation 2 Diabetes (BARI 2D) used a 2 by 2 factorial design in a sample of participants with type 2 diabetes mellitus and angiographically documented stable coronary artery disease. BARI 2D compared revascularization combined with aggressive medical treatment versus aggressive medical treatment alone, and simultaneously, two glycemic control strategies, insulin sensitization versus insulin provision [1, 2].

The trial group randomly assigned 2368 patients with both type 2 diabetes and heart disease to undergo either prompt revascularization with intensive medical therapy or intensive medical therapy alone and to undergo either insulin-sensitization or insulin-provision therapy. There were two primary end points: the rate of death and a composite of death, myocardial infarction, or stroke (major cardiovascular events). Randomization was stratified according to the choice of percutaneous coronary intervention (PCI) or coronary artery bypass grafting (CABG) as the more appropriate intervention.

The protocol included as part of its statistical analysis plan to test for interaction effects for the two factors. The statistical interactions between the cardiac study groups and the glycemic study groups for rates of death and major cardiovascular events were tested overall and within the PCI and CABG strata at a two-sided alpha level of 0.05. The interactions were found not to be statistically significant, which allowed the group to compare the revascularization and medical-therapy groups (regardless of the diabetes treatment) and vice versa.

At 5 years, rates of survival did not differ significantly between the revascularization group (88.3%) and the medical-therapy group (87.8%, $P = 0.97$) or between the insulin-sensitization group (88.2%) and the insulin-provision group (87.9%, $P = 0.89$). The rates of freedom from major cardiovascular events also did not differ significantly among the groups: 77.2% in the revascularization group and

75.9% in the medical-treatment group ($P = 0.70$) and 77.7% in the insulin-sensitization group and 75.4% in the insulin-provision group ($P = 0.13$).

The Physician's Health Study

Another use of a factorial design when it can be assumed there is no interaction, is to create an efficient trial which is one trial overlayed on another trial, each asking different questions. The Physician's Health Study used this approach [3–5].

A total of 22,071 physicians were randomly assigned, according to a 2 by 2 factorial design, to one of four treatment groups: aspirin and beta carotene, aspirin and placebo beta carotene, placebo aspirin and beta carotene, or placebo aspirin and placebo beta carotene. There were two primary outcome measures: The study was designed to test two primary-prevention hypotheses in a population of healthy male physicians: whether aspirin in low doses (325 mg every other day) reduces mortality from cardiovascular disease, and whether beta carotene (50 mg on alternate days) decreases the incidence of cancer.

The trial design assumed no interaction between low-dose aspirin and beta carotene for either outcome measure. The study design is depicted in Fig. 8.2.

The design was somewhat controversial at the time because it made an assumption of no interaction between low-dose aspirin and beta carotene. While it appeared to be acceptable to make that assumption for the cardiovascular outcome, it was less clear that it was safe to assume no interaction for the cancer outcome.

The trial's Data and Safety Monitoring Board stopped the aspirin component of the trial early when it became clear that aspirin had a significant effect on the risk of a first myocardial infarction. At that time, there were too few strokes or deaths upon which to draw conclusions about the effect of aspirin on stroke or cardiovascular

Cancer Prevention Objective

		Beta - Carotene	Placebo	Outcome Measure
Cardiovascular Disease Prevention Objective	Low Dose Aspirin	Low Dose Aspirin + Beta-Carotene	Low Dose Aspirin + Placebo	Cardiovascular Mortality
	Placebo	Beta-Carotene + Placebo	Placebo + Placebo	
	Outcome Measure	Cancer Incidence		

Fig. 8.2 Figure design of the Physician's Health Study

mortality, but the DSMB felt the study should not continue to provide more definitive information about those endpoints since the benefit for myocardial infarction was now established. The beta carotene component continued to completion. It was concluded that 13 years of supplementation with beta carotene produced neither benefit nor harm regarding cancer incidence.

Conclusion

Factorial designs can be very useful in large-scale trials to assess the effects of multiple treatments and how they influence each other.

References

1. Brooks MM, Frye RL, Genuth S, Detre KM, Nesto R, Sobel BE, Kelsey SF, Orchard TJ. Bypass angioplasty revascularization investigation 2 diabetes (BARI 2D) trial investigators. Hypotheses, design, and methods for the bypass angioplasty revascularization investigation 2 diabetes (BARI 2D) trial. Am J Cardiol. 2006;97(12A):9G–19G.
2. BARI 2D Study Group, Frye RL, August P, Brooks MM, Hardison RM, Kelsey SF, MacGregor JM, Orchard TJ, Chaitman BR, Genuth SM, Goldberg SH, Hlatky MA, Jones TL, Molitch ME, Nesto RW, Sako EY, Sobel BE. A randomized trial of therapies for type 2 diabetes and coronary artery disease. N Engl J Med. 2009;360(24):2503–15. doi:10.1056/NEJMoa0805796.
3. Hennekens CH, Buring JE. Methodologic considerations in the design and conduct of randomized trials: the U.S. physicians' health study. Controlled Clin Trials. 1989;10:142S–50S.
4. The Steering Committee of the Physicians' Health Study Research Group. Belanger C, Buring JE, Cook N, Eberlein K, Goldhaber SZ, Gordon D, Hennekens CH, Mayrent SL, Peto R, Rosner B, Stampfer M, Stubblefield F, Willett W. Final report on the aspirin component of the ongoing physicians' health study. N Engl J Med 1989;321:129–35.
5. Hennekens CH, Buring JE, Manson JE, Stampfer M, Rosner B, Cook NR, Belanger C, LaMotte F, Gaziano JM, Ridker PM, Willett W, Peto R. Lack of effect of long-term supplementation with beta-carotene on the incidence of malignant neoplasms and cardiovascular disease. N Eng J Med. 1996;334:1145–9.

Chapter 9
Cross-over Trials

Domenic J. Reda

Description

In a cross-over trial, each study participant serves as their own control. Although non-randomized cross-over trials can be conducted, it is preferable to randomly assign treatments. Let us assume that it is desired to compare two treatments A (control) and B (experimental) in a cross-over trial. In a non-randomized cross-over, all participants may receive treatment A first and then treatment B. In a randomized cross-over trial, all participants would receive both treatments in sequence, but the sequence order is randomized. Thus, half would receive treatment A followed by treatment B and half would receive treatment B followed by treatment A. Figure 9.1 shows the design layout for such a trial.

A full cross-over design would assign each participant to receive all treatments in a randomly selected order. Here the number of trial periods would equal the number of treatments being evaluated in the trial. An incomplete cross-over design would randomly assign participants to a sequence of treatments, but they would not receive all treatments. Thus, a 3-group 2-period cross-over design, as illustrated in Fig. 9.2, would be considered an incomplete design.

Advantages of Cross-over Designs

Cross-over trials have two advantages over parallel-group trials. The first is that precision is increased, which generally results in a reduction in the required sample size. The gain in precision is due to two factors. Since each patient serves as their

D.J. Reda (✉)
Department of Veterans Affairs, Cooperative Studies Program Coordinating Center (151K), Hines VA Hospital, Building 1, Room B240, Hines, IL 60141, USA
e-mail: Domenic.Reda@va.gov

© Springer International Publishing AG 2017
K.M.F. Itani and D.J. Reda (eds.), *Clinical Trials Design in Operative and Non Operative Invasive Procedures*, DOI 10.1007/978-3-319-53877-8_9

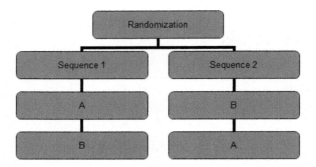

Fig. 9.1 Standard 2-group 2-period cross-over design

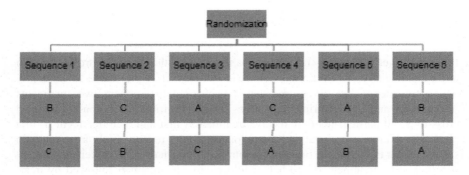

Fig. 9.2 Incomplete cross-over design 3 treatments, 2 periods

own control, then the sample size is reduced by 50%, albeit at the expense of a longer trial since participants must complete all rounds of treatment before they exit the trial.

In addition, since pre- and post-treatment responses tend to be correlated, the magnitude of the correlation will reduce the sample size requirement further.

As an example, Dunbar et al. [1] conducted a single-site randomized double-blind cross-over trial to determine if confocal laser endomicroscopy with optical biopsy and targeted mucosal biopsy (CLE-TB) improves the diagnostic yield of endoscopically inapparent Barrett's Esophagus (BE)-associated neoplasia compared to standard endoscopy with a 4-quadrant random biopsy (SE-RB) protocol.

Patients with biopsy-proven BE or biopsy-proven BE with suspected non-localized, endoscopically inapparent high-grade dysplasia (HGD) were randomly assigned to receive standard endoscopy first and CLE with TB 2–6 weeks later or to receive the two procedures in the reverse sequence. At the end of the second endoscopic procedure, the study co-investigator was allowed to unblind the endoscopist and disclose the prior pathologic diagnoses and the location of any areas of biopsy-proven HGD. An endoscopic mucosal resection could be performed at that time if a mucosal lesion was highly suspicious for HGD or early cancer.

To obtain the target sample size, the expected yield for neoplasia of standard endoscopy with a four-quadrant random biopsy (SE-RB) protocol was estimated to be 10% and the neoplasia yield for CLE-TB was estimated to be 40%. Using an alpha of 0.05 and power of 90%, 37 patients were needed using a paired design. If this had been designed as a parallel-group trial, the target sample size would have been 47 per treatment group, or 94 in total.

The diagnostic yield for neoplasia with CLE-TB was 33.7% (95% CI 15.2–52.2%), while the diagnostic yield for neoplasia during SE-RB was 17.2% (95% CI 6.2–28.2%).

The other advantage of cross-over designs is that it may enhance recruitment to the trial, especially when one of the treatment groups is placebo. A cross-over design guarantees that all participants will receive an active treatment some time during their participation in the trial.

Period Effects

Because each person serves as their own control, one potential problem with interpretation of results in a cross-over trial is the potential for responses to change over time, independent of the treatment given. For example, if a medical condition has a seasonal component, the difference in effect from the first treatment to the second could be due to a period effect rather than a true difference in effectiveness of the two treatments. When the order of receiving the treatments is randomly assigned, for example when half the patients receive treatment A in the first period and half receive treatment A in the second period, then the period effects are balanced by the random assignment of treatment sequence.

Carry-over Effects

Another potential problem is the carry-over effect. If treatment A has some residual effect after the participant stops receiving treatment A and then the participant immediately receives treatment B, the residual effect of treatment A cannot be separated from the effect of treatment B. In this instance, random assignment of the order of receiving the treatments may not resolve the issue. It is possible that the length and magnitude of residual effects differs among different treatments. If treatment B has no residual effect, but treatment A does, then the group that receives A second will not have their response to A affected by the earlier treatment B, while those who receive treatment B second will have their response to B affected by the carry-over effect of A.

Wash-out

One strategy to address the problem of carry-over effects is to incorporate a wash-out period in between treatments. Of course, the wash-out period needs to be long enough to allow wash-out of any of the potential treatments.

Drop-Outs

As suggested earlier, if a participant leaves a trial early, then the effect of the missing data has a greater impact than when a participant leaves a parallel-group trial early. In a cross-over trial, data collected for the participant for any of the treatments they received before leaving the study have limited utility since the design is dependent on each participant serving as their own control.

Analysis

The problems with carry-over effects and drop-outs can be seen in the following statistical model for a 2-group 2-period cross-over trial. Assume the following parameters for the model:

π = the period effect: the expected secular difference between period 2 and period 1

τ = the treatment effect: the expected difference due to treatment between treatments A and B

λ_a = carry-over due to treatment A

λ_B = carry-over due to treatment B

μ_i = effect due to patient i: the response we should expect of patient i were we to treat the patient in period 1 with B

In the presence of cross-over, the model can be expressed in the following 2 by 2 box:

	Expected Response	
Group	Period 1	Period 2
AB	$\mu_j + \tau$	$\mu_j + \pi + \lambda_A$
BA	μ_K	$\mu_K + \pi + \tau + \lambda_B$

It can be shown that in the presence of carry-over effects the model cannot be solved for the treatment effects. When carry-over effect can be ignored, the responses can be modeled as follows:

	Expected Response	
Group	Period 1	Period 2
AB	$\mu_j + \tau$	$\mu_j + \pi$
BA	μ_K	$\mu_K + \pi + \tau$

Now the treatment effects of A and B can be estimated. As an alternative, the mixed-effects model, a flexible statistical model often used for the analysis of longitudinal data, can be used to estimate carry-over effects [2].

When the outcome measure is continuous, then repeated measures analysis of variance can be used. For a binary outcome measure, such as complication within 30 days of the procedure (yes, no), then a more sophisticated form of repeated measures analysis using generalized estimating equations (GEE) can be used. For studies where the outcome measure is survival or some other time to event outcome, survival analysis methods are not useful because once a participant has an event (such as mortality) before all treatments have been received, there is no opportunity to observe the event again on the remaining treatments.

When a Cross-over Design Is Not Useful

Thus, cross-over designs have important limitations that limit their utility in trials of procedures, especially invasive procedures. Cross-over trials are not useful when one or more of the treatments will result in a permanent change to the participant, such as curing the condition. Similarly, cross-over designs are generally not useful for acute conditions because of the potential that the condition may resolve before the participant completes the full sequence of treatments, such as influenza. Finally, any medical condition or treatment that carries a significant likelihood that the patient will be unable to continue in the trial is not suitable for a cross-over trial.

Example: The NIDCD/VA Hearing Aid Trial

One example of a trial for which the medical condition and the treatments being evaluated was suitable for a cross-over design was the VA/NIDCD Hearing Aid Trial [3]. The objective of the trial was to compare the benefits provided to patients with sensorineural hearing loss of 3 commonly used hearing aid circuits. It was designed as a 3-period, 3-treatment cross-over trial. The study was conducted at eight audiology laboratories in Department of Veterans Affairs medical centers across the USA in a sample of 360 patients with bilateral sensorineural hearing loss.

Patients were randomly assigned to 1 of 6 sequences of linear peak clipper (PC), compression limiter (CL), and wide dynamic range compressor (WDRC) hearing aid circuits. All patients wore each of the 3 hearing aids, which were installed in identical casements, for 3 months. Thus, the trial was double-blind.

Outcome measures included results of tests of speech recognition, sound quality, and subjective hearing aid benefit, administered at baseline and after each 3-month intervention with and without a hearing aid. At the end of the experiment, patients ranked the 3 hearing aid circuits.

The investigators concluded that each circuit provided significant benefit in quiet and noisy listening situations. The CL and WDRC circuits appeared to provide superior benefits compared with the PC, although the differences between them were much less than the differences between the aided and unaided conditions.

Note that this trial was a nearly ideal setting in which to conduct a cross-over trial. Sensorineural hearing loss is a chronic condition that changes very slowly over time, especially during the nine-month treatment period (3 months per device) for each patient. Thus, period effects were not expected. In addition, the effect of wearing a hearing aid was not expected to change the participant's unaided hearing acuity. Thus, no carry-over effects were expected. Finally, the withdrawal rate was expected to be low given the nature of the condition and the treatments.

Example: Epinephrine and Thoracic Epidural Anesthesia

Niemi and Breivik conducted a double-blind randomized cross-over trial in 12 participants that assessed the effectiveness of epinephrine combined with a small-dose infusion of ropivacaine and fentanyl after major thoracic or abdominal surgery [4].

Patients scheduled for major thoracic or upper abdominal surgery were selected for the study. After titration to optimal epidural analgesia with a triple component mixture on the day of surgery, patients were randomly allocated to receive one of the two trial epidural analgesic mixtures on the first postoperative day and the alternative epidural mixture on the second postoperative day.

Patients were excluded if they had any contraindications to insertion of an epidural catheter, such as infection, anatomical abnormalities of the spine, or full anticoagulation. Also excluded were patients with incomplete or unstable analgesia caused by technical epidural catheter problems, including epidural catheter insertions that were too high or too low.

Before the induction of general anesthesia, an epidural catheter was inserted at an appropriate level between the 6th and 12th thoracic interspace, depending on the site of surgery. All patients received a standard anesthesia protocol during surgery and a standard epidural infusion post surgery. The patients were allowed to self-administer one 4-mL bolus of the epidural analgesic mixture, up to twice per hour. All patients received rectal acetaminophen 1 g, every sixth hour.

For each patient, two coded 100-mL plastic bags containing ropivacaine 1 mg/mL and fentanyl 2 µg/mL, with and without epinephrine 2 µg/mL, were prepared by the hospital pharmacy. At 8:00 am on the first postoperative day, the epidural infusion was changed, as determined by the randomization procedure, from the triple mixture to one of the two coded epidural mixtures. This was infused at the same rate as the triple epidural mixture for up to 3 h, or for as long as the patient could tolerate any increased pain after receiving the predetermined rescue medication. At this time, the epidural infusion was changed back to the ropivacaine–fentanyl–epinephrine mixture, a bolus of 5 mL was given, and the infusion continued at the same rate as before the blinded study period started. The patients were observed for another 5 h for pain intensity and side effects. On the second postoperative day at 8:00 am, if the patient still had optimal analgesia with the same infusion rate of the ropivacaine–fentanyl–epinephrine epidural mixture, the study was repeated with the alternative, coded epidural mixture.

Whenever the patients were dissatisfied with pain relief, they were allowed to self-administer one 4-mL bolus of the epidural analgesic mixture infused at the time, up to twice per hour. When pain intensity increased to severe pain when coughing, despite the epidural bolus doses, morphine 1–5 mg was added and titrated intravenously by one of the investigators. If pain when coughing remained severe, the epidural infusion was changed back to the unblinded epidural infusion with epinephrine. The amounts of epidural mixture actually administered and any IV morphine were recorded hourly.

For pain at rest and when coughing, pain intensity remained low and unchanged during the blinded test period with epinephrine. Without epinephrine and as soon as after 2 h, there was a highly significant difference in pain intensity from baseline ($P < 0.001$) and between the periods with and without epinephrine ($P < 0.001$). This difference increased as long as the mixture without epinephrine was infused. When the epidural infusion was changed back to the mixture with epinephrine, the pain intensity decreased within the next 15 min so that after 1 h there was no difference in pain intensity compared with baseline.

Conclusion

Cross-over trials are generally not an acceptable design for trials of procedures, especially invasive procedures and those that will result in a permanent change in the participant's medical condition. However, because of their efficiency, they can be useful when the assumptions that allow a cross-over design are met. They may be useful for trials in surgical patients where an aspect of care is being evaluated, such as choice of anesthesia regimen.

References

1. Dunbar KB, Okolo P 3rd, Montgomery E, Canto MI. Confocal laser endomicroscopy in Barrett's esophagus and endoscopically inapparent Barrett's neoplasia: a prospective, randomized, double-blind, controlled, crossover trial. Gastrointest Endosc. 2009;70(4): 645–54. doi:10.1016/j.gie.2009.02.009.
2. Laird NM, Skinner J, Kenward M. An analysis of two-period crossover designs with carry-over effects. Stat Med. 1992;11(14–15):1967–79
3. Larson VD, Williams DW, Henderson WG et al. Efficacy of 3 commonly used hearing aid circuits A crossover trial. JAMA. 2000;284(14):1806–13. doi:10.1001/jama.284.14.1806.
4. Niemi G, Breivik H. Epinephrine markedly improves thoracic epidural analgesia produced by a small-dose infusion of ropivacaine, fentanyl, and epinephrine after major thoracic or abdominal surgery: a randomized, double-blinded crossover study with and without epinephrine. Anesth Analg. 2002;94(6):1598–605.

Chapter 10
Cluster Randomized Clinical Trials

William G. Henderson

Introduction

Cluster randomized clinical trials (CRCTs—also called group randomized trials or community trials) are randomized clinical trials in which the units randomized are groups of patients rather than individual patients. This type of trial is conducted when the interventions being studied are applied to groups of patients at a time rather than individual patients. However, in both types of trials the outcomes of interest are recorded for each patient individually. CRCTs are frequently used in health services research, an area of health research involving the organization, delivery, and financing of health services. They often involve studies of behavior, lifestyle modification, educational programs, and healthcare models.

Some examples of CRCTs in surgery include:

1. A cluster randomized trial in which 20 general surgeons in Ontario, Canada, were randomly assigned to use decision aids or not to help the surgeons inform their patients with breast cancer about different treatment options. Patients were clustered within surgeons. Patient outcomes included knowledge scores about the treatment options, measures of decisional conflict and satisfaction with decision-making, and frequency of choosing breast conservation therapy [1].

2. The Quality Initiative in Rectal Cancer (QIRC) trial, in which hospitals in Ontario, Canada, were randomized to a knowledge translation strategy involving workshops, use of opinion leaders, operative demonstrations, a postoperative questionnaire, and audit and feedback to teach surgeons a new technique of mesorectal excision (experimental group) versus the normal practice environ-

W.G. Henderson (✉)
Adult and Child Consortium for Outcomes Research and Delivery Science (ACCORDS),
Department of Biostatistics and Informatics, Colorado School of Public Health, University
of Colorado Denver, 13199 E. Montview Blvd, Suite 300, Aurora, CO 80045, USA
e-mail: William.Henderson@ucdenver.edu

© Springer International Publishing AG 2017
K.M.F. Itani and D.J. Reda (eds.), *Clinical Trials Design in Operative
and Non Operative Invasive Procedures*, DOI 10.1007/978-3-319-53877-8_10

ment (control group) to improve patient outcomes (rate of permanent colostomy and rate of local recurrence of cancer) [2]. Patients were clustered within surgeons and hospitals.

3. The PEDUCAT trial, in which groups of patients defined by hospital ward and weeks of the year were randomized to a preoperative seminar and standard information brochure to learn how best to behave after surgery versus the standard brochure only in the prevention of postoperative complications [3]. Patients were clustered within hospital ward and weeks of the year.

4. The QUARISMA (Quality of Care, Obstetrics Risk Management, and Model of Delivery) trial, in which 32 hospitals in Quebec, Canada, were randomized to an intervention involving audits of indication for cesarean delivery, provision of feedback to health professionals, and implementation of best practices versus usual care to try to reduce the rate of cesarean delivery, and major and minor neonatal morbidity [4]. Patients were clustered within hospitals; and

5. The FIRST trial, in which 117 general surgery residency programs were randomized to current Accreditation Council for Graduate Medical Education (ACGME) duty-hour policies (standard-policy group) or more flexible policies that waived rules on maximum shift lengths and time off between shifts (flexible policy group) for general surgery residents. Outcomes included 30-day rate of patient postoperative death or serious complications, other postoperative complications, resident perceptions, and satisfaction regarding resident well-being, education, and patient care [5]. Patients and residents were clustered within general surgery residency programs.

Some advantages of CRCTs include the ability to study interventions that are naturally applied at the cluster level, ability to produce results that are generalizable and relevant to real world decisions, and a greater possibility of avoiding contamination (i.e., the intervention under study "spilling over" into the control group). Some disadvantages include the need for a large number of clusters and a larger overall sample size compared to a trial performing randomization at the patient level; increased training, monitoring, and statistical complexity; and increased cost and the need for a large funding source.

Intraclass Correlation and Sample Size Determination in a CRCT

CRCTs tend to be less efficient than RCTs that randomize at the patient level because often patients within a cluster are more correlated than are patients from different clusters. This correlation is called the "intraclass correlation" (ICC) and can range between 0 and 1, although in practice in most CRCTs the ICC ranges between 0.001 and 0.05. The ICC is defined as:

ICC = ρ = (Between cluster variance)/(Between cluster variance + Within cluster variance), or the proportion of the total variance that is attributable to the clustering effect. When ρ is close to 0, this means that the between cluster variance is low compared to the within cluster variance; in other words, the individuals within a cluster are not necessarily very much alike (large variance of individuals within a cluster). When ρ is close to 1, this means that the between cluster variance is large compared to the within cluster variance; in other words, the individuals within a cluster tend to be much more alike (not much variance between them). In the design of CRCTs, the ICC for the primary outcome variable is often unknown, and assumptions must be made about the ICC in order to plan sample size for the study.

Sample size determination for the CRCT and final analysis of the CRCT require that the clustering of the patients in the clinical trial is taken into account. Failure to account for the clustering effect (i.e., ignoring the grouping) in the sample size determination of the clinical trial will result in an underpowered study; failure to account for the clustering effect in the final analysis of the clinical trial will result in a larger Type I error in the clinical trial compared to the nominal Type I error, usually $\alpha = 0.05$ (i.e., the investigator will underestimate the variance of the estimates in the clinical trial and will find more results that are statistically significant than should be found).

The sample size for a CRCT (i.e., the total number of participants in the trial) is very sensitive to the value of the ICC. To calculate the sample size for a CRCT, one can calculate the sample size for the trial assuming that randomization is at the patient level using standard methods and then apply an "inflation factor" which is IF = $[1 + (m - 1) \times \rho]$, where m = cluster size (i.e., the number of patients in each cluster, assuming a constant cluster size across all clusters), and ρ = ICC. Inflation factors for various combinations of ICC and cluster sizes are given in Table 10.1. Total sample sizes for trials randomizing at the patient level only need to be increased by 2–10% for cluster sizes of 20–100 when $\rho = 0.001$, but they need to be increased by 19–99% when $\rho = 0.01$ and by twofold to sixfold when $\rho = 0.05$. For example, using standard methods to calculate a sample size for a clinical trial randomizing at the patient level that achieves 90% power to detect a success rate of 40% versus 30% as statistically significant with a two-sided test at $\alpha = 0.05$, we obtain a sample size of 956 patients. If we instead designed a CRCT with cluster sizes of 20 patients, we would require 975 (956 × 1.02) patients (48–49 clusters of 20 patients each) if $\rho = 0.001$; 1319 (956 × 1.38) patients (66 clusters of 20 patients each) if $\rho = 0.02$; and 1864 (956 × 1.95) patients (93–94 clusters of 20 patients each) if $\rho = 0.05$. Investigators planning a CRCT need to have a good estimate of the ICC. Some groups have tried to report ICCs for various settings, populations, and endpoints to help inform study design and analysis [6]. Whenever a new CRCT is published, it should be required that the ICCs be reported, in addition to the main results of the study, to enhance the accurate planning of future studies.

Table 10.1 Inflation factors for CRCT sample sizes for various combinations of intraclass correlations (ICCs) and cluster sizes

Cluster sizes					
ICC	$N = 20$	$N = 40$	$N = 60$	$N = 80$	$N = 100$
0.001	1.02	1.04	1.06	1.08	1.10
0.01	1.19	1.39	1.59	1.79	1.99
0.02	1.38	1.78	2.18	2.58	2.98
0.05	1.95	2.95	3.95	4.95	5.95
0.10	2.90	4.90	6.90	8.90	10.90
0.15	3.85	6.85	9.85	12.85	15.85
0.20	4.80	8.80	12.80	16.80	20.80

There are two sample size choices in a CRCT, the number of clusters to use and cluster size, or number of patients per cluster. Generally, increasing the number of clusters is a more efficient way to increase statistical power than increasing cluster size. From the previous example with $\rho = 0.02$, we saw that 66 clusters of 20 patients each would yield a total sample size of about 1320 patients to give 90% power to detect a success rate of 40 vs. 30% using an $\alpha = 0.05$ two-sided test. The IF was $[1 + 19 \times 0.02] = 1.38$. If instead we designed a CRCT with 20 clusters of 66 patients each, the corresponding IF $= [1 + 65 \times 0.02] = 2.30$, and keeping total sample size of 1320 would yield a test with statistical power of only 71%. Generally, it is unusual for a CRCT to have adequate statistical power with fewer than 8–10 clusters per treatment arm.

Choice of Design and Balancing in a CRCT

There are three designs that have commonly been used in a CRCT: (1) A completely randomized design involving no prestratification or matching of clusters; (2) stratification of clusters and then randomization of clusters within the strata; and (3) matching of clusters and then randomization within the matched pairs. With a completely randomized design, it is very easy to have imbalance between treatment groups on important baseline patient variables because the number of clusters in a typical trial is small. Some prestratification of clusters is usually desirable to reduce the chances of important baseline imbalances. Prestratification factors might include varying cluster sizes, geographical area, or some overall measure of socioeconomic status. The advantage of stratifying on cluster size and then randomizing within strata is that this helps to guarantee that total sample size in the treatment arms will be relatively equal. One-to-one matching might be useful if the total number of clusters available is not too small. However, if one of the clusters in a matched pair withdraws from the trial, data from the other cluster in the pair cannot be used in the analysis.

Once the clusters in a CRCT are defined, the investigators should think about whether all patients within each cluster should be included in the clinical trial, or whether certain patient inclusion/exclusion criteria are needed. If a sample of patients from each cluster is used, active steps should be taken (e.g., taking a random sample of the patients) to reduce potential selection biases. Blinding or masking issues should also be considered. In a CRCT, it is often not possible to blind the treatments given to the patients, but perhaps the people doing the outcome evaluations could be blinded to treatment condition.

Analysis Issues

Two types of statistical models are widely used for individual-level analyses of CRCTs that account for the ICCs: (1) conditional or subject-specific models, also called mixed-effects models, and (2) marginal or population-averaged models that use the generalized estimating equations (GEE) approach. In the subject-specific model, the treatment effect estimate is specific to a given cluster because the treatment effect estimate is conditional on the specific characteristics of that cluster. In the population-averaged model, the treatment effect estimate is the average change across the entire population under different intervention conditions. For large numbers of clusters, both models tend to converge to yield similar results. Baseline covariates (cluster or patient characteristics) can be incorporated into either model. Application of GEE generally requires that a total of 40 or more clusters be included in the study. Several papers have recommended conditional models for CRCTs focused on change within participants (e.g., preintervention vs. postintervention) and marginal models for CRCTs focused on differences between participants (e.g., intervention condition vs. control condition) [7].

Ethical and Regulatory Issues in CRCTs

CRCTs pose distinct ethical and regulatory challenges for several reasons. First, the units of randomization, intervention, and outcome measurement may involve different organizations and people, so that the identification of the "research subjects" and issues of informed consent are challenging. Second, since the interventions are often administered at the cluster level, many people within each cluster are affected even though some of them (even "vulnerable" people) might not be formal participants in the CRCT and have consented to the CRCT. Third, randomization of clusters often occurs before recruitment and consent of individual participants into the CRCT. And fourth, CRCTs often involve organizations, and it is sometimes unclear what permissions are necessary from these organizations in order to participate.

The 2012 Ottawa Statement on the Ethical Design and Conduct of Cluster Randomized Trials [8] is a consensus statement developed from a meeting of a multidisciplinary expert panel held in November, 2011, to provide guidance on the ethical design and conduct of CRCTs in health research primarily intended for researchers and research ethics committees (RECs). Fifteen recommendations were made and organized by seven identified ethical issues (see Table 10.2). The consensus statement was the product of a transparent and detailed process, including the publication in the open-access journal, *Trials,* of the study protocol [9] and selected background papers on clinical equipoise [10], identifying the research subjects [11], the role and authority of gatekeepers [12], and when informed consent is required [13]. A follow-up workshop meeting of the NIH Health Care Systems Research Collaboratory was held in 2013 to consider the different aspects of the Ottawa statement particularly pertaining to issues of relevance in the US regulatory environment [14].

Data Monitoring

A data monitoring committee (DMC) should be appointed for a cluster randomized trial as it would be for a clinical trial randomizing at the patient level. These DMCs are independent expert panels who undertake regular reviews of the data as the trial progresses to safeguard the interests of the study participants and preserve the integrity of the trial.

Although many data monitoring issues are the same for CRCTs as they are for RCTs that randomize at the patient level, there are some monitoring issues that might be different between the two kinds of randomized trials related to patient eligibility, protocol adherence, consistency of measurement across sites, outcomes, follow-up, early termination of the trial, monitoring of the ICC, and composition of the DMC (see Table 10.3) [15].

Reporting of CRCTs

The Consolidated Standards of Reporting Trials (CONSORT) statement was developed to improve the design and reporting of randomized controlled trials. It was first published in 1996 and further updated in 2001 and 2010. The statement includes a checklist of items that should be reported in the major manuscript from every randomized clinical trial. The statement also recommends including a flow diagram that enumerates all patients screened, randomized, treated, and followed up in a RCT. In 2012, these standards were updated for cluster randomized trials [16]. Table 10.4 summarizes the CONSORT reporting items that were updated for cluster randomized trials.

Table 10.2 Recommendations from the 2012 Ottawa statement on the ethical design and conduct of cluster randomized trials

Ethical issue	Recommendation number	Recommendation
Justify the CRCT design	1	Researchers should provide clear rationale for use of CRCT and adopt statistical methods appropriate for the design
REC review	2	Researchers must submit CRCT for REC review before commencing
Identifying research participants	3	Researchers should clearly identify research participants using 4 published criteria [11]
Obtaining informed consent (IC)	4	Researchers must obtain IC, unless waiver is granted by REC
	5	If IC is not possible before randomization of clusters, it should be obtained ASAP after cluster randomization and before study intervention and data collection
	6	A REC may approve waiver or alteration of IC when research not feasible without waiver and interventions and data collection are minimal risk
	7	Researchers must obtain IC from service providers who are research participants unless there is IC waiver or alteration
Gatekeepers	8	Gatekeepers should not provide proxy consent for individuals in their cluster
	9	When a CRCT may affect cluster or organization interests, the researcher should obtain the gatekeeper's permission, but this does not replace IC of participants
	10	When CRCT interventions substantially affect cluster interests, researchers should seek cluster consultation on study design, conduct, and reporting
Assessing benefits and harms	11	Researchers must ensure that study intervention is adequately justified and consistent with competent practice in the field
	12	Researchers must adequately justify choice of control condition; when control is usual practice, control participants must not be deprived of effective care to which they would have access, if there were no trial
	13	Data collection should be adequately justified, minimized consistent with sound design, and be in reasonable relation to knowledge to be gained
Protecting vulnerable participants	14	Clusters may contain vulnerable participants; researchers and RECs must consider whether additional protections are needed

(continued)

Table 10.2 (continued)

Ethical issue	Recommendation number	Recommendation
	15	When individual IC is required and there are vulnerable participants, RECs should pay special attention to recruitment, privacy, and IC procedures for those participants

REC research ethics committee; *IC* informed consent

Table 10.3 Differences in monitoring considerations by a data monitoring committee (DMC) for a RCT randomizing at the patient level versus a cluster randomized trial (CRCT)

Aspect of the trial	RCT randomizing at the patient level	Cluster randomized clinical trial (CRCT)
Patient eligibility	Monitored closely by the DMC	Very few eligibility criteria; close monitoring probably not needed
Protocol adherence	Monitored closely by the DMC	Mostly irrelevant since level of adherence should reflect treatment use in everyday practice
Consistency of measurement across sites	Largely defined in detailed operations manual, so consistency across sites should be high	Should be closely monitored by DMC since consistency of measurement could be quite variable across sites
Outcomes	Outcomes are generally objective, clinical/biological measures such as mortality, disease progression, biomarkers	Outcomes are often subjective, assessed by treating clinicians, EHR-derived or from claims data, and have more site variability
Follow-up	Usually standardized in protocol and monitored by DMC	Follow-up intervals might differ considerably by site and should be closely monitored by DMC
Early termination for efficacy or futility	Often very important in patient-level randomized RCTs, particularly when outcomes are mortality or major morbidity	Less important in CRCTs, because treatment arms are often accepted treatments used in practice, and outcomes are not usually life-threatening
Monitoring of ICC	Not applicable in patient-level randomized RCTs	Important to monitor in CRCTs, because sample size and power of trial are very sensitive to ICC
Composition of DMC	Clinicians expert in field of study, biostatisticians, bioethicists	Additional members with expertise in medical setting, bioinformatics, and patient representatives

ICC intraclass correlation

Table 10.4 Extension of CONSORT statement to cluster randomized trials

CONSORT Item number	Standard checklist item	Extension for cluster designs
1a	Title and abstract—identification as a randomized trial in title	Identification as a cluster randomized trial in the title
2a	Scientific background and explanation of rationale	Rationale for using a cluster design
3a	Description of trial design including allocation ratio	Definition of cluster and how design features apply to clusters
4a	Eligibility criteria for participants	Eligibility criteria for clusters and participants
5	Interventions for each group, including how and when administered	Whether interventions pertain to cluster level, individual participant level, or both
6a	Primary and secondary outcomes, including how and when assessed	Whether outcomes pertain to cluster level, individual participant level, or both
7a	How sample size was determined	Method of calculation, number of clusters, equal or unequal cluster sizes, assumed ICC
8b	Type of randomization, stratification, blocking, and block size	Details of stratification or matching of clusters if used
9	Allocation concealment mechanism	Whether allocation concealment was at cluster level, individual participant level, or both
10	Who generated randomization, enrolled participants, assigned them to intervention	Who generated randomization, enrolled clusters, assigned clusters to interventions; mechanism by which individuals were included (complete enumeration or random sampling); from whom consent sought and whether before or after randomization of clusters
12a	Statistical methods used to compare groups	How clustering was taken into account in analysis
13a	For each group, number of participants randomized, received intended treatment, analyzed for primary outcome	Number of clusters and participants randomized, received treatment, analyzed for primary outcome
13b	Losses and exclusions after randomization, and reasons	Losses and exclusions for both clusters and individual members
16	For each group, number of participants in analysis, and whether analysis is by assigned groups	For each group, number of clusters and participants in each analysis

(continued)

Table 10.4 (continued)

CONSORT Item number	Standard checklist item	Extension for cluster designs
17a	Results for each group, estimated effect size and precision	Results at the individual or cluster level and ICC for each primary outcome
21	Generalizability of trial findings	Generalizability to clusters and/or individual participants

The Stepped Wedge Cluster Randomized Clinical Trial (SW-CRCT)

The SW-CRCT involves a sequential rollout of the intervention to all clusters over a number of time periods or "steps," with the clusters randomly assigned to the steps. The advantages of this type of design is that eventually all of the clusters will receive the intervention rather than having some clusters only in the control condition throughout the study, and it is often logistically and financially easier to roll out the intervention rather than having to provide the intervention to a large number of clusters at the beginning of the study. Each cluster will usually have one or more time periods of measurement in the control condition and in the intervention condition (i.e., periods after the intervention is introduced). Once a cluster starts the intervention, it remains in that condition until the end of the study.

Analysis of stepped wedge CRCTs can be based on "horizontal" and "vertical" comparisons. "Horizontal" comparisons are based on outcome measurements taken before and after the intervention for each cluster and are unbiased if there are no secular trends. "Vertical" comparisons are based on outcome measurements from clusters that have switched to the intervention and clusters that have yet to switch to the intervention (i.e., clusters that are still in the control condition) and are unbiased due to the randomization of clusters to the steps. Many stepped wedge CRCTs are analyzed with a mixed model, including a random effect for cluster and fixed effects for time period to account for a secular trend [17].

Summary

CRCTs are most useful when interventions are applied at the cluster level and there is concern about the possibility of contamination if the intervention is applied to individual patients. In CRCTs, it is very important to account for the intraclass correlation when determining sample size and analyzing data from the CRCT. CRCTs tend to be less efficient and require larger sample sizes compared to clinical trials that randomize at the patient level. CRCTs have special requirements with regard to ethical and regulatory considerations, data monitoring, and in reporting the trials in the literature. The stepped wedge cluster randomized trial is a special type of CRCT that is useful when interventions are thought to be effective and it is desirable that all clusters eventually receive that intervention.

References

1. Whelan T, Levine M, Willan A, et al. Effect of a decision aid on knowledge and treatment decision making for breast cancer surgery. A randomized trial. JAMA. 2004;292:435–41.
2. Simunovic M, Goldsmith C, Thabane L, et al. The quality initiative in rectal cancer (QIRC) trial: study protocol of a cluster randomized controlled trial in surgery. BMC Surg. 2008;8:4.
3. Fink C, Diener MK, Bruckner T, et al. Impact of preoperative patient education on prevention of postoperative complications after major visceral surgery: study protocol for a randomized controlled trial (PEDUCAT trial). Trials. 2013;14:271.
4. Chaillet N, Dumont A, Abrahamowicz M, et al. A cluster-randomized trial to reduce cesarean delivery rates in Quebec. N Engl J Med. 2015;372:1710–21.
5. Bilimoria KY, Chung JW, Hedges LV, et al. National cluster-randomized trial of duty-hour flexibility in surgical training. N Engl J Med. 2016;374:713–27.
6. Adams G, Gulliford MC, Ukoumunne OC, et al. Patterns of intra-class correlation from primary care research to inform study design and analysis. J Clin Epidemiol. 2004;57:785–94.
7. Murray DM, Varnell SP, Blitstein JL. Design and analysis of group-randomized trials: a review of recent methodological developments. Am J Publ Health. 2004;94:423–32.
8. Weijer C, Grimshaw JM, Eccles MP, et al. The Ottawa statement on the ethical design and conduct of cluster randomized trials. PLOS Med. 2012;9:11.
9. Taljaard M, Weijer C, Grimshaw J, et al. Study protocol: ethical and policy issues in cluster randomized trials: rationale and design of a mixed methods research study. Trials. 2009;10:61.
10. Binik A, Weijer C, McRae AD, et al. Does clinical equipoise apply to cluster randomized trials in health research? Trials. 2011;12:118.
11. McRae AD, Weijer C, Binik A, et al. Who is the research subject in cluster randomized trials in health research? Trials. 2011;12:183.
12. Gallo A, Weijer C, White A, et al. What is the role and authority of gatekeepers in cluster randomized trials in health research? Trials. 2012;13:116.
13. McRae AD, Weijer C, Binik A, et al. When is informed consent required in cluster randomized trials in health research? Trials. 2011;12:202.
14. Anderson ML, Califf RM, Sugarman J. Ethical and regulatory issues of pragmatic cluster randomized trials in contemporary health systems. Clin Trials. 2015;12:276–86.
15. Ellenberg SS, Culbertson R, Gillen DL, et al. Data monitoring committees for pragmatic clinical trials. Clin Trials. 2015;12:530–6.
16. Campbell MK, Piaggio G, Elbourne DR, et al. Consort 2010 statement: extension to cluster randomized trials. BMJ. 2012;345:19–22.
17. Rhoda DA, Murray DM, Andridge RR, et al. Studies with staggered starts: multiple baseline designs and group-randomized trials. Am J Publ Health. 2011;101:2164–9.

Chapter 11
Adaptive Trial Designs

Joshua S. Richman and Judy C. Boughey

The nature of any experiment is that its outcome is uncertain. Due to their great expense and logistical challenges, key aspects of clinical trials including treatments, interventions, definition and measurement of outcomes and sample size must be carefully planned in advance. Because the parameters required for precise planning are often not completely known, it follows that clinical trials are almost always planned with incomplete information. While simple trial designs like the parallel two-arm trial with fixed recruitment goals and equal randomization between groups remain common, the fact that their design is fixed from the beginning may result in an inefficient or even an unethical use of resources. One approach to minimize these concerns is the use of an adaptive trial design. Adaptive designs respond to these limitations by carefully building pre-specified decision points or rules into the trial design which allows for the ongoing conduct of a trial to be informed and changed by data collected during the trial. The crucial element of adaptive designs is that these changes and decision points must be pre-specified. The pre-specification allows full control at the design stage of the probability of type-one errors (false positives). This contrasts with 'flexible' designs that allow for changes in the trial conduct that are not fully specified in advance [1, 2]. The key point is that adaptive trials are not flexible because the possibility of changes and the decision points have

J.S. Richman (✉)
Department of Surgery, University of Alabama at Birmingham
and the Birmingham VAMC, Kracke 217C, 1922 7th Ave South,
Birmingham, AL 35203, USA
e-mail: jrichman@uabmc.edu

J.C. Boughey
Division of Subspecialty General Surgery, Mayo Clinic,
200 First Street SW, 55905 Rochester, MN, USA
e-mail: Boughey.judy@mayo.edu

© Springer International Publishing AG 2017   99
K.M.F. Itani and D.J. Reda (eds.), *Clinical Trials Design in Operative
and Non Operative Invasive Procedures*, DOI 10.1007/978-3-319-53877-8_11

been made in advance to be determined by the data and the protocol rather than being left to the researchers' discretion. Although adaptive trials can be quite complicated, because of careful planning their statistical properties can be understood in advance. The same is not true of flexible trials, which makes their interpretation more difficult. Discussion in this section will be limited to pre-planned adaptive trials.

General Considerations

Potential Advantages

Adaptive designs can use resources more efficiently because they can allow a trial to be stopped early due to inferiority, superiority or futility, or can focus a study on the most promising treatments. For example, a multi-arm adaptive design may allow for less promising therapeutic arms to be dropped early in the study, allocating more of the remaining patients and resources to the more promising study arms. In response to early data, adaptive enrichment designs can change the enrollment criteria to target subgroups that have the greatest chance of benefitting from the treatment. This helps not only increase the success rate of the study, but also increase the chances patients are receiving an effective intervention. Designs that include sample size re-estimation, often with an internal pilot design, can help ensure that studies have sufficient sample size and thus a high probability for success. Studies with an internal pilot can also progress more rapidly from stage II to stage III without the need to obtain separate funding between a pilot study and a larger definitive trial.

Potential Disadvantages

Trials with adaptive designs are more complicated than traditional trials and require increased effort to ensure that they are properly designed. The complexity and possibility that the trial procedures will change at various points during the trial increases the amount of training required and adds logistical challenges for the conduct and monitoring of the study. Improper designs can introduce bias or result in findings that are difficult to interpret. Adaptive designs may also result in greater expense than standard designs.

Sequential Group Designs

Many trials are designed to include interim testing during the course of the trial, often as part of the data and safety monitoring plan. Group sequential designs specifically include interim testing at pre-defined points during a trial. The points for interim analyses can be determined by patient accrual, number of events observed, or the amount of time since the trial commenced.

This type of trial can be considered to be an adaptive design when stopping rules are set to identify whether the trial should be stopped early due to inferiority or superiority of the experimental treatment. If either superiority or inferiority of the experimental procedure can be conclusively demonstrated at an interim analysis, a compelling ethical argument can be made that there is no longer equipoise and continuing the randomized trial is unethical. Trials can also be stopped due to futility—the case where based on data already collected, it is determined that there is a very small probability of observing a significant effect at the trial's conclusion. In this scenario, the argument can also be made that continuing the trial is unethical because the additional data are unlikely to provide useful information.

The primary concern with sequential analyses is that testing outcomes at multiple time points inflates the probability of a type-one error, or α. Several strategies for defining the stopping rules are well documented in the literature. In general, the stopping rules are defined in terms of the p value required for significance at each point designed to preserve the overall α-level. The trade-off among the methods is between making it easier to stop a trial early (larger p value required for interim analyses) and more difficult for a final analysis to be significant (smaller p value required for the final analysis). One of the simplest is the Pocock boundary which, for a given number of planned tests, sets a single p value for stopping the trial. [3] For example, to preserve an overall α of 0.05 with four planned tests (three interim and one final), the trial will be considered conclusive if the test, at any point, has a p value <0.0182. A disadvantage of this method is that it requires pre-specifying the number of planned analyses and the p value allowed for the final analysis is the same as for the interim time points. A similar approach called the Haybittle–Peto stopping rule sets the stopping rule to be a p value less than 0.001 for interim analyses and then tests the final analysis at whichever p value maintains the desired overall α-level. [4, 5] This has the advantage of preserving the nominal α-level for the final analysis, but the potential disadvantage of requiring very extreme results to stop a trial early.

A more popular approach uses O'Brien-Fleming boundaries with very small p values for stopping rules at early analyses. The p values for stopping rules at subsequent tests increase gradually so that final test can have an α-level close to the overall level (e.g., 0.045).

Both of these methods require specifying the number of interim tests and the point at which they will be conducted in advance, usually in terms of recruitment or the number of events observed. A more flexible method introduced by Lan and DeMets rests on the idea of α spending, where each test 'spends' a certain amount of the overall α-level [6]. By using a pre-specified spending function, it allows for boundaries to be calculated when analyses are desired rather than being specified in advance. This approach also allows for an increase in the number of interim 'looks' at the data, for example, due to study extensions. The choice of spending function will determine whether they look more like an O'Brien-Fleming or Pocock boundary.

Multi-arm Adaptive Designs (Drop-the-Losers; Pick-the-Winners)

In the early stages of research, there may be considerable uncertainty about which of several procedures or treatments is best and a full-scale multi-arm trial to evaluate multiple options concurrently may be prohibitively expensive. An appropriate adaptive design would be a multi-arm drop-the-losers (alternatively, pick-the-winner) approach. These designs are typically for a two-stage study with multiple arms included at the initial stages in the study [7]. At the end of the initial phase, the least promising treatments are dropped while recruitment and data collection are continued only for the most promising treatment(s). Typically, these trials only have power for the definitive analysis at the conclusion of data collection. Thus, the selection of the best treatments after the initial phase is often not based on statistically significant differences between groups and the selection is therefore more susceptible to chance. Nevertheless, it can be a useful strategy for efficiently screening multiple treatments to more narrowly focus a definitive study. Designs that include data from the first phase are also vulnerable to bias if the effect of the best performing intervention in the first phase was higher than its actual expected value.

Adaptive Randomization

Classically, study participants are randomized to their study group with fixed probabilities that remain constant throughout the study. In contrast, adaptive randomization methods change these probabilities throughout the study according to data already collected. There are two types of adaptive randomization: covariate-adaptive randomization and response-adaptive randomization [1].

In a large study, classical randomization with constant allocation probabilities is very likely to balance most covariates across study arms. However, there is no guarantee that every covariate will be balanced, and the likelihood of observing large differences in covariates between groups due to chance is higher in small studies. Covariate-adaptive randomization methods assess the balance between groups for key covariates as enrollment accrues and randomization probabilities are changed to promote balance. Covariate-adaptive randomization may be desirable when there are particular covariates known in advance for which balance is particularly important. Balance on these covariates could be important either because they are linked to the outcome of interest, for example age and mortality after surgery, or because they are needed for planned subgroup analyses, like analyses within each gender or within races. While stratified randomization may be appropriate for balancing a few categorical characteristics, adaptive methods are more likely to be successful for simultaneously balancing several covariates including continuous characteristics [8–10]. An effective and accepted technique for adaptive randomization is called minimization. After randomizing the first few patients, the method calculates a measure of imbalance based on the chosen covariates. As new participants are enrolled, this imbalance measure along with their covariates is used to adaptively alter randomization probabilities to minimize the overall imbalance in characteristics between study groups [8].

Using adaptive randomization methods does require careful attention be paid to the study's randomization protocol. In particular, the covariates that are the focus of the adaptive randomization must be captured reasonably quickly around the time of enrollment to ensure that they can inform future randomizations. Fortunately, the availability of centralized and web-based randomization makes coordinating covariate-adaptive randomization practical even across multi-site studies.

The second major type of adaptive randomization is response-adaptive randomization, where randomization probabilities change in relation to observed study outcomes increasing the probability of being randomized to the more successful treatment, often referred to as 'play-the-winner.' The canonical example was a prospective trial of extracorporeal membrane oxygenation (ECMO) neonatal respiratory failure [11]. The first patient had an equal chance of being randomized to receive ECMO or not. Afterward, probability of randomization to a treatment was increased according to how successful the treatment had been. Ultimately, a single neonate did not receive ECMO and died, while 11 received ECMO and survived.

The play-the-winner design was justified in that case because, although ECMO for neonates had not been tested in a randomized trial, there were ethical concerns about randomizing patients to receive standard therapy when ECMO was promising and potentially lifesaving. As a practical matter with the gravely ill patient population, an unsuccessful outcome, mortality, was known to be common with standard treatment and would be observed soon after randomization and would inform future randomizations. It follows that this design would be inappropriate for a study of long-term survival, but it could be used for a trial where the outcome was both common and proximal like discharge home vs. an acute-care facility.

Adaptive randomization allows multiple interventions to be compared in the same trial against one control group—allowing fewer patients to receive standard therapy and more patients to receive experimental agents. This decreases the cost of the clinical trial. For example, if the one adaptive trial has a control group and intervention A, intervention B and intervention C being compared, the patients enrolled in the study have higher chance of receiving one of the novel interventions. From the cost of the trial, fewer patients are treated in the control group, keeping study costs lower than if this was run as three independent trials of intervention A versus control, intervention B versus control and intervention C versus control.

Another example is the ISPY2 trial which evaluates multiple experimental treatments for breast cancer. The number of experimental agents in the study varies over time all compared to one control arm. The objective is to accelerate oncology drug testing and expedite approval. The adaptive design is based on biomarker subtypes with the endpoint being complete eradication of disease at time of surgery.

Enrichment Designs

Clinical trials often have specific inclusion and exclusion criteria that serve to 'enrich' the study sample with the type of patients who the investigators believe are most likely to benefit from the experimental therapy. Specifying a narrow study cohort prior to the trial risks including patient subgroups that benefit very little, if at all, or has a chance of excluding subgroups that may benefit the most. Adaptive enrichment designs begin by enrolling a broad range of patients for the initial phase [1, 12]. After the first phase of the trial, planned interim analyses are used to identify which subgroups in the trial appear most or least likely to benefit from the intervention. Following this determination, enrollment criteria are shifted to include the most promising subgroups and exclude the least promising.

The potential advantage of this approach is that it allows data to identify the best patient groups for a definitive trial and then efficiently targets recruitment to those groups. In this sense, it is very similar to the pick-the-winners approach with a broad early phase that is then more narrowly focused for the remainder of the trial. It also shares similar limitations due to the variability of early analysis with limited data. The groups showing the largest benefit in early analyses may regress toward the mean and show a smaller benefit in the final analysis. This can also occur if the identification of the subgroups is the result of exploratory data analysis. In that case, large effects for a particular subgroup may not generalize to a larger sample. Similarly, subgroups that are dropped after the first phase may have ultimately showed a larger effect in the final analysis if that group had continued to be enrolled.

Sample Size Re-estimation and Internal Pilot Designs

Typically, trials have fixed sample sizes designed to maintain adequate statistical power. However, sample size calculations are based on many unknowns such as the size of the hypothesized treatment effect, or 'nuisance parameters' that are of less interest like variability in measures or outcome rates. These nuisance parameters are not the main focus of the study but are nevertheless critical for determining sample size. Some estimates can be drawn from data in the literature on similar populations, and others are extrapolated from limited data or are informed, and hopefully conservative, estimates. Given the high cost of clinical trials, there is pressure to design the trial with a sample size just large enough to provide a definitive answer. Underestimating the necessary sample size risks having inadequate statistical power, while overly large sample sizes can become prohibitively expensive. Inaccurate estimates of any of the parameters at the design stage can result in a trial that does not have an appropriate sample size.

An adaptive design approach to overcome some of the uncertainty in sample size estimation is to incorporate early data to re-estimate the required sample size. In theory, any of the unknown parameters needed to calculate sample size could be used for re-estimation, including the main effect between treatment and control groups, or variability in measures and rates of outcomes [7]. Many authors are critical of sample size re-estimation methods that consider the observed differences between control and intervention groups at an interim time point in the study on the grounds that they can increase type-one error or treatment bias and that they convey early information to investigators about treatment effects that can compromise blinding. For example, knowing that the sample size has been increased may imply that in early observations the treatment effect is not as large as was hoped and this knowledge may influence the ongoing conduct of the trial. In contrast, while interim analyses in group sequential designs also provide some information, the actions taken are to continue the study as planned (i.e., no action) or to stop the study early. In neither case is important information given that may alter the conduct of the study going forward [1].

The most accepted sample size re-estimation practices consider estimating parameters that pool measurements across study groups providing no information about differences between groups. Using early data to estimate the variance can provide more precise estimates and allow for a corrected sample size going forward. Similarly, calculating event rates can be important for studies whose outcomes are survival or other discrete events because their statistical power relies on the number of observed events rather than the number of participants. Information that the events rates are lower than projected can lead to increasing enrollment or prolonging follow-up to maintain statistical power. Usually, these methods only allow for increasing sample size beyond the initial target. Estimates of parameters from early data may not be precise, and revising the sample size downward based on an underestimate of the variance (or over-estimate of the event rate) may ultimately result in an under-powered study.

Formally, internal pilot designs are a specific form of sample size re-estimation conceived as two-stage studies where the initial phase is planned as a pilot study without hypothesis testing [1, 13]. These avoid the potential pitfalls of considering group differences and inflating the type-one error with multiple testing. The final analysis includes data from both the initial pilot phase and the second phase. Regardless of interim testing, there is a small penalty in terms of type-one error from the sample size re-estimation itself. However, a properly designed internal pilot can limit and control this impact [14–16].

As with other adaptive designs, sample size re-estimation methods add complexity to a clinical trial. A key decision is at which point to do the re-estimation. If done too early, parameter estimates may include very little information and be very imprecise, while waiting too long could make expanding the sample size impractical. At the very least, sample size re-estimation should be done at a point in the accrual period when there is still enough time to get the necessary IRB and regulatory approvals in place before recruitment are scheduled to end. The importance of including sample size re-estimation can vary widely depending on circumstances, though in general it becomes more important with studies that are initially planned with small sample sizes and with relatively large uncertainty about the variability in outcomes or the hypothesized study effect [17]. From the budgetary standpoint, this design may not be appealing because it explicitly allows for greater expenses than initially planned. Overall sample size re-estimation can provide a method to help ensure that a study will have adequate power or to decide that a properly powered study would not be feasible.

Summary and Further Reading

Given that studies are designed with uncertain outcomes, adaptive designs offer the opportunity to use data collected early in the trial to inform the conduct of the rest of the study. Careful planning of the scope and decision points of adaptations is critical to avoid compromising the integrity of the trial. Adaptive trials do inevitably add statistical and logistical complexity and can be more difficult to explain and interpret. For further reading, more extensive reviews of adaptive methods are available, including the report 'Adaptive Designs for Medical Device Clinical Studies' issued by the FDA [18] and 'Standards for the Design, Conduct, and Evaluation of Adaptive Randomized Clinical Trials' from the Patient Centered Outcomes Research Institute. [19].

References

1. Kairalla JA, Coffey CS, Thomann MA, Muller KE. Adaptive trial designs: a review of barriers and opportunities. Trials. 2012;13:145.
2. Brannath W, Koenig F, Bauer P. Multiplicity and flexibility in clinical trials. Pharm Stat. 2007;6(3):205–16.
3. Pocock SJ. Group sequential methods in the design and analysis of clinical trials. Biometrika. 1977;64(2):191–9.
4. Haybittle JL. Repeated assessment of results in clinical trials of cancer treatment. Br J Rad. 1971;44(256):526–793.
5. Peto R, Pike MC, Armitage P, et al. Design and analysis of randomized clinical trials requiring prolonged observation of each patient. I. Introduction and design. Br J Cancer. 1976;34(6):585–612.

6. DeMets DL, Lan KK. Interim analysis: the alpha spending function approach. Stat Med. Jul 15–30 1994;13(13–14):1341–1352; discussion 1353–1346.
7. Chow SC, Chang M. Adaptive design methods in clinical trials—a review. Orphanet J Rare Dis. 2008;3:11.
8. Rosenberger WF, Sverdlov O, Hu F. Adaptive randomization for clinical trials. J Biopharm Stat. 2012;22(4):719–36.
9. Rosenberger WF. Handling covariates in the design of clinical trials. Stat Sci. 2008;23 (3):404–19.
10. Antogninin AB, Zagoraiou M. The covariate-adaptive biased coin design for balancing clinical trials in the presence of prognostic factors. Biometrika. 2010;98(3):519–35.
11. Bartlett RH, Roloff DW, Cornell RG, Andrews AF, Dillon PW, Zwischenberger JB. Extracorporeal circulation in neonatal respiratory failure: a prospective randomized study. Pediatrics. 1985;76(4):479–87.
12. Wang SJ, Hung HM, O'Neill RT. Adaptive patient enrichment designs in therapeutic trials. Biometrical J Biometrische Z. Apr 2009;51(2):358–374.
13. Wittes J, Brittain E. The role of internal pilot studies in increasing the efficiency of clinical trials. Stat Med. 1990;9(1–2):65–71; discussion 71–62.
14. Kieser M, Friede T. Re-calculating the sample size in internal pilot study designs with control of the type I error rate. Stat Med. 2000;19(7):901–11.
15. Coffey CS, Muller KE. Controlling test size while gaining the benefits of an internal pilot design. Biometrics. 2001;57(2):625–31.
16. Coffey CS, Kairalla JA, Muller KE. Practical Methods for Bounding Type I Error Rate with an Internal Pilot Design. Commun Stat Theory Meth. 2007;36(11).
17. Guoqiao W, Kennedy RE, Cutter GR, Schneider LS. Effect of sample size re-estimation in adaptive clinical trials for Alzheimer's disease and mild cognitive impairment. Alzheimer's Dement Transl Res Clin Interventions. 2015;1(1):63–71.
18. Health and Human Services, Food and Drug Administration. Adaptive Designs for Medical Device Clinical Studies: Guidance for Industry and Food and Drug Administration Staff. 2016; http://www.fda.gov/downloads/medicaldevices/deviceregulationandguidance/guidance documents/ucm446729.pdf. Accessed (Issued July, 2016).
19. Detry MA, Lewis RJ, Broglio KR, Conner JT, Berry SM, Berry DA. Standards for the Design, Conduct, and Evaluation of Adaptive Randomized Clinical Trials. 2012; http://www. pcori.org/assets/Standards-for-the-Design-Conduct-and-Evaluation-of-Adaptive-Randomized-Clinical-Trials.pdf.

Chapter 12
Pragmatic Trials

Ryan E. Ferguson and Louis Fiore

The Case for Pragmatic Trials

Reports from the Institute of Medicine, the Federal Coordinating Council for Comparative Effectiveness Research, and the Congressional Budget Office cite the lack of evidence to support a given course of treatment as a significant obstacle to improving the quality and lowering the cost of health care [1–4]. Also recognized is the inability of current models of evidence generation to meet this need fully. Widespread gaps in evidence-based knowledge result from a paucity of randomized clinical trials of comparative effectiveness [5]. Reliable evidence of this type is needed to improve health-care quality and to support the efficient use of limited resources [5].

Pragmatic Trials: One End of the Spectrum

Randomized controlled trials have traditionally been viewed as a dichotomy, either as effectiveness trials or as efficacy trials [6]. Current thinking places trials on a spectrum between "explanatory trials" which attempt to test causal hypotheses and "pragmatic trials" which attempt to help clinicians choose between treatment

R.E. Ferguson (✉)
Boston Cooperative Studies Program Coordinating Center, Massachusetts Veterans Epidemiology Research and Information Center, VA Boston Healthcare System
150 South Huntington Ave (151-MAV), Boston, MA 02130, USA
e-mail: ryan.ferguson@va.gov

L. Fiore
Department of Veterans Affairs Boston Healthcare System,
150 South Huntington Avenue, Boston, MA 02130, USA
e-mail: lfiore@bu.edu

© Springer International Publishing AG 2017
K.M.F. Itani and D.J. Reda (eds.), *Clinical Trials Design in Operative and Non Operative Invasive Procedures*, DOI 10.1007/978-3-319-53877-8_12

options [7]. Explanatory trials focus on the efficacy of an intervention under "ideal conditions." In contrast, pragmatic trials are designed to determine the effects of an intervention under the usual condition(s) in which it is delivered in a health-care setting [7]. Few trials are purely pragmatic or explanatory and, as a result, we are "left with a multi-dimensional continuum rather than a dichotomy where a particular trial may display varying levels of pragmatism across [many] dimensions" [7].

Explanatory trials are a necessary component of the research process as they are required for the introduction of novel therapeutics into clinical care. Most pre-approval trials of health-care interventions are on the explanatory end of the trials spectrum [8] and are intended to demonstrate benefit under ideal circumstances in an ideal patient population. Failure in this mode, where there is the greatest perceived chance of success, warrants future effectiveness trials unnecessary [8]. If, however, efficacy is demonstrated, an effectiveness trial may be helpful in determination of the utility of the intervention to a more generalized patient population being treated in everyday practice. Thus, demonstrated success in an efficacy trial is an important prerequisite for progression to an effectiveness trial [9].

Pragmatic trials assessing the effectiveness of an intervention in a setting that resembles usual care informs health-care practitioners and health-care planners on the best treatment options for their patients [10]. A key issue for pragmatic studies is the balance between internal validity (reliability and accuracy of the results) and external validity (generalizability of the results). Explanatory trials seek to create an environment that will maximize internal validity by rigorous and stringent control of factors that may obscure or diminish the ability to measure the utility of an intervention. (e.g., inclusion criteria, exclusion criteria, and protocol-defined treatments). Pragmatic trials seek instead to maximize external validity so that the trial results can be widely generalized and hence integrated into clinical care. Pragmatic trials must balance internal and external validity such that treatment effects are preserved, but are observed across a greater diversity of patients treated by processes extant in the more relaxed clinical environment [10].

Karanicolas et al. [11] point out that the usefulness and generalizability of results of pragmatic trials are dependent on the context (i.e., the distinctive features of the trial setting, population, and investigative staff) in which the trial was performed. Consider a clinical trial comparing web-based self-help for problem drinking where inclusion criteria required the participants to have internet access [8]. Treweek and Zwarenstein [8] point out that this is likely less an issue in the Netherlands where internet penetration was close to 88% in 2007, than in Poland where internet penetration was just under 30% in the same year. Thus, the context of a pragmatic trial will directly impact both interpretation of the effectiveness of the intervention and its external validity. Balance of internal and external validity and the context of the trial are inextricably linked design issues for pragmatic trials.

Key Design Features of Pragmatic Trials

Features of both explanatory and pragmatic trials are presented in Table 12.1. Gartlehner et al. [12] and Thorpe et al. [7] independently built tools to help investigators assess the degree to which their trial is pragmatic or explanatory to assure that the design is optimized for the intended purpose. These tools focus on the design features in Table 12.1 and help investigators understand the design features that contribute to the validity balance. Below, we focus on design decisions that enhance external validity or internal validity.

External validity, or generalizability, is maximized by limiting exclusion criteria and keeping inclusion criteria broad. Enrolled subjects will then more closely resemble the heterogeneity of the general patient population as reflected by their comorbidities and medications usage patterns. External validity is further improved when the treatment protocol allows for flexibility in the management of the subject by allowing the health-care provider the freedom to deviate from the study protocol

Table 12.1 Comparison of pragmatic and explanatory trial designs

	Pragmatic trials	Explanatory trials
Objective	To compare the effectiveness of health care and delivery	To assess the efficacy of the intervention
Setting	Routine clinical care	Research/experimental care
Patient population	Heterogeneous to mimic real world; little or no selection	Homogeneous to minimize bias; highly selected
Investigators; stakeholders	health-care providers; CEO and CFO of health-care institution	Scientists and clinical trialists; sponsor
Interventions	Complex intervention; applied flexibility with treatment regime; mimics routine care	Standardized intervention; protocol strictly enforced; regime often simpler than pragmatic trials
Outcomes	Direct impact on clinical care and practice guidelines (e.g., QOL; function)	Impact understanding of action; indirect (or no real) impact on clinical care (e.g., biomarker, range of motion)
Design issues	• High external validity • Low internal validity • Randomized • Large sample Size • Unblinded • Not placebo controlled • Long-term follow-up	• Low external validity • High internal validity • Randomized • Large sample Size • Blinded • Placebo controlled • Short-term follow-up
Sponsor	health-care systems; ACOs; NIH	Pharmaceutical industry; NIH; government
Funding	$$$	$$$
Example trial	Comparative effectiveness of two diuretics for the prevention of MACE outcomes (CSP 597)	Investigational new drug application for a third-generation oral hypoglycemic agent

[Based on data from Ref. 8 & 14]

if it is in the best interest of the patient. This freedom is "fundamentally pragmatic and has to be permitted if the results are to be accepted as generalizable" [10].

Internal validity is instead maximized by features such as restriction of enrollment and randomization and blinding. Restriction as operationalized in inclusion and exclusion criteria assures a tightly controlled and highly selected homogeneous study population that reduces bias and confounding by comorbid conditions, treatment indication, etc. Randomization further ensures that the remaining diversity of the patient population is equally distributed between treatment allocations by balancing known and unknown baseline confounders. The assumption of equal distribution is not absolute, and further control may be required in the secondary analyses of the trial. Finally, blinding of participants and/or the providers helps ensure that opportunities for information bias are reduced.

Analysis of Pragmatic Trials

Analysis of pragmatic trials follows the "intent-to-treat" principle (i.e., once randomized always analyzed) where study groups are analyzed according to the treatment group to which they were *originally* assigned. Intention to treat analysis becomes problematic for pragmatic studies when subjects' treatments are changed in the course of usual care to that of the non-assigned study arm. The downstream result of this is an observed dilution of the treatment effect. Although dilution effect is often viewed as a weakness of pragmatic trials, as it is for explanatory trials, it does reflect the expected results when the treatment is used in the "real-world setting" and, as such, is informative for clinical care. Explanatory trials, on the other hand, impose protocol-defined restrictions on patient care that more successfully maintain treatment fidelity and reduce the dilution effect, at the expense of perhaps misrepresenting the benefit when the treatment is applied to a non-study setting.

Strengths and Limitations of Pragmatic Trials

Strengths

The greatest strength of pragmatic trials is the evidence of effectiveness in everyday clinical contexts [13]. Explanatory trials are often restricted in their patient populations under study and in the treatment regimens followed. For this reason, the results are often poorly translated into clinical care. The broad inclusion criteria and the flexible treatment guidelines of pragmatic trials ensure greater generalizability of the results to real-world settings. Economic impact and quality of life are also better studied in a pragmatic trial [14]. The results will contribute to a better understanding of the acceptability of interventions to patients, providers, and health-care systems.

Limitations

Pragmatic trials focus on the clinical and comparative effectiveness of interventions in routine care settings where considerable variability in patient care can result in obscuring the effect attributed to the treatment under study [14]. Another important consideration is that for practical reasons pragmatic studies often lack blinding as a design feature, thus increasing the risk of bias and decreasing internal study validity. Importantly, the reduced interval validity of pragmatic studies is balanced by increased external validity that allows study results to generalize better to normal clinical settings [14]. Pragmatic trials conducted in the clinical care ecosystem have design limitations based on what trial related activities can and cannot be carried out in this setting given time commitment and cost considerations. Kent and Kitsios [9] argue that extrapolating the results of broadly inclusive pragmatic trials to the care of real patients may often be as problematic as extrapolating the results of narrowly focused explanatory or efficacy trials. For example, a null explanatory trial will provide definitive evidence that a therapy is not of value while a null pragmatic trial will not provide similar definitive evidence. As discussed above, dilution of the effect may reduce the observed difference in effect such that a treatment proven successful in an explanatory trial has no demonstrated utility in a pragmatically designed study. Moreover, the relaxed inclusion and exclusion criteria of pragmatic trials result in greater heterogeneity of baseline risks of enrolled subjects and difficulty in interpreting the trial result for a "typical" patient [9]. Instead, a negative effectiveness trial will underscore the caution that physicians must use when generalizing the results of a positive efficacy trial. Kent and Kitsios emphasize: "that while both types of trials yield useful information, pragmatic trials do not provide a more accurate measure of the "true" treatment effect, since the concept of a true effect is fundamentally illusory. While extrapolating the results of efficacy trials to the care of individual patients in the real world can be problematic, and requires careful physician judgment and decision-making, the same is unfortunately true for the results of effectiveness trials. Unless more attention is paid to these underappreciated limitations, pragmatic trials run the risk of driving harmful policies" [9].

Conclusion

Pragmatic studies are designed to address an evidence gap in health-care delivery. Such trials often have a mixture of efficacy and effectiveness outcomes and should carefully balance issues related to internal and external validity. Care should be taken in interpretation of pragmatic trials. Pragmatically designed trials have a host of limitations that are often underappreciated, and extrapolating results from such limited studies can lead to the implementation of "harmful" policies.

References

1. Institute of Medicine. Learning what works best; the nation's need for evidence on comparative effectiveness in health care. Washington DC, USA: Institute of Medicine of the National Academies; 2007.
2. Institute of Medicine. Initial national priorities for comparative effectiveness research. Washington DC, USA: Institute of Medicine of the National Academies; 2009.
3. Congressional Budget Office. Research on the comparative effectiveness of medical treatments: issues and options for an expanded federal role. Washington, DC, USA: Congress of the United States, Congressional Budget Office; 2007.
4. Federal coordinating council for comparative effectiveness research. Report to the President and the Congress: U.S. Department of Health and Human Services. Washington DC, USA: US Department of Health and Human Services, 2009.
5. Tunis SR, Stryer DB, Clancy CM. Practical clinical trials: increasing the value of clinical research for decision making in clinical and health policy. JAMA. 2003;290(12):1624–32. doi:10.1001/jama.290.12.1624.
6. Schwartz D, Lellouch J. Explanatory and pragmatic attitudes in therapeutical trials. J Chronic Dis. 1967;20(8):637–48.
7. Thorpe KE, Zwarenstein M, Oxman AD, Treweek S, Furberg CD, Altman DG, Tunis S, Bergel E, Harvey I, Magid DJ, Chalkidou K. A pragmatic–explanatory continuum indicator summary (PRECIS): a tool to help trial designers. J Clin Epidemiol. 2009;62(5):464–75.
8. Treweek S, Zwarenstein M. Making trials matter: pragmatic and explanatory trials and the problem of applicability. Trials. 2009;10(1):1.
9. Kent DM, Kitsios G. Against pragmatism: on efficacy, effectiveness and the real world. Trials. 2009;10(1):48.
10. Godwin M, Ruhland L, Casson I, MacDonald S, Delva D, Birtwhistle R, Lam M, Seguin R. Pragmatic controlled clinical trials in primary care: the struggle between external and internal validity. BMC Med Res Methodol. 2003;3(1):28.
11. Karanicolas PJ, Montori VM, Devereaux PJ, Schünemann H, Guyatt GH. A new "mechanistic-practical" framework for designing and interpreting randomized trials. J Clin Epidemiol. 2009;62(5):479–84.
12. Gartlehner G, Hansen RA, Nissman D, Lohr KN, Carey TS. A simple and valid tool distinguished efficacy from effectiveness studies. J Clin Epidemiol. 2006;59(10):1040–8.
13. Medical Research Council. A framework for the development and evaluation of RCTs for complex interventions to improve health. London: MRC; 2000.
14. MacPherson H. Pragmatic clinical trials. Complement Ther Med. 2004;12(2):136–40.

Chapter 13
Point-of-Care Clinical Trials

Mary T. Brophy and Ryan E. Ferguson

Background

When discussing with a patient the indication, risk and benefits of an operative or non-operative invasive procedure, the physician must assess multiple factors that may influence the expected outcome and formulate individualized recommendations for the individual patient. This assessment requires a number of clinical decisions as how best to optimize every aspect of care, from presentation to recovery, minimizing the potential for unexpected complications, morbidity and mortality. Patients expect this personalized treatment plan to be based upon the best and most up to date scientific evidence applied to their specific situation.

The problem clinicians face is a scarcity of the highest quality scientific evidence to guide most of these treatment decisions [1]. Healthcare policy makers similarly suffer from a lack of data as they attempt to create systems that produce the most cost-effective, highest quality care [2]. These knowledge gaps lead to decision making that is arbitrary, based on clinician impressions and bias rather than on evidence, and result in variability in practice across clinicians with delivery of suboptimal care and inefficient use of valuable resources [3].

The randomized controlled clinical trial is the gold standard for medical evidence generation. Rigorous traditional clinical trials enroll a homogeneous patient population and attempt to control to the extent possible for variations in clinical practice. As such these trials are considered 'explanatory' in that they determine treatment superiority in an idealized setting and form the basis of FDA approval of

M.T. Brophy (✉) · R.E. Ferguson
Boston Cooperative Studies Program Coordinating Center, Massachusetts Veterans
Epidemiology Research and Information Center, VA Boston Healthcare System,
150 South Huntington Ave (151-MAV), Boston, MA 02130, USA
e-mail: mary.brophy@va.gov

R.E. Ferguson
e-mail: ryan.ferguson@va.gov

© Springer International Publishing AG 2017
K.M.F. Itani and D.J. Reda (eds.), *Clinical Trials Design in Operative
and Non Operative Invasive Procedures*, DOI 10.1007/978-3-319-53877-8_13

new therapeutics or label changes in already-marketed drugs. The idealized experimental environment of explanatory clinical trials and the highly selected patient population accounts for the skepticism of clinicians to adopt recommendations based on their findings and accounts for the lag between publication of study results and acceptance by the medical community (the T2 translation gap).

In contrast to explanatory clinical trials, pragmatic studies are designed to inform clinical decision making and typically compare the effectiveness of two or more treatment interventions in settings that more closely reflect usual care. Study selection criteria and procedures mandated by the study protocol are relaxed and lead to enrollment of a more diverse patient population whose treatment more closely resembles that delivered in usual care. Pragmatic clinical trials vary considerably in the extent to which they are integrated into clinic practice, and studies comparing treatment options already in widespread use (comparative effectiveness studies) fit best into the pragmatic framework [4]. It is important to point out that even pragmatic clinical trials can be overly 'operationalized' and lose many of the benefits (efficiency, scalability) that this design type offers [4–6].

Widespread adoption of electronic health record systems has made possible a transformational change in pragmatic clinical trial design—the point-of-care (POC) clinical trial. These trials embed clinical trial processes such as subject randomization and ascertainment of outcomes unobtrusively into the electronic health record to the fullest extent possible [7]. The ability to embed clinical trial operation seamlessly into the clinical care ecosystem minimizes the distinctions between clinical care and research and generates more generalizable results that can be rapidly implemented. Other features of POC studies include reduced cost (no need for a separate clinical trial apparatus to treat patients) and greater scalability (from less stringent selection criteria) that allows for rapid iteration of clinical trials and incorporation of findings directly and efficiently into clinical practice as decision support, creating an integrated environment of research-based care that defines a learning healthcare system [8] (Figs. 13.1, 13.2 and 13.3).

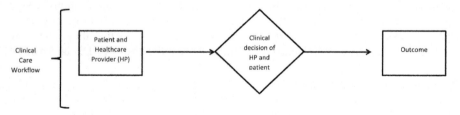

Fig. 13.1 Panel A. Traditional clinical workflow: choice of intervention is selected by the healthcare provider and the patient is followed for outcomes

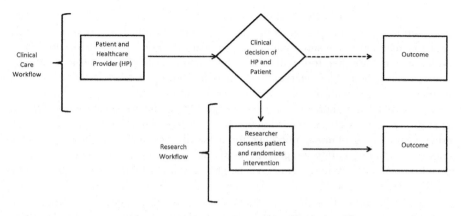

Fig. 13.2 Panel B. Traditional research silo: clinical care and research operate independently. Healthcare provider is in equipoise, and the choice of an intervention is randomized. Defined subset of patients enters the research workflow for structured follow-up. Outcomes often not fed back into clinical workflow

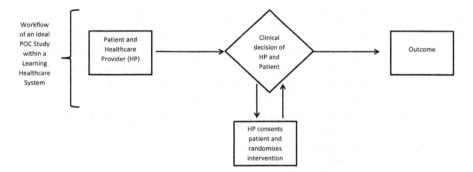

Fig. 13.3 Panel C. Integrated learning: clinical care and research operate together to create a learning healthcare system. Healthcare provider is in equipoise, and the choice of an intervention is randomized. Patient is randomized but stays in the traditional clinical workflow

Definition and Trial Design Characteristics for POC Clinical Trials

POC clinical trials provide a mechanism to perform large, simple and clinically integrated randomized trials to answer a plethora of compelling clinical questions. As stated, the defining feature that distinguishes POC trials is the use of EHR systems to embed the trial in routine clinical care to the maximum extent possible. Ideally, the possibility of randomization should be presented to the provider and patient when a treatment decision needs to be made, with confirmation of eligibility and the informed consent process being the only perturbations from usual care.

Trials best suited to POC methodology address clinician's uncertainty in the use of common clinical interventions that lack comparative effectiveness data to guide decision making and where healthcare providers do not have a strong treatment preference and are therefore willing to allow randomization (referred to as having clinical equipoise). The interventions studied should be used in an open-label manner consistent with the intervention's usual and intended practice, and not for new or expanded indications. The safety profile of the treatment, procedure or device should be well known allowing for risk-based monitoring, and exclusion criteria should be minimal allowing for a broad and easily identifiable eligible patient population. Follow-up procedures should follow usual care with minimal or no additional study requirement or visits, and all required data elements should be readily accessible and resident in the electronic health systems databases. Finally, outcomes should be clinically important and to the extent possible ascertained from structured data elements in the EHR [7, 9]. Linkage of multiple health databases (e.g., inpatient and outpatient) can improve capture and confirmation of endpoints and facilitate long-term follow-up [9, 10].

An exemplar point-of-care interventional study is the Thrombus Aspiration during ST-Segment Elevation Myocardial Infarctions in Scandinavia (TASTE) trial [11]. This multicenter open-labeled trial identified and obtained oral informed consent for participants presenting with ST-segment elevation myocardial infarctions (SEMI) to be randomized to manual coronary artery aspiration prior to percutaneous coronary intervention (PCI) or PCI alone. The primary endpoint of the study, all-cause mortality at 30 days, was not reduced by thrombus aspiration. One year follow-up continued to show no difference in mortality [12].

The design and conduct of TASTE demonstrates many of the key features of POC design and conduct. The study addressed a clinically relevant question in which there was equipoise in both the literature and in clinical practice. The outcome was important to patients and providers garnering a willingness to participate. TASTE study procedures were seamlessly integrated into the clinical workflow through minor modifications of the electronic health record system that facilitated study execution. The modifications allowed providers to confirm patient eligibility and document that oral informed consent was obtained from patients. Documentation of these events triggered randomized treatment assignment to thrombus aspiration or usual care study arms. No extra study-specific activities were required, and there was no attempt to blind treatment allocation. Because complications of the study procedures (clot aspiration and PCI) are well established, monitoring of adverse events proceeded as they would for usual care. The outcome of all-cause morality at 30 days was easily captured and confirmed by linkage to national death registries.

Electronic Health Record Systems Requirements

Implementation of POC trials involves a multidisciplinary team, including clinicians, researchers and informatics personnel. Execution of a randomized clinical trial within the clinical care ecosystem is facilitated by an electronic health record system with sufficient flexibility to allow for adaptations required for the study. The best systems are modular and generalizable to allow customizable workflows and data objects.

Essential functionalities include the ability to identify, enroll, randomly assign and implement the study intervention and track all necessary data elements from all participants. Creation of workflows outside of clinicians' usual clinical care interaction with the electronic health record and use of additional complimentary information systems should be avoided. Not only is development of new software or additional functionality to existing systems resource intensive, the addition of unfamiliar workflows and applications reduces the willingness of clinicians to participate in the program [6, 10].

There are inherent trade-offs that come with using electronic health system-generated databases in point-of-care trials. Data resident in electronic healthcare data systems are easy to access but are primarily collected in nonstandard formats and with varying degrees of accuracy depending on the intention and sophistication of the stakeholder entering the information. Additionally, data aggregated from other sources such as registries and quality assurance databases introduce additional variability in data quality. An understanding of the provenance of all data elements, how and by whom the data elements were collected and some assessment of internal validity is critical to designers of embedded clinical trials and has important ramifications on all aspects of study design such as selection of inclusion and exclusion criteria and definition of study endpoints and adverse events. Outcomes that require data contained only in free text or that require additional adjudication add to the cost and complexity of the trial and should be avoided when possible. Finally, centralized data monitoring systems need to be in place to assure that there is no disruption or change in data availability or structure over the lifetime of the study [9, 10].

Analytical Considerations

The heterogeneity introduced by inclusion of a more diverse study population and real-world implementation in the clinical ecosystem used by POC methodology presents issues when using frequentist analytic approaches. Techniques used to account for this variability result in trials with increased sample sizes, increased time to reach accrual targets, subsequent delays in trial completion and increase in cost.

Use of Bayesian adaptive approaches has been touted as a more efficient statistical method for use in pragmatic comparative effectiveness research [3]. The dynamic features of Bayesian and adaptive approaches tolerate uncertainty and allow for change in trial design as information accumulates during trial conduct. This approach allow for changes such as alteration of the randomization allocations based on information that accumulates during trial conduct, the ability to incorporate new interventional arms and adaptively dropping arms for futility thereby enriching enrollment in surviving options. The capability to produce informative results sooner using smaller samples sizes in a more cost-effective scalable manner has led to increased adoption of Bayesian adaptive approaches by pharmaceutical, device and biotechnology products research and development programs [3].

Decision Support and Creation of a Knowledge Base

Optimally, the electronic health record system used to conduct a POC trial can be adapted to implement the findings of the comparative effectiveness research as decision support. Clinician buy-into transition from pragmatic trial to decision support is facilitated by the nature of the trial—that it was executed within the healthcare system itself and studied the extant patient population. While findings from pragmatic trials may be readily adopted locally (locally selfish research), they may or may not be relevant for other healthcare systems with different patient populations and practice patterns, that is they may lack generalizability [7].

Results from POC trials embedded in clinical care can be combined with relevant background eternal knowledge to create a customized prediction model for individual patients. Creation of such a knowledge base is described by the VA Point of Care Precision Oncology Program [13].

Real-Time Implementation of Trial Results

Pragmatic clinical trials embedded in a healthcare system offer a unique opportunity to close the so-called implementation gap. This is accomplished by a hybrid approach, using frequentist operating characteristic and Bayesian adaption of randomization allocation as proposed in a Department of Veteran Affairs POC trial comparing methods for inpatient insulin administration [7]. The study analysis plan uses adaptive randomization modifying the assignment probability, after accrual of a fixed number of patients, preferentially to the winning therapy using a stopping rule with the acceptable frequentist Type 1 error of an efficiency trial. As a result, if a superior treatment exists by the time the study winner is determined, the majority of patients would have been randomized to the better treatment, thereby having implemented the finding as it was determined. The inferior treatment could then be more easily shut off without significant numbers of patients receiving the inferior treatment. Alternatively if the study fails to reach its efficiency boundary by study termination, then no substantial therapeutic difference exists and other factors such as cost, ease of use or clinician preference come into play in determining the clinical recommendation.

Summary

Point-of-care methodology is well suited for experimental comparative effectiveness research in the conduct of operative or non-operative invasive procedures [14]. Since labeling approval of devices and technology do not require comparative trials (21 CFR860.7(c)2), as required for drug approval, new devices, hardware, robotics, imaging and operational techniques are continuously evolving and can be quickly adopted into practice with little or no comparative evidence showing either improvement in meaningful clinical outcomes or quality of care. POC trials provide a mechanism to compare their use impact on clinically important outcomes such as death, infection or organ failure in an open-label manner within clinical practice. These important outcomes are often routinely captured with some degree of validation in quality assurance and improvement program electronic databases. Bayesian and adaptive designs are also particularly useful in the field as outcomes often occur in a shorter time period following the procedure allowing for adaptive randomization allocation [3] and therefore continuous evaluation. In addition, optimization of peri-procedural management, such as use of anticoagulant, antiplatelet therapy, infection prophylaxis, renal protection from dye load, can be evaluated as new drugs and formulations are adopted into practice.

The principle advantages of using POC trials include lower cost and generation of research results that are more likely to be implemented by the providers who have generated the evidence. This methodology provides a means to institutionalize a process where learning from each patient encounter can help determine the best care for the next patient—an integrated environment of research based care. There are important limitations on the questions that POC trials can address and on the outcomes that can be used as endpoints. Clinical equipoise is a hard requirement, and the questions asked need to be considered important to clinicians and patients. There is an operational dependency on electronic health record systems that are configurable and that have some capacity for incorporation of work flows.

An additional challenge to future expanded use of point-of-care trials methodology is the reexamination of regulatory governance and ethical oversight that has become the norm for human subjects' research [4, 9]. In particular should the same degree of human subject protection be required for experimental comparative effectiveness research comparing approved treatments, as that used for drugs or devices that are under development? A rethinking of the regulations regarding research consent and engagement, recognizing the different order of human experimentation in comparative effectiveness trials of widely used treatments, is required to facilitate dissemination of POC clinical trials and accelerate the transformation in healthcare that the methodology can provide.

References

1. Tricoci P. Scientific evidence underlying the ACC/AHA clinical practice guidelines. JAMA. 2009;301:831–41.
2. Tunis SR, Stryer DB, Clancy CM. Practical clinical trials increasing the value of clinical research for decision making in clinical health policy. JAMA. 2003 Sept 24;290:1624–1632.
3. Luce BR, Kramer JM, Goodman SN, Connor JT, Tunis S, Whicher D, Schwartz JS. Rethinking randomized clinical trials for comparative effectiveness research: the need for transformational change. Ann Intern Med. 2009;15(3):206–9.
4. Fiore LD, Lavori PW. Integrating randomized comparative effectiveness research with patient care. N Engl J Med. 2016;374(22):2152–8.
5. Peto R, Baigent C. Trials: the next 50 years. Large scale randomized evidence of moderate benefit. Br Med J. 1998;317:1170–1.
6. van Staa TP, Goldacre B, Gulliford M, Cassell J, Pirmoharmed M, Taweel A, et al. Pragmatic randomized trials using routine electronic health records: putting them to the test. BMJ. 2012;7(44):e55–61.
7. Fiore LD, Brophy M, Ferguson RE, D'Avolio LD, Hermos JA, Lew RA, et al. A point-of-care clinical trial comparing insulin administration using sliding scale versus a weight-based regimen. Clin Trials. 2011;8:183–95.
8. Olsen L, Aisner D, McGinnisJM. The learning healthcare system: workshop summary (IOM Roundtable on Evidence Based Medicine): Washington, DC: National Academies Pr; 2007.
9. van Staa TP, Dyson L, McCann G, Padmanabhan S, Belatri R, Goldacre B, et al. The opportunities and challenges of pragmatic point-of-care randomized trials using routinely collected electronic records: evaluation of two exemplar trials. Chapter 12: Discussion, recommendations and guidance. Health Technol Assess 2014 July;18(43):99–123.
10. D'Avolio LD, Ferguson RE, Goryachev S, Woods P, Sabin T, O'Neil J, et al. Implementation of the department of veterans affair first point-of-care trial. J Am Med Inform Assoc. 2012;19: e170–8.
11. Frobert O, Lagerqvist B, Olivecrona GK, Omerovic E, Gudnason T, Maeng M, et al. Thrombus aspiration during ST-segment elevation myocardial infarction. N Engl J Med. 2013;24(369):1587–97.
12. Lagerqvist B, Frobert O, Olivecrona GK, Gudnason T, Maeng M, Aistrom P, et al. Outcomes 1 tear after thrombus aspiration for myocardial infarction. N Engl J Med. 2014 Sept 18;371:1111–20.
13. Fiore LD, Brophy MT, Turek S, Kudesia V, Ramnath N, Shannon C, Ferguson R, et al. The VA point-of-care precision oncology program; balancing access with rapid learning in molecular cancer medicine. Biomarkers Cancer. 2016;8:1–8.
14. Vickers AJ, Scardino PT. The clinical-integrated randomized trial: proposed novel method for conducting large trials at low cost. Trials. 2009;10:14.

Part III
Statistical Considerations

Chapter 14
Basic Statistical Considerations

Eileen M. Stock and Kousick Biswas

Introduction

In recent years, significant strides in medical research have led to improvements in disease treatment and patients' quality of life. In any research, it is critically important to formulate a research question that adequately addresses the aims of a study. An example of a research question might be "Does laparoscopic cholecystectomy differ from open cholecystectomy in hospital length of stay" (ACTIVE trial) [1]. This research question will ultimately dictate the study design and methodology that will be employed. The reliability and validity of the results will depend on the proper selection of a research approach and design.

Hypothesis Testing

Following the establishment of a research question, a *null* and *alternative* hypothesis, denoted H_0 and H_a, should be formulated. The hypotheses will be determined by the research question, what groups and how many groups are to be compared, and at what time points an outcome will be measured such as cross-sectional occurring at one point in time or longitudinal to measure differences over time as in a prospective clinical trial. The alternative (research) hypothesis

E.M. Stock (✉) · K. Biswas
Cooperative Studies Program Coordinating Center, Office of Research
and Development, U.S. Department of Veterans Affairs, VA Medical Center,
5th Boiler Street, Perry Point, MD 21902, USA
e-mail: Eileen.Stock@va.gov

K. Biswas
e-mail: Kousick.Biswas@va.gov

© Springer International Publishing AG 2017
K.M.F. Itani and D.J. Reda (eds.), *Clinical Trials Design in Operative
and Non Operative Invasive Procedures*, DOI 10.1007/978-3-319-53877-8_14

corresponds to the primary purpose of the trial and what the researcher is trying to prove. The null hypothesis is the hypothesis being tested, the complement of H_a, always contains equality, and assumed to be true until it is decided to either *reject* or *fail to reject* H_0.

The usual scenario in hypothesis testing is demonstration of a difference (between two procedures). For example, if testing for a difference in the mean hospital length of stay for open cholecystectomy (μ_1) versus laparoscopic cholecystectomy (μ_2), the hypothesis is $H_0 : \mu_1 = \mu_2$ vs. $H_a : \mu_1 \neq \mu_2$. For a one-sided upper or lower tail test, $H_a : \mu_1 > \mu_2$ or $H_a : \mu_1 < \mu_2$. Here μ_1 and μ_2 represent the unknown "true" mean hospital length of stay for treatment group 1 and treatment group 2. Depending on the scientific hypothesis, the design of a trial can be superiority, non-inferiority, or equivalence. The objective of a superiority trial is to find a procedure to be better than the established alternative and was the framework proposed for the original randomized clinical trials. The objective of a non-inferiority trial is to find a new procedure that is not inferior to another procedure. Lastly, an equivalence trial aims to determine whether a new procedure is neither worse nor better than the established intervention.

Study Design

While RCTs are the gold standard for establishing safety and efficacy of a therapeutic intervention, there are many challenges in the design of trials assessing a procedure. Barriers forfeiting the reliability of trials, hence clinical evidence influencing surgical practice, can entail areas related to planning and design, eligibility criteria, choice of treatment comparator, benefit-to-harm ratio, as well as experience of the study team [2, 3]. Unfortunately, only about 15% of trials are in surgery of which nearly half are discontinued (43% vs. 27% in medicine), mostly for slow recruitment (18%) [4, 5], wasting already scarce resources, and raising ethical concerns if results are never reported to inform practice. An unexpected lower recruitment can result from the approach for obtaining consent, the randomization scheme, or the treatment comparator.

Recruitment Approach and Consent

There are numerous reasons why recruitment in a RCT may be low. First, patients may be completely unaware of an ongoing trial applicable to their ailment. Also, providers may be unaware and not mention a trial because of time constraints in explaining the trial, treatments, risks, benefits, and alternatives [6]. Additionally, affecting recruitment is the added burden on medical staff along with regular clinical duty, especially if facilities are already understaffed.

The subject area may influence recruiting. When informed of a new malady or needed surgery, patients may feel overwhelmed, alone, and be hesitant to participate. The complexity of the enrollment process involving extensive screening of eligibility criteria, difficult terminology, travel expenses, insurance coverage, and an unknown or experimental treatment can be daunting.

The method of recruitment can also impact participation. For seven varying recruitment strategies of 1562 cancer patients and their caregivers, two were the most effective—online recruitment by researchers of patients waiting for radiotherapy and mailing study information with routine care letters to patients scheduled to receive radiotherapy that were later contacted by telephone if opted out [7]. Less effective approaches included those relying on hospital providers, recruitment at a rehabilitation center, newspaper advertising, flyers, internet, and social media.

Equally important is ensuring patients' understanding of the material provided during consent, which tends to be the most common element absent from the process [6]. Among 141 consent discussions for an orthopedic surgical intervention, only 12% evaluated patients' understanding [8]. While pamphlets, diagrams, videos, and audio may improve comprehension, it should not be a substitute for open dialogue between the patient and provider [9].

Treatment Comparator and Randomization

One aspect of the design that can largely influence patient accrual to the point where the desired sample size is not attainable or findings are so biased they are deemed unreliable is the choice of a treatment comparator. In a traditional two-arm RCT, patients are assigned to one of two arms. One arm may comprise a new experimental treatment and the other standard care or a sham (placebo). If a patient finds they are not randomized to the new treatment, they may react negatively and refuse participation. In a trial with equal allocation to a surgical procedure versus sham, patients may be reluctant to participate because of the high likelihood (50%) of not receiving treatment (Table 14.1). Ideally, treatment allocation should not be known in advance in order to preserve randomness and prevent potential manipulation and bias [2, 3]. This poses an additional challenge when comparing an operative and non-operative procedure.

When treatments differ greatly, patient preferences are likely to influence the balance of patient accrual in each arm [3] as was observed in the MIMOSA trial comparing two distinct initial treatment approaches (surgical vs. pharmacological and behavioral therapy), for women with mixed urinary incontinence despite both being standard therapy [10]. An unbalanced benefit-to-harm ratio may lead patients to favor one treatment more. Operative procedures may require multiple preoperative and postoperative visits, adding burden on the patient. In such trials, a feasibility phase should be considered.

Table 14.1 Challenges to the planning and conduct of randomized trials comparing a surgical procedure with different types of comparators

	Surgical versus sham (placebo)	Surgical versus similar procedure	Surgical versus different procedure	Surgical versus non-surgical
Patients reluctant to participate	Yes	Unlikely	Likely	Yes
Randomize in operating theater	Yes	Yes	Likely	No (providers vary)
Imbalanced surgical experience	No	Unlikely	Likely	No (providers vary)
Poor compliance with allocation	Yes	Unlikely	Yes	Yes
Contamination, lack fidelity	Unlikely	Yes	Unlikely	No

[Based on data from Ref. 2]

Randomization should occur as close to the time of the intervention as possible to avoid the effects of patients' preferences and knowledge of allocation leading to withdrawal [2, 3] such as in the operating theater for two surgical procedures. For substantially different treatments, participants may have to be informed of their randomization [2]. For multicenter trials, stratified randomization is important to offset variability (site-specific or surgeon-related) [3]. A number of alternative randomization approaches have been utilized to overcome difficulty in recruiting and meeting sample size, including the use of unequal treatment allocation ratios to account for dropouts and adaptive randomization in which the allocation ratio changes during the course of the trial [11, 12]. However, these methods still remain less commonly used in practice.

Blinding

Blinding of participants, investigators, physicians, or other caregivers plays a significant role in the removal of potential bias that might otherwise skew results and deem a RCT inferior and of poor quality. There are three types of blinding—*single* (participants), *double* (participants and physician), and *triple* (participants, physician, and others determining eligibility, compliance, or evaluating endpoints) [13]. The absence of blinding can result in several forms of bias. The first is *performance bias*, which refers to differences in the delivery of care between groups attributable to behavioral responses by caregivers or participants from knowledge of treatment allocation. The comparison is confounded by the characteristics and preferences of caregivers and patients if one treatment is preferred over another; though, masking of surgeons, patients, and other caregivers is difficult and often impossible in surgical trials [2]. Another form of bias is *attrition bias*, resulting from differential withdrawal rates across groups. A surgical arm involving a waiting list or additional postoperative follow-up assessments is an example [2]. Lastly, *detection bias* refers to differences between groups in how outcomes are determined due to subjective evaluation of assessors such as self-reported outcomes when participants are unmasked [2].

Surgeon Characteristics

Most RCTs involve randomization administered by the same clinician, which is not possible when treatments are from different specialties (e.g., operative vs. non-operative) [3]. The delivery of a surgical procedure is influenced by attributes of the surgeon (e.g., skill, experience, preferences, decision-making ability), other team members (e.g., anesthesiologist, technicians, nurses), and those involved in preoperative and postoperative care (e.g., ED, ICU, imaging, recovery, rehabilitation) [2]. The learning curve for a procedure can confound results [3]. Outcomes such as symptomatology and functioning may be measured by surgeons and physicians differently (e.g., subjective assessments, unstandardized definitions). This variability in practice is unavoidable and, if great, can influence outcomes. To avoid criticism, the surgical procedure and care-practice measures should also be evaluated [2]. Comparing endoscopic versus open carpal tunnel release is an example of a non-operative and operative procedure with multiple interacting components and requiring a specific level of experience and training among surgeons [14]. Trials involving a varied benefit-to-harm ratio are sometimes difficult to recruit surgeons [15].

Analysis

When initially developing the idea for a RCT, a statistician should be consulted to help identify specific aims, hypotheses, the study design, analysis plan, and sample size. Hypotheses should focus on what the research is intended to demonstrate, clearly stating the outcomes of interest, groups to be compared, and the time period involved. Justification supportive of the hypotheses, such as pilot data, should also be included. Finally, it should be discussed how contingencies, such as missing data, which could bias findings will be handled.

Sample Size

For a clinical trial to be successful, sufficient planning is needed that should include sample size determination. This entails estimating how many participants should be enrolled in the study. The feasibility of the trial should also be assessed, identifying whether the proposed time and resources seem reasonable. Finally, a sample size should be estimated that achieves sufficient power to detect a specific treatment effect, factoring in the size or magnitude of the effect and its variability.

Outcome Measure

While a continuous outcome tends to result in improved statistical power (or alternately smaller sample size for the same level of power), a binary outcome is more easily interpretable. Most basic science and translational science studies use continuous outcomes, whereas RCTs usually involve binary or time-to-event outcomes. Observational studies may have either type of outcome. In a two-group parallel trial using a continuous outcome, the difference between groups is tested by comparing the means at some point in time using the t-test for two independent samples. For a binary outcome, the difference between groups is tested by comparing the proportion having the outcome at some point in time using the chi-square test for homogeneity of proportions or Fisher's exact test.

Baseline Assessment

While non-randomized studies try to account for pretreatment disparities between groups, the prospective design of a RCT helps provide some protection against biases resulting from baseline differences [2]. Although randomization on average produces homogeneity between groups, it does not guarantee balance. Accordingly, patient data should be collected at baseline before randomization during screening and after randomization prior to treatment. This information can then be used to check for balance [16]. Keep in mind that an insignificant association does not necessarily imply imbalance is not present. It merely suggests it was not detected (e.g., small sample size, low power). Furthermore, unless sample sizes are very large, rejecting the null hypothesis implies an imbalance that should be addressed in the analysis. These data may additionally be used to stratify (e.g., stratified randomization, subgroup analyses).

Intention-to-Treat Analysis

Under the intent-to-treat (ITT) principle ("once randomized, always analyzed"), patients remain in their assigned treatment group for the primary analysis, regardless of compliance or dropout. Even when a surgeon decides that a surgical procedure is inappropriate or unsafe after randomization, in which the patient may receive a different treatment from that originally assigned, these patients remain in their assigned treatment group regardless of receiving the alternative treatment. ITT analysis reflects the practical clinical scenario and allows generalizability by maintaining prognostic balance generated from the original random treatment allocation, producing an unbiased estimate of the treatment effect. Sample size is preserved, ensuring statistical power, and type I error is minimized [17]. Otherwise, the exclusion of non-compliant participants and dropouts from the final analysis may introduce bias. If allocation is disrupted, the study may no longer be considered a RCT. On the other hand, ITT analysis has been criticized for being too conservative (susceptible to type II error) and fails to answer the study question of whether the treatment works if used as intended.

Kaplan–Meier Estimator and Survival Curves

In RCTs, the outcome measure is typically binary or a time-to-event measure. Survival analysis is the branch of statistics for analyzing "time-to-event" data. Examples include time until a particular event (death), recurrence (revascularization), or time to a response (10% decrease in weight). Components necessary for the analysis include whether the event occurred (dichotomous) and the length of time from the start of follow-up to a precise endpoint, either when the event occurred or last known follow-up (censored). Censoring is when a participant does not experience the event prior to study closure, withdrawal, or loss to follow-up. Right-censoring is most common, i.e., the event has not been observed yet but might occur in the future. Left-censoring and interval-censoring are less common. The latter type of survival analysis applies when the time of the event is less-precisely known. When an event is noted to have occurred, it is assumed to have occurred in some interval since the last time event status was determined [18, 19].

Survival curves are estimated with Kaplan–Meier estimators to determine the probability of a patient surviving (or event-free) past a specified time. Curves are monotonically decreasing and stepwise (step-for-each event). When stratified by treatment arm, curves are estimated for each group separately and compared using a test for equality (parametric likelihood ratio test or nonparametric log-rank or Wilcoxon test). Rejection of equality indicates that the event rates differ between groups. However, these tests are less reliable when curves cross.

References

1. Catena F, Ansaloni L, Di Saverio S, et al. The ACTIVE (Acute Cholecystitis Trial Invasive Versus Endoscopic) study: multicenter randomized, double-blind, controlled trial of laparoscopic (LC) versus open (LTC) surgery for acute cholecystitis (AC) in adults. Trials. 2008;9:1.
2. Ergina PL, Cook JA, Blazeby JM, et al. Challenges in evaluating surgical innovation. Lancet. 2009;374:1097–104.
3. Cook JA. The challenges faced in the design, conduct and analysis of surgical randomised controlled trials. Trials. 2009;10:9.
4. Rosenthal R, Kasenda B, Dell-Kuster S, et al. Completion and publication rates of randomized controlled trials in surgery: an empirical study. Ann Surg. 2015;262:68–73.
5. Kasenda B, von Elm E, You J, et al. Prevalence, characteristics, and publication of discontinued randomized trials. JAMA. 2014;311:1045–51.
6. Cordasco KM. Chapter 39 obtaining informed consent from patients: brief update review. Evidence Reports/Technology Assessments, No. 211. Rockville (MD): Agency for Healthcare Research and Quality (US), 2013.
7. Sygna K, Johansen S, Ruland CM. Recruitment challenges in clinical research including cancer patients and their caregivers. A randomized controlled trial study and lessons learned. Trials. 2015;16:428.
8. Braddock C 3rd, Hudak PL, Feldman JJ, Bereknyei S, Frankel RM, Levinson W. Surgery is certainly one good option: quality and time-efficiency of informed decision-making in surgery. J Bone Joint Surg Am. 2008;90:1830–8.
9. Zuckerman MJ, Shen B, et al. Informed consent for GI endoscopy. Gastrointest Endosc. 2007;66:213–218.
10. Brubaker L, Moalli P, Richter HE, et al. Challenges in designing a pragmatic clinical trial: the mixed incontinence—medical or surgical approach (MIMOSA) trial experience. Clin Trials. 2009;6:355–64.
11. Dumville JC, Hahn S, Miles JN, Torgerson DJ. The use of unequal randomisation ratios in clinical trials: a review. Contemp Clin Trials. 2006;27:1–12.
12. Berry DA. Adaptive clinical trials: the promise and the caution. J Clin Oncol. 2011;29:606–9.
13. Bridgman S, Engebretsen L, Dainty K, Kirkley A, Maffulli N, Committee IS. Practical aspects of randomization and blinding in randomized clinical trials. Arthroscopy. 2003;19:1000–6.
14. Macdermid JC, Richards RS, Roth JH, Ross DC, King GJ. Endoscopic versus open carpal tunnel release: a randomized trial. J Hand Surg Am. 2003;28:475–80.
15. McCulloch P, Kaul A, Wagstaff GF, Wheatcroft J. Tolerance of uncertainty, extroversion, neuroticism and attitudes to randomized controlled trials among surgeons and physicians. Br J Surg. 2005;92:1293–7.
16. Senn S. Testing for baseline balance in clinical trials. Stat Med. 1994;13:1715–26.
17. Gupta SK. Intention-to-treat concept: a review. Perspect Clin Res. 2011;2:109–12.
18. Singh R, Mukhopadhyay K. Survival analysis in clinical trials: basics and must know areas. Perspect Clin Res. 2011;2:145–8.
19. Prinja S, Gupta N, Verma R. Censoring in clinical trials: review of survival analysis techniques. Indian J Community Med. 2010;35:217–21.

Chapter 15
Methods and Timing of Randomization

Robert George Edson

Reasons to Conduct Randomized Trials

In randomized control trials comparing a control group and an intervention group, each trial participant has the same chance (most often 1 to 1) of being assigned to the respective groups. Some trials, especially Phase I or II drug trials, have uneven assignment such as two for intervention to every one for control to collect more information on participants' response to the intervention. It is important to consider what type of blinding will be used in the trial, either single blind (where the participant does not know the assignment, to eliminate subjective bias or the "placebo effect," but the physician does) or double blind (where neither knows the assignment). Drug trials usually are double blind, while invasive trials often use single blind since it is difficult if not impossible to blind the treating physician.

The randomized design for choosing controls has several advantages over other options [1].

1. Use of a randomization procedure under which the assignment to group cannot be anticipated avoids the potential for bias in making group assignments.
2. Randomization tends to balance the groups on important prognostic factors and participant characteristics, even on variables which are unknown and unmeasured.
3. Randomization assures the validity of statistical tests of significance, by allowing the assignment of a probability distribution to the difference in outcome between groups receiving equally effective treatments.

R.G. Edson (✉)
VA Palo Alto Health Care System, Cooperative Studies Program Coordinating Center,
701-B North Shoreline Blvd, Mountain View, CA 94043-3208, USA
e-mail: bob.edson@va.gov

© Springer International Publishing AG 2017
K.M.F. Itani and D.J. Reda (eds.), *Clinical Trials Design in Operative and Non Operative Invasive Procedures*, DOI 10.1007/978-3-319-53877-8_15

Randomization Procedures

Prior to randomization, the potential study participant must be identified by the study staff, provide informed consent, meet the eligibility criteria, and agree to be randomized [2]. There are numerous methods for performing randomization; the description below follows Chap. 6 of [3].

With a *fixed allocation randomization* procedure, the probability of being assigned to the intervention or control is the same for each participant throughout the study. Fixed allocation procedures include the following.

1. Simple randomization, which uses a fair process (e.g., use of an unbiased coin or random number generator) to make assignments.
2. Blocked randomization, where assignments are made for multiple participants based on blocks with an equal number of assignments for each group (e.g., if there are two groups A and B, a block of size 4 would be any of the six possible orderings with two A's and two B's). Two refinements of blocked randomization may be implemented to reduce the likelihood of knowing the treatment assignment pattern. The first is permuted block randomization, in which the randomization sequence varies from one block to the next. The second is permuted block randomization with random block sizes, which employs a second level of randomization to randomly determine the size of the next permuted block.
3. Stratified randomization, under which the assignment is done independently within each combination of levels for characteristics deemed to be correlated with the primary study outcome. For example, if you want to stratify on sex, and age <60 or not, you would have 2*2 or 4 strata. Stratified randomization can be applied to simple or blocked (and permuted block) randomization.
4. For these randomization methods, the randomization codes for the study can be determined prior to starting recruitment using a computer program. The code list should be created and maintained by someone not involved in recruitment or follow-up of study participants.

Under an *adaptive randomization* procedure, the probability of assignment to group changes as the study proceeds. Some adaptive randomization procedures are described below.

1. Baseline adaptive randomization, where the goal is to balance the number of participants in each group. There are common techniques for performing baseline adaptive randomization, described below; however, these are less frequently used in randomized clinical trials.

    (a) The biased coin method [4] is based on assignments made for already randomized participants when making the assignment for the next participant but it does not consider the participants' responses. If the counts by group are equal or nearly so, then the next assignment is made with equal probability. If the count imbalance is greater than a pre-specified amount, the group with the lower count has a better than equal chance of being assigned.

(b) The urn design [5–8] refers to randomly selecting a ball from an urn filled with balls of different colors with each color representing a treatment group. Say red balls are for Group A and black balls are for Group B. For the first assignment there are an equal number of balls by color. If the first ball selected is red, that participant is assigned to Group A, and the red ball is returned to the urn and one or more black balls are added. If the first selection is a black ball, the participant is assigned to Group B and the black ball is returned to the urn and one or more red balls are added. Repeat this process for each assignment.

2. The minimization method [9] strives to balance overall assignments between groups for a set of baseline characteristics. This method is often employed when the number of combinations of baseline characteristics is large relative to the planned sample size for the study, which makes stratified randomization impractical. However, this method requires a computer program to be run for each randomization. For the example described above for stratified randomization, minimization would tend to balance counts by group for males (regardless of age category or enrolling site), females, age <60, and age $\geq$ 60. The assignment for the next participant is based on the counts by group of similar participants already randomized. Say for the example above the study already has ten participants randomized and the counts by group and stratification factor are given in Table 15.1. If the next participant is female and 58 years old, tallying by group the numbers in the female and <60 rows results in a count of 1 + 3 = 4 for Group A and 2 + 4 = 6 for Group B. Since the count is smaller for Group A, the assignment for the eleventh randomization is Group A.

3. Response adaptive randomization considers the participants' responses to the study treatment when making the assignment for the next participant. Common models for response adaptive randomization are described below, each of which assumes there are one or two treatment groups, and the participants' response to treatment can be ascertained quickly relative to the length of the study.

(a) Under the play-the-winner model [10], after the first assignment, the second participant receives the same assignment if the first participant's response

Table 15.1 Randomization counts by group and stratification factor in example

Stratification factor	Level	Number randomized by group		Characteristics of next participant
		A	B	
Sex	Male	4	3	
	Female	1	2	X
Age	<60	3	4	X
	$\geq$ 60	2	1	

was successful; otherwise, the second participant is assigned to the other group. The process continues where the next assignment is based on the successful or unsuccessful response of the immediately preceding participant.

(b) For the two-armed bandit model [11], the probability of success is updated as soon as the response is known for each participant, and group assignment probabilities are adjusted so that the treatment currently deemed "better" would be assigned to a higher proportion of future participants.

For the randomization methods cited above, Table 15.2 summarizes the advantages and disadvantages and provides recommendations on when the method should be used in a given study.

Mechanism and Timing of Randomization

Whichever randomization method is used, it should be implemented in the proper manner (e.g., to avoid revealing treatment assignment to blinded participants or site staff). It is common to have an independent entity (e.g., a data coordinating center or a biostatistician or clinician not involved in participant care) be responsible for developing the randomization procedures and making treatment assignments. The enrolling site staff may contact the independent entity or use a study website to get the assignment, and part of the process should be to have site staff verify that the participant meets eligibility criteria before receiving the group assignment.

It is important to have randomization performed as closely as possible to the time when the participant is deemed eligible and ready to begin treatment; if randomized before this, the participant may decide to withdraw, the participant's medical condition may change so they no longer meet the eligibility criteria, or the physician may feel the participant is no longer a good study candidate before the participant starts treatment. The withdrawal of participants between the time of randomization and start of therapy may lead to biased study results unless the analysis follows the intent-to-treat principle and includes data for all randomized participants [12].

Even when randomization is well timed with the start of treatment, problems may occur. For example, say the results of an invasive procedure are needed to determine whether the participant is eligible, and the process is to obtain the randomized assignment while the participant is on the operating table, and then perform the assigned treatment. The interruption of the operative procedure to get the treatment assignment may be disruptive, especially if it takes a while to get the assignment or if the randomization system is not available. The physician must always put the highest priority on the patient's safety and welfare, even if that means not randomizing that participant.

Table 15.2 Advantages, disadvantages, and usage recommendations for various randomization methods

Method	Advantages	Disadvantages	Usage recommendations
Simple	1. Simple to perform 2. Each assignment cannot be predicted	1. May lead to large relative imbalance, especially if sample size is small	1. Not used often 2. Only consider if sample size is over 200 [2]
Blocked	1. Avoids serious group imbalance and ensures imbalance is never large and at times there is no imbalance	1. If block size does not vary and is known, last assignment in each block known 2. Data analysis more complicated than Simple	1. Use if study has more than several hundred participants 2. Often used in combination with Stratified 3. If blocked and stratified, include baseline variables used to determine assignments as covariates in analyses
Stratified	1. Ensures group balance in prognostic factors 2. Power of study is increased if stratification is accounted for in the analysis	1. Must decide which prognostic factors will influence treatment response 2. Must be able to easily and reliably obtain participant's status on stratification factors	1. Use when prognostic factors are so important that you do not want to risk randomization producing imbalanced groups 2. More useful for small studies since large samples increase chance of groups having similar characteristics 3. Control number of stratification factors to avoid small number of participants in any given stratum. Often some factors considered are highly correlated so many may be dropped without affecting the balance of assignments by group 4. Enrolling sites may have important differences (e.g., patient characteristics, methods and quality of treatment, available equipment, degree to which they follow the protocol) [12], so consider having site as a stratification factor

(continued)

Table 15.2 (continued)

Method	Advantages	Disadvantages	Usage recommendations
Baseline adaptive	1. Less susceptible than blocked to selection bias	1. Blocked controls group balance more closely 2. More complicated than Simple, Blocked, Stratified 3. Population needs to be stable throughout study enrollment (e.g., if entry criteria changed, adaptive methods may not be able to fix imbalance existing before change)	1. Often used in conjunction with stratified
Minimization	1. Better balance than Blocked and Stratified when there are lots of prognostic factors and a small sample 2. Provides unbiased estimates of treatment effect and slightly increased power compared to Stratified [13]	1. More complicated than Simple, Blocked, Stratified 2. Population needs to be stable throughout study enrollment 3. Only time assignment determined randomly is when group counts are the same	1. Include baseline variables used to determine assignments as covariates in analyses [14, 15]
Response adaptive	1. Maximizes proportion of participants on "better" treatment	1. Limited to studies with one or two groups 2. Primary response variable must be measurable quickly relative to study length 3. May have several important response variables so it is difficult to choose the most important 4. Population needs to be stable throughout study enrollment 5. Possible imbalance likely to result in loss of power and larger sample size than fixed allocation randomization with equal assignment probabilities [16]	1. Procedures are complicated, so not often used

Mechanics of Randomization

There are various ways to inform the recruiting site of the participant's treatment assignment (for an unblinded or single-blind trial) or coded assignment (for a double-blind study), including the following.

1. Transferring the randomization list to a series of cards in sealed envelopes with envelopes numbered sequentially to follow the order of the list and instructing the site staff to open the next envelope in series with the next participant are ready to be randomized. Pocock [2] suggests using this method only if randomization is not done centrally and there is no one else for the site to consult with for randomization. Also, this method is not compatible with the adaptive randomization procedures described above.
2. Having the site contact (via telephone, email, etc.) a staff member at the centralized office who goes through the process to produce the randomization assignment and communicate it to the site staff. One drawback of this option is randomization may only occur when the centralized office is staffed.
3. Having the site staff contact a voice response system connected to a computer which takes the place of the centralized office in Option 2 above. With this method, sites may randomize at any time as long as the voice response system and computer are functioning properly.
4. Having the site staff use a web-based system in a manner similar to Option 3 above.

Since none of these options are totally reliable, it is a good idea to have one or more backup randomization methods in place for the study. For example, your primary method could be web-based with the option to call or email the centralized randomization staff if the website is down or otherwise unavailable to the site staff.

References

1. Byar DP, Simon RM, Friedewald WT, et al. Randomized clinical trials: perspectives on some recent ideas. N Engl J Med. 1976;295:74–80.
2. Pocock SJ. Clinical trials—a practical approach. Chichester: Wiley; 1983.
3. Friedman LM, Furberg CD, DeMets D. Fundamentals of clinical trials. 5th ed. Cham: Springer; 2015.
4. Efron B. Forcing a sequential experiment to be balanced. Biometrika. 1971;58:403–17.
5. Wei LJ. An application of an urn model to the design of sequential controlled clinical trials. J Am Stat Assoc. 1978;73:559–63.
6. Wei LJ, Smythe RT, Smith RL. K-treatment comparisons with restricted randomization rules in clinical trials. Ann Stat 1986;265–274.
7. Wei LJ, Lachin JM. Properties of the urn randomization in clinical trials. Control Clin Trials. 1988;9:345–64.
8. Wei LJ, Smythe RT, Lin DY, Park TS. Statistical inference with data-dependent treatment allocation rules. J Am Stat Assoc. 1990;85:156–62.

9. Pocock SJ, Simon R. Sequential treatment assignment with balancing for prognostic factors in the controlled clinical trial. Biometrics. 1975;31:103–15.
10. Zelen M. Play the winner rule and the controlled clinical trial. J Am Stat Assoc. 1969;64:131–46.
11. Robbins H. Some aspects of the sequential design of experiments. Bull Am Math Soc. 1952;58:527–35.
12. Armitage P, Colton T, editors. Encyclopedia of biostatistics, vol. 5. Chichester: Wiley; 1998.
13. Birkett NJ. Adaptive allocation in randomized controlled trials. Control Clin Trials. 1985;6:146–55.
14. Forsythe AB, Stitt FW. Randomization or minimization in the treatment assignment of patient trials: validity and power of tests. Health Sciences Computing Facility: University of California; 1977.
15. Kahan BC, Morris TP. Improper analysis of trials randomised using stratified blocks or minimisation. Stat Med. 2012;31:328–40.
16. Simon R, Weiss GH, Hoel DG. Sequential analysis of binomial clinical trials. Biometrika. 1975;62:195–200.

Chapter 16
Sample Size Calculation

Eileen M. Stock and Kousick Biswas

Introduction

Every clinical trial should be planned in advanced. This plan should include the study's objectives, primary and secondary endpoints, data collection, inclusion and exclusion criteria, required sample size with scientific justification, statistical methodology, and an approach to handle missing data [1]. A sample size calculation is used to determine the minimum number of participants needed in a clinical trial in order to be able to answer the research question under investigation. During the planning phase of a clinical trial, sample size estimation should be one of the very first and key components to consider in the design of a study. Knowing the anticipated sample size allows investigators to determine whether a study is feasible and to develop an appropriate budget and identify needed resources to carry out the study. The calculation of sample size with a sufficient level of significance and power is essential to the success of a trial.

Requirements for Sample Size Calculation

The estimation of sample size involves the consideration of multiple components, including the study's objective and primary hypothesis, type of endpoint to be analyzed, expected treatment effect and variability, treatment allocation ratio if it is

E.M. Stock (✉) · K. Biswas
Cooperative Studies Program Coordinating Center,
Office of Research and Development, U.S. Department of Veterans Affairs,
VA Medical Center, 5th Boiler Street, Perry Point, MD 21902, USA
e-mail: Eileen.Stock@va.gov

© Springer International Publishing AG 2017   141
K.M.F. Itani and D.J. Reda (eds.), *Clinical Trials Design in Operative
and Non Operative Invasive Procedures*, DOI 10.1007/978-3-319-53877-8_16

desirable to have more randomized to one group than another, anticipated recruitment rate, and the estimated number of dropouts. Other parameters influencing sample size calculation include types of error (I and II) and power [1, 2].

Types of Error and Power

Consider the multisite randomized clinical trial comparing operative and nonoperative treatment using accelerated functional rehabilitation for acute Achilles tendon ruptures [3]. For the primary outcome of rerupture, the *null hypothesis*, denoted H_0, would be that there exists no difference between the two population proportions of rerupture. That is, there is no difference in the rate of rerupture between those with acute Achilles tendon rupture undergoing surgical repair and those treated nonoperatively. The *alternative hypothesis* (for a two-sided test; typically denoted H_a) is that there is a difference in the rate of rerupture. A *Type I error*, commonly referred to as *significance level* and denoted as α, is defined as the probability of erroneously rejecting the null hypothesis when it is in fact true. In this example, a Type I error would be concluding a difference in the rate of rerupture between treatment procedures that is unlikely to actually exist, i.e., a false positive. A *Type II error*, denoted as β, is the probability of failing to reject a false null hypothesis. That is, erroneously missing an actual difference in rerupture rates between treatment procedures, a false negative. *Power* (equal to $1 - \beta$) is the probability of rejecting the null hypothesis when it is false and should be rejected (Table 16.1) [1, 2].

Study's Primary Hypothesis

The primary purpose of a clinical trial, written as a scientific hypothesis, guides the design of the trial. Traditionally, a two-arm parallel-group design is employed to look for a difference between treatments (two-sided). Two-sided *p-values* provide the probability that the results are compatible with the null hypothesis (H_0 true).

Table 16.1 Summary of type I and II errors

	True state	
Statistical decision	H_0 true (No treatment benefit) Should fail to reject H_0	H_0 false (Treatment benefit) Should reject H_0
Fail to reject H_0 (No treatment benefit)	Correct decision	Type II error (β)
Reject H_0 (Treatment benefit)	Type I error (α)	Correct decision, power ($1 - \beta$)

When the p-value is small (say, *p-value* <0.05), the null hypothesis is rejected (reject H_0) and there is evidence to support a difference in treatment effects. The direction of the test statistic establishes whether the new treatment is superior or inferior to the control treatment. In some instances, there is no interest in rejecting a null hypothesis in both directions (i.e., there is no interest in an inferiority results) and a superiority trial may be preferred to examine whether a new treatment is superior (better) than the established alternative (one-sided) [4].

While the traditional approach is intended to determine whether there is a difference between the experimental treatment and control, this may not be the relevant approach when the control is known to be effective and it is hoped that the experimental treatment can be shown to be as effective. In this instance, it is usually the case, that the experimental treatment may offer other advantages to the control treatment, such as convenience or tolerability, if it can be shown to be as effective to the control. Equivalence trials are designed to establish that the new procedure cannot be worse nor better than the conventional procedure if the null hypothesis is rejected. It requires that the two treatment approaches be identical within some acceptable range, δ (normally $\pm 20\%$) [5]. Lastly, for a non-inferiority trial, the aim is to show that the new treatment is as good as or better (no worse) than the established treatment [4]. Each of the mentioned designs will be selected according to the study's primary hypothesis and rely on prior information about the effects of the new procedure on a specific endpoint [1].

Study Design Considerations

Various study designs, such as a parallel-group, crossover, factorial, or cluster, may be employed to address a study's objectives and ensure the required sample size is achieved. Each design will vary in their approach for sample size calculation. In the case of rare events, the need for a multisite trial is higher.

Study Endpoint Expected Response

A study's endpoint, whether continuous, dichotomous, or time-to-event, will govern the type of model and sample size calculation. In the case of multiple comparisons, an adjustment to the significance level may be necessary. For a continuous endpoint, information on the expected central tendency (mean score) and variability (standard deviation) of the new procedure and its comparator are needed to more precisely estimate the sample size. The greater the variation within groups or the smaller the expected difference between groups, the larger the sample size will need to be in order to produce the same result. For a dichotomous variable, the proportion of participants achieving success in each group is needed. Most importantly, the expected treatment effect, as compared to its comparator, should be clinically meaningful [1].

Participant Retention Rates and Treatment Allocation

While sample size calculations determine the required number of participants for specific analyses, other aspects of recruitment should also be considered such as screen-failures, dropouts, and patients who are lost to follow-up. A trial should enroll more subjects to account for potential dropouts and those lost to follow-up. Attrition rates can vary tremendously, where $\leq 5\%$ is of little concern but $\geq 20\%$ poses serious threats to the validity of the trial [6]. Most RCTs (60–89%) published in leading journals have missing endpoint data, with complete case analysis the most frequently used strategy for handling this missing data [7, 8]. For many of these trials (18%), dropout rates exceeded 20% [8, 9]. For this reason, the number of enrollments, in trials where the primary outcome measure is continuous or binary, can be determined using an adjustment to the sample size and estimated dropout rate in the formula, *Enrollment = Sample Size/(1 − dropout rate)* [1]. For time-to-event, or survival data, the adjustment for dropout rate is more involved. In some instances, interim analyses may be requested to monitor treatment effects and ensure enrollment follows a specific trajectory [10, 11].

If one treatment arm is anticipated to have a greater dropout rate than its comparator, an unequal treatment allocation may be employed to ensure a balanced distribution at the end of the trial. Additionally, varied allocation and enrollment can occur in cases where it is unethical to assign an equal number of patients to each arm (e.g., placebo or sham treatment) [1]. Thus, sample size is adjusted in these scenarios. Note that departures form 1:1 randomization will increase the sample size requirement.

Conventional Guidelines

In sample size calculations, the level of significance (α) for a study is typically assumed to be 0.05 (or 5%) [12]. However, 1% or less may be used for larger samples and 10% for smaller samples. Also, the minimum power for which sample size is calculated is 80%. Larger power may be used to estimate sample size in order to provide a more conservative estimate in case treatment effects or recruitment are less than anticipated.

Calculation of Sample Size

There are many approaches to sample size estimation, with some of the more common calculations involving the comparison of two means, proportions, or a time-to-event measure and testing for a difference between groups. The next few sections describe these in more detail.

Comparing Two Means

The formula for calculating sample size comparing the mean of two treatment arms is

$$n_1 = \kappa n_2; \quad n_2 = \left(1 + \frac{1}{\kappa}\right)\left[\frac{\left(z_{\alpha/2} + z_\beta\right)^2}{d^2}\right] = \left(1 + \frac{1}{\kappa}\right)\left[\frac{\left(z_{\alpha/2} + z_\beta\right)^2 \left(\sigma_1^2 + \sigma_2^2\right)}{2\left(\bar\mu_1 - \bar\mu_2\right)^2}\right],$$

where $z_{\alpha/2}$ is the critical value of the standard normal distribution at $\alpha/2$ (e.g., 1.96 for a 95% confidence interval with Type I error $\alpha = 0.05$), z_β is the critical value of the standard normal distribution at β (e.g., 0.84 for 80% power and Type II error $\beta = 20\%$), κ is the matching ratio, μ_i is the population mean of the endpoint in group i, σ_i^2 is the population variance of the endpoint in group i, and d is Cohen's effect size [13]. For studies with 1:1 randomization, $\kappa = 1$.

Comparing Two Proportions

The formula for calculating sample size comparing two proportions is

$$n_1 = \kappa n_2; \quad n_2 = \left[\frac{p_1(1 - p_1)}{\kappa} + p_2(1 - p_2)\right]\left(\frac{z_{\alpha/2} + z_\beta}{p_1 - p_2}\right)^2,$$

where p_i is the population proportion of group i, and $p_1 - p_2$ is the effect size or difference desired to be detected [13].

Comparing Time-to-Event

The formula for calculating sample size for a time-to-event analysis (Cox proportional hazards model) is

$$n = \frac{1}{p_1 p_2 p_A} \left(\frac{z_{\alpha/2} + z_\beta}{\ln(\theta) - \ln(\theta_0)} \right)^2,$$

where p_i is the proportion with the event in group i, p_A is the overall event rate, θ is the hazard rate, θ_0 is the hypothesized hazard rate under the null hypothesis, and $\ln(\theta) - \ln(\theta_0)$ the regression coefficient (treatment indication) [13, 14]. Note that sample size formulae accounting for the length of the recruitment and follow-up periods, and drop-outs, are more sophisticated.

Available Software

Statistical software packages with tools for sample size and power analysis calculations include SAS (SAS Institute, Inc.; Cary, NC), G*Power (Faul, Erdfelder, Lang, & Buchner, 2007), PASS (NCSS, LLC.; Kaysville, Utah), R (The R Foundation for Statistical Computing; Auckland, New Zealand), M*plus* (Muthén & Muthén; Los Angeles, CA), and PS available online at Vanderbilt University (Dupont & Plummer, 1990) [15]. Several of these packages are available at no cost.

Common Pitfalls Related to and Affecting Sample Size

Sample size calculations pose several challenges, including obtaining an accurate estimate of treatment effects, selecting an appropriate power and significance level, and even selecting the correct formula to be used [16]. As a result, sample size underestimation or overestimation may occur.

Sample Size Underestimation

Sample size underestimation refers to a sample size for a trial that was calculated to be less than that required [16]. This results in lower power than is needed and may lead to misleading results such as the determination of no treatment effect (*p-value* > α) when one really existed. The treatment effect was not statistically significant even though it was clinically significant. That is, recruiting too few participants can lead to inconclusive results because of the low likelihood of finding a clinically relevant difference statistically significant.

Revisiting the Achilles Tendon Rupture trial, small sample size was a limitation of the study (72 participants per each arm), and therefore was underpowered to definitively make a conclusion about rerupture rates [3]. A meta-analysis had shown rerupture rates to be approximately 2.8% following operative repair and 11.7% for nonoperative treatment [17]. ConsequentlyH, the Rupture trial underestimated the sample size required. Instead, rates of 2.8% and 4.2% for operative and nonoperative treatment, respectively, were observed. The former would require a sample size of 104 participants in each group using a one-sided 2-sample independent proportions test, assuming a significance level of $\alpha = 0.05$. The latter would require 2148 participants per arm (Fig. 16.1). Although the actual power for comparing rerupture rates was 12% (Fig. 16.2), with a Type II error of 88%, this study was the largest to date of its kind and findings would provide clinical insight and pilot data should a larger trial be pursued.

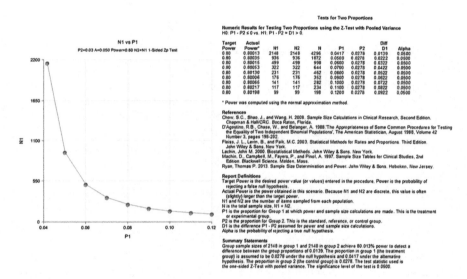

Fig. 16.1 Sample size estimation for comparing rerupture rates, varying rates in the nonoperative group [created through the use of: PASS 14 Power Analysis and Sample Size Software (2015). NCSS, LLC. Kaysville, Utah, USA, ncss.com/software/pass]

```
> power.prop.test(n=72, p1=(2/72), p2=(3/72), sig.level=0.05, power= , alternative="one.sided")

    Two-sample comparison of proportions power calculation

              n = 72
             p1 = 0.02777778
             p2 = 0.04166667
      sig.level = 0.05
          power = 0.1169202
    alternative = one.sided

NOTE: n is number in *each* group
```

Fig. 16.2 Power analysis for observed difference in rerupture rates [created through the use of: R (The R Foundation for Statistical Computing; Auckland, New Zealand)]

Sample Size Overestimation

On the contrary, a sample size selected to be much larger than was required describes *sample size overestimation* [16]. Studies that are too large are also problematic for at least two reasons. This scenario may be evident from an exceptionally strong statistical significance (very small *p-value*), which raises ethical concerns if more subjects were exposed to an inferior treatment than were required or resources wasted. Additionally, for larger sample sizes, smaller differences can be detected and be statistically significant even when the difference is not clinically meaningful. In trial design, each assumption may be made too conservatively, to avoid the risk of failure, and the analysis of the study's primary objective becomes overpowered as a result.

Selecting a Clinically Meaningful Difference

Determining the clinically meaningful difference for which a study is powered to detect is generally the most difficult task of the sample size calculation process. A very thorough literature search should be conducted to obtain any available data on the potential effect of the proposed new treatment. This may include published abstracts, results of phase II trials or pilot studies, and subgroup analyses from a previously conducted trial. If enough publications are available, meta-analysis techniques can be used to obtain an estimate of the potential treatment effect.

Often data are limited to help inform the potential treatment effect estimate. In those cases, an investigator might look to other published studies in this area to determine the magnitude of effect that was used when that study was designed. Often, FDA has determined the degree of treatment effect needed to establish efficacy and their guidelines may be useful as a resource. Additionally, a panel of experts in the area of investigation can be convened to develop a consensus estimate of treatment effect.

Available Databases

There are multiple databases available for use in obtaining estimates for sample size calculations. In 1994, the VA established a VA National Surgical Quality Improvement Program (NSQIP) in which all medical centers performing major surgery participated [18]. The database contains 135 variables collected preoperatively and up to 30 days postoperatively. Data is categorized as demographic, surgical profile, preoperative, intraoperative, or postoperative. Each hospital submits an average of 1,600 major operations per year into the database [19]. While the aim of NSQIP was initially quality improvement in surgical care through periodic reports and assessments of performance, VA investigators can also query the database for scientific research purposes and to obtain estimates of event rates for a power analysis such as mortality, cardiac and noncardiac complications, postoperative pneumonia, intubations, pulmonary embolism and venous thrombosis, renal dysfunction, and infections. Similarly, the American College of Surgeons National Surgical Quality Improvement Program (ACS NSQIP) can be used for sample size estimation as in the comparison of postoperative complication rates for regional versus general anesthesia among surgical patients with chronic obstructive pulmonary disease [20, 21]. Other useful available databases include the Society of Thoracic Surgeons (STS) National Database including separate databases for adult cardiac, general thoracic, and congenital heart surgery [22], and the Centers for Disease Control (CDC) Cancer Registry [23].

References

1. Sakpal TV. Sample size estimation in clinical trial. Perspect Clin Res. 2010;1:67–9.
2. Jones SR, Carley S, Harrison M. An introduction to power and sample size estimation. Emerg Med J. 2003;20:453–8.
3. Willits K, Amendola A, Bryant D, et al. Operative versus nonoperative treatment of acute Achilles tendon ruptures: a multicenter randomized trial using accelerated functional rehabilitation. J Bone Joint Surg Am. 2010;92:2767–75.
4. Christensen E. Methodology of superiority vs. equivalence trials and non-inferiority trials. J Hepatol. 2007;46:947–54.
5. Steinijans V, Hauschke D. International harmonization of regulatory bioequivalence requirements. Clin Res Regul Aff. 1993;10.
6. Fewtrell MS, Kennedy K, Singhal A, et al. How much loss to follow-up is acceptable in long-term randomised trials and prospective studies? Arch Dis Child. 2008;93:458–61.
7. Akl EA, Briel M, You JJ, et al. LOST to follow-up information in trials (LOST-IT): a protocol on the potential impact. Trials. 2009;10:40.
8. Wood AM, White IR, Thompson SG. Are missing outcome data adequately handled? A review of published randomized controlled trials in major medical journals. Clin Trials. 2004;1:368–76.
9. Bell ML, Kenward MG, Fairclough DL, Horton NJ. Differential dropout and bias in randomised controlled trials: when it matters and when it may not. BMJ. 2013;346:e8668.
10. Floriani I, Rotmensz N, Albertazzi E, et al. Approaches to interim analysis of cancer randomised clinical trials with time to event endpoints: a survey from the Italian National Monitoring Centre for Clinical Trials. Trials. 2008;9:46.
11. Broglio KR, Stivers DN, Berry DA. Predicting clinical trial results based on announcements of interim analyses. Trials. 2014;15:73.
12. Kadam P, Bhalerao S. Sample size calculation. Int J Ayurveda Res. 2010;1:55–7.
13. Chow S, Shao J, Wang H, editors. Sample size calculations in clinical research. 2nd ed. Boca Raton: Chapman & Hall/CRC; 2008.
14. Wang H, Chow S. Sample size calculation for comparing time-to-event data. In: D'Agostino R, Sullivan L, Massaro J, editors. Wiley encyclopedia of clinical trials. New York: Wiley; 2007.
15. Dupont WD, Plummer WD. Power and sample size calculations: a review and computer program. Control Clin Trials. 1990;11:116–28.

16. Noordzij M, Tripepi G, Dekker FW, Zoccali C, Tanck MW, Jager KJ. Sample size calculations: basic principles and common pitfalls. Nephrol Dial Transplant. 2010;25:1388–93.
17. Lo IK, Kirkley A, Nonweiler B, Kumbhare DA. Operative versus nonoperative treatment of acute Achilles tendon ruptures: a quantitative review. Clin J Sport Med. 1997;7:207–11.
18. Khuri SF, Daley J, Henderson WG. The comparative assessment and improvement of quality of surgical care in the Department of Veterans Affairs. Arch Surg. 2002;137:20–7.
19. Fuchshuber PR, Greif W, Tidwell CR, et al. The power of the National Surgical Quality Improvement Program–achieving a zero pneumonia rate in general surgery patients. Perm J. 2012;16:39–45.
20. ACS National Surgical Quality Improvement Program (ACS NSQIP). Participant Use Data Files. Available from https://www.facs.org/quality-programs/acs-nsqip. American College of Surgeons.
21. Hausman MS Jr, Jewell ES, Engoren M. Regional versus general anesthesia in surgical patients with chronic obstructive pulmonary disease: does avoiding general anesthesia reduce the risk of postoperative complications? Anesth Analg. 2015;120:1405–12.
22. The Society of Thoracic Surgeons. STS National Database. Available from http://www.sts.org/national-database.
23. Centers for Disease Control and Preventions. National Program of Cancer Registries (NPCR). Available from http://www.cdc.gov/cancer/npcr/.

Chapter 17
Principles of Analysis

Gary R. Johnson and Tassos C. Kyriakides

Introduction

The analysis plans for data from clinical trials involving operative procedures are driven by the special design features and definitions of study outcomes that arise for these types of studies. In this section, we will discuss some of the nuances and precautions for planning and conducting the analysis of clinical trials comparing operative procedures or devices and for clinical trials comparing operative procedures to other nonoperative procedures.

Developing the Analysis Plan

An analysis plan should be prespecified in the protocol and finalized prior to conducting any scheduled interim analyses or final analysis. The analysis plan must include measures to avoid bias in the comparison of the trial interventions. Two major concerns are to ensure that: (a) the periods of risk are handled equally and (b) the study population to be included in the primary analysis is defined by the randomization assignment. This is usually handled by the following recommended practices:

G.R. Johnson (✉) · T.C. Kyriakides
VA Cooperative Studies Program, Office of Research and Development,
VA Connecticut Healthcare System, Cooperative Studies Program
Coordinating Center (151A), 950 Campbell Avenue,
West Haven, CT 06516, USA
e-mail: gary.johnson4@va.gov

T.C. Kyriakides
e-mail: tassos.kyriakides@va.gov

© Springer International Publishing AG 2017   151
K.M.F. Itani and D.J. Reda (eds.), *Clinical Trials Design in Operative
and Non Operative Invasive Procedures*, DOI 10.1007/978-3-319-53877-8_17

1. Define that the follow-up time for surveillance for study outcomes begins at the time of randomization, and define the parameters for the duration of that observation period such that the observation period is balanced for each intervention and occurrences of unexpected events are counted equally for all intervention groups.
2. Define what will be counted as an outcome for each intervention; this may be a single measure, for example, all-cause mortality, or may be a composite outcome, for example, graft failure, reoperation, and late sequelae.
3. Define the methodology to be used to compare outcomes (e.g., hazard ratios from life table regression, odds ratios from logistic regression, or the use of general linear models for comparison of means for a repeated measure of treatment effect).
4. Perform analyses using the intent-to-treat principle including all randomized participants. This will avoid bias that might occur by excluding participants who do not adhere to the assigned intervention. Problems with this type of non-adherence can also be reduced by designing the trial to minimize the time period between randomization and the completion of the assigned intervention or operative procedure.
5. Consider prespecified stratification factors to balance pre- and perioperative risk factors between interventions; these might be included as stratification factors in the randomization scheme or as planned covariates in the primary analysis.

Important elements to consider for inclusion in the statistical analysis plan beyond what is described in the initial study protocol are (Abridged from VA Cooperative Studies Program SAP guidance):

- Definitions of all primary and secondary endpoints
- Statements of hypotheses to be tested and the parameter estimation
- Levels of clinical and statistical significance (one-tailed or two-tailed)
- Description of the methods of analysis and presentation of results:

  - Rules for handling intervals in which study visits or assessments are scheduled to occur
  - Decision rules for the inclusion/exclusion of data in special cases
  - Definitions of compliance and adherence
  - Methods for handling multiple comparison methods
  - Use of baseline measurements in stratification or in adjustment of treatment effects
  - Specification of fixed or random effects models
  - Approaches for handling covariables or associated risk factors in the analyses
  - Rules for the calculation of derived variables
  - Rules for potentially early-stopping of the trial
  - Methods for handling missing data
  - Methods for handling outliers
  - Methods for handling withdrawals and protocol deviations

  – Methods for point and interval estimation
- Description of any interim analyses, and specifications for any sample size reestimation
- Description of the content of what will be identified as the final statistical report (e.g., mock-up or templates of tables that summarize the planned interim monitoring and final analyses).

Analytical Approaches for Studies Evaluating Effectiveness of Operative Procedures

Intent-to-Treat Principle: The primary analysis should proceed directly from the randomized assignment of individuals to the treatments being compared. This analytic strategy, known as intent to treat (ITT), requires that all randomized participants be included in the analysis according to their originally assigned treatment, regardless of what happens after the random assignment. Any analysis that either drops randomized participants from the analysis or, in the case they receive a different treatment than originally assigned, analyses them according to the treatment actually received and thus has the potential to introduce bias.

In some instances, a modified intent-to-treat analysis may be defendable for the primary analysis. A Modified Intent-to-Treat (MITT) plan may allow for dropping from analysis participants who never received the randomized treatment or received partial or very limited treatment. In these instances, the reason for not receiving the assigned treatment must be independent of the study intervention. Trials involving surgical procedures are usually not suitable for a modified intent-to-treat analyses. For example, a trial that compares two different surgical interventions where it is discovered after randomization that a patient is not a suitable candidate for the assigned intervention (but may have been able to receive the other intervention) would not be appropriate for a modified intent-to-treat analysis. Such a plan would introduce bias into the comparison of the interventions.

The primary analysis of a well-designed and well-conducted randomized trial may be very straightforward or very complex. A trial comparing 30-day complication rates for two surgical interventions could use a chi-square test for homogeneity to compare the proportion of participants who developed complications within 30 days in the two groups, or a more complex intervention trial might have the modeling of repeated measurements of intra- or perioperative markers of clinical risk as the primary analysis.

A common approach to evaluation of the success or failure of a procedure is to use survival or failure time analyses that compare the probability of survival or being event free during a follow-up period after randomization to a study intervention or procedure. Methodologies for analysis of survival data include test statistics for the comparison of survival distributions [1–3] and life table regression methods [4].

Short-term outcomes: When comparing two operative procedures or devices a time-to-event analysis may still be appropriate if the objective of the study is to assess the occurrence and time of peri- and postoperative events.

Long-term outcome: Survival analysis is more typically planned for comparing the long-term outcomes after a procedure where the outcome measure would include not only the short-term outcomes, but also late postoperative events and sequela and possibly recurring events.

Repeated measures over time: A trial may be designed to evaluate changes in repeated measurements over a specific time period. For example, repeated measurements of functional status, markers of clinical risk, severity of post-procedure pain or other symptoms, or measures of health-related quality of life may be used as primary or secondary outcomes. These types of data collected longitudinally and prospectively can be analyzed as dependent variables in mixed effects models. The analysis plan should identify the time points to be included in the analysis.

Example: Carpal tunnel syndrome: Participants randomized to endoscopic versus open procedures were assessed for postoperative pain (primary outcome) and other measures of functional status and quality of life at three weeks, six weeks, and three months, with additional assessments at 12 months [5]. While this study does not provide a good example of estimating an overall intervention effect over 12 months, it does demonstrate how repeated patient-reported outcomes can be analyzed to compare interventions.

Secondary and Supportive Analyses

Subgroups

Complete the analysis of the comparison of intervention outcomes in prespecified subgroups by calculating the relative hazards ratios from models including the intervention and subgroup parameter and an interaction term. Presentation of these estimates of relative risk (e.g., relative risk estimate and 95% confidence intervals) in a table or a forest plot on the log scale will provide an easy way to assess the relative effects in different subgroups. The subgroups may be risk factors identified by previous research or observation. Prespecifying subgroups and specifying adjustments that will be made for multiple comparisons will help in the acceptance of study results, otherwise will be viewed as exploratory.

Safety

Adverse events for an operative procedure may overlap with events that have also been reported as study outcomes. For example, a complication of a surgical procedure may be a component of a composite outcome [e.g., readmission for reoperation due to postoperative complication might be counted as a treatment-related hospitalization in a composite outcome].

Supportive Analyses

Supportive analyses should be included in the analysis plan such as analysis of cause-specific death in addition to all-cause mortality, and the analysis components of a composite outcome. The supportive analyses also include sensitivity analyses for alternatives to the primary intent-to-treat approach where the effect of operative interventions are assessed in a modified intent-to-treat population or other approaches that select a subset of the randomized population to be included in the analyses based in treatment assigned or received.

The analytic strategy known as a per-protocol analysis limits the analysis to participants who actually received or adhered to the randomly assigned intervention or strategy. The results of this type of analysis would not take precedence over the primary intent-to-treat analysis, but could provide additional supportive information that investigates the degree to which the intent-to-treat results may have been impacted by noncompliance with the randomized treatment assignment. Another approach is an as-treated analysis where the analysis groups are formed according to those who actually received the intervention, rather than according to the randomly assigned intervention. In this case participants who get the alternative intervention (crossovers) are grouped with those who adhered to the treatment per-protocol. Similar to per-protocol analysis, the as-treated analysis strategy is not based on the randomized intervention assignment and is inherently biased. These sensitivity analyses may not always produce results that are aligned with the primary analysis but if not done will leave a gap in the interpretation of the results. Of course, any potential biases in these supportive analyses should be recognized in any presentation.

Example: REFLUX Trial [6]

In this trial, participants were randomized to laparoscopic fundoplication surgical procedure or long-term medical treatment for gastroesophageal reflux disease. Main outcomes were disease-specific and general health-related quality of life measures and surgical complications. In the publication of the trial results, both the intent-to-treat and the per-protocol results were presented together with the justification of the large proportion of participants randomized to laparoscopic fundoplication (38%) who did not get the procedure. The adjusted treatment effect was greater in the per-protocol group (15.4, 95% confidence interval [CI]: 10.0, 20.9) than the intent-to-treat population comparison (11.2, 95% CI: 6.4, 16.0), and even greater when the analysis was performed according to the treatment received (16.7, 95% CI: 9.7, 23.6) although with a wider confidence interval. In this example, the results were fortunately consistent for the three approaches and the supportive analyses were clearly identified and discussed as biased.

Thus, in a well-controlled randomized clinical trial, the intent-to-treat is considered the most conservative approach in the comparison of the study interventions and minimizes bias. Per-protocol and as-treated analyses provide a more direct comparison of the treatments actually received, but have more potential for bias because the randomized design is compromised.

Although intent-to-treat is theoretically an unbiased strategy, bias can still be introduced after the randomization. Outcome evaluation can be biased, especially if the outcome is subject to interpretation or subjective assessment with knowledge of the intervention assigned. Blinding of the treatment assignment protects against biased outcome evaluation, although this is often difficult to achieve in a study involving devices or operative procedures. Drop-outs or withdrawals of participants may occur during the follow-up and result in missing data, which can also introduce bias. This problem is not specific to trials of surgical procedures. Statistical methods to address the problem of bias due to missing data are the subject of another chapter in this book.

Cost-Effectiveness Analysis

The protocol may plan for a cost-effectiveness analysis. Unless the study is completed in a setting where all costs can be identified (e.g., within one institution) these analyses usually are conducted on direct costs for the procedure and any complications or sequelae and do not include all indirect costs. The protocol may plan for only completing this exercise when a treatment effect has been found in the experimental arm, but such a comparison can be of value even when there is no significant difference. The active comparator group may be less costly than the control or standard of care group.

Interim Analyses

Standard techniques can be applied for scheduling interim analyses. However, there should be special consideration for timing the analyses at a point when the necessary proportion of study events (information) defined a priori in the analysis plan has been observed, rather than at an enrollment or study duration milestone. For example, if the primary study outcome is postoperative status two years after randomization, enough two-year events need to be accrued before completing the analysis.

Special Considerations and Cautions

Non-proportional Hazards

The primary analysis can be conducted using a nonparametric approach such as the Kaplan–Meier method for calculating survival curves; this allows for a comparison of the interventions using the log-rank test without the assumption of proportional hazards. The events are weighted equally relative to the number of participants at risk no matter when the event occurs during follow-up. However, covariate adjusted analyses are usually planned and even with nonparametric approach, the results of the study can be misinterpreted. Therefore, an evaluation of possible time-dependent treatment effects and an assessment of hazard ratios over time should be undertaken. An extreme example of non-proportional hazards occurs when survival curves cross or hazard ratios change direction (relative to 1.0). In this case time-dependent effects need to be accounted for as well as the consideration of baseline hazard rates for risk factors [7]. In some cases, a piecewise analysis of segments of follow-up time might help explain the results.

Examples

D1 versus D2 dissection for gastric cancer. Several trials on the treatment of gastric cancer demonstrate the problem of non-proportional hazards. The Dutch Gastric Cancer Trial [8] first presented the results of D1 versus D2 methods of dissection as having no difference in mortality with some early benefit of the D1 method, though acknowledging the non-proportional hazards. The survival curves crossed at approximately 4 years, with the subsequent hazard ratios in favor of D2. Long-term follow-up in this same population showed a long-term benefit of the D2 method [9] (see Fig. 17.1). Similarly, a concurrent study by the MRC comparing D1 to D2 showed non-proportional hazards. A methodology paper assessing the proportional hazards in the Dutch Gastric Cancer Trial demonstrated several methods for approaching this problem including time-dependent treatment and covariate effects and accounting for baseline hazards [7].

Learning Curve

If the intervention trial is evaluating a new procedure or device, then the possibility of learning curve effects should be taken into account in the analysis, especially if the new procedure is being compared to a well-established procedure [10].

In addition, it is possible that during the course of a trial, multiple versions or modifications of the investigational device or procedure may be used in the same

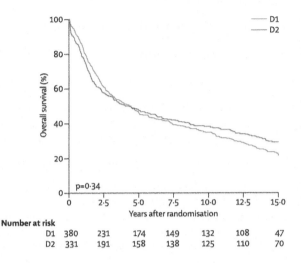

Fig. 17.1 Overall survival in patients treated with curative intent (N=711). D1=standard limited lympadenectomy. D2=standard extended lymphadenectomy. Reprinted from [9] Example of non-proportional hazards. Reprinted From The Lancet Oncology with permission from Elsevier

study by intervention, by design, or by necessity to adapt trial interventions to changing technology. Some devices go through manufacturing revisions during the intervention phase of the trial, some might be withdrawn from the market, and each device might have a different period that it has been available for use. Thus, some consideration should be given to this in subsequent/sensitivity analyses. Major changes in device technology could introduce bias into a trial, especially in a watchful-waiting trial where an intervention group that gets the device or procedure early would not be a good comparator group if the group receiving the intervention later received a different version of the device or procedure.

Analyses when multiple sites treated within one subject: This needs to be considered when the randomization unit is one participant, but the procedure or intervention may be administered to many sites (e.g., multiple coronary grafts or stents or angioplasty to many vessels, or dental implants). The approach used by many trials is to rely on randomization or stratified randomization to balance the extent of disease in treatment groups, and to define the main outcomes as occurrence in any site (e.g., artery). Depending on the disease and possibility of varying outcomes depending on site, the analysis plan may need to take into account the measurement of outcomes for multiple interventions per randomized unit.

Example: PREVENT IV Trial

In this trial, two methods of preventing graft failure were compared in patients undergoing coronary bypass surgery (CABG) [11]. Vein grafts were treated ex vivo with either edifoligide or placebo in a pressure-mediated delivery system. The primary endpoint was all-cause mortality or 75% or greater stenosis of any graft.

Since patients were randomized and not arteries, the analysis may have been biased if there was an imbalance in number and which arteries were grafted. In secondary analyses both by patient and by graft, the generalized estimating equation (GEE) methods were used to adjust for the within-subject correlation among grafts.

Operative Versus Nonoperative Comparisons

As discussed in other chapters, the comparison of an operative procedure to a nonoperative procedure needs to be carried out with precautions and special considerations in the analysis plan. Risks related to operative procedures are likely to be perioperative and early in the postoperative period, while the risks of not operating may be much later. Therefore, in the study protocol, the main hypothesis and objectives of the trial need to be explicitly stated over what time period the intervention comparisons will be made. To balance risk between operative and nonoperative interventions, a period after randomization equivalent to the operative-risk period can be defined for the nonoperative intervention for the surveillance of safety or effectiveness outcomes.

Example: ADAM Study

Time to death after abdominal aortic aneurysm (AAA) repair scheduled within 6 weeks after randomization compared to watchful waiting for symptoms of AAA growth or rupture before operating. [12]. In this trial, the secondary outcome of AAA-related death included deaths that occurred within 30 days after randomization for those randomized to surveillance, as well as deaths directly or indirectly caused by AAA rupture, AAA surgery, preoperative evaluation, late graft failure or complication, death related to recurrence of AAA after grafting, or any death occurring within 30 days after AAA surgery or any death.

Alternatively, another way to balance risk between operative and nonoperative interventions is to prespecify in the analysis plan that the initial procedure will not be counted as an outcome. In a trial randomizing one group to implantation of a device or a procedure, the hospitalization for the planned procedure might be excluded for the adverse experience analysis while the repeat of that operation is included.

Example: COURAGE Study

In this trial, time to death or nonfatal myocardial infarction after PCI procedure compared to intensive medical treatment only [13]. The secondary outcome of revascularization, did not count the initial percutaneous coronary intervention (PCI) in the PCI group as revascularization, and compared the number or patients requiring subsequent revascularization in the PCI group with all revascularization in the medical group.

Additional considerations for adherence to assigned intervention group:

In the case of watchful-waiting design studies and other intervention versus nonintervention analyses where measures must be taken to help reduce bias against penalizing the operative intervention over the nonintervention group, adherence to the assigned intervention should be considered for supportive analyses. If there is poor adherence to one or more interventions there may be poor separation of treatments. This might be due to a larger portion of randomized participants not receiving the intervention or a large proportion of the nonintervention participants crossing-over into the intervention arm. Adherence to per-protocol assigned intervention should be included in the presentation of results even though the primary analysis is by intention-to-treat.

Example

In the ADAM Study of open repair of AAA (described above), randomization was to immediate AAA repair or to surveillance of changes in AAA size (growth to 5.4 cm) and symptoms of AAA rapid growth or symptoms of AAA rupture, and scheduling AAA repair when study criteria were met [14]. The cumulative proportion of immediate AAA repair participants operated on within 6 weeks was monitored for adherence to the study criteria, as well as AAA repairs that occurred later in follow-up. At 6 weeks, 72.7% of the immediate surgery group had AAA repair and by the end of the study 92.6% were repaired. In the surveillance group, 61.6% had AAA repair over the nearly 8 year of follow-up period (mean 4.9 years). Most repairs in the surveillance group were by protocol criteria, but the proportion of off-protocol repairs was also reported. These were where AAA repair was completed for AAA that did not meet the surveillance group criteria for repair; and occurred in 9.0% of the surveillance participants. In this example, there was good separation of intervention rates under protocol conditions, with a low crossover rates (low failure to have repair in the immediate surgery group, and low rate of AAA repair in the surveillance group prior to meeting criteria for repair). Even though this was a strategy trial of comparative effectiveness, the results of the trial would have been questioned had there not been a clear separation of interventions rates. (see Fig. 17.2).

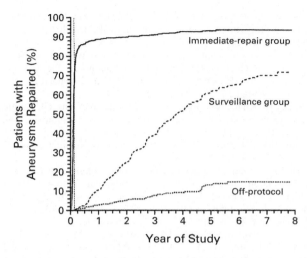

Fig. 17.2 Cumulative rate of repair of Abdominal Aortic Aneurysm, According to Treatment Group [14]. With permission from Massachusetts Medical Society

Example VA CSP Study on Transurethral Resection of the Prostate (TURP) [15]

Another example of separation of interventions in a watchful-waiting design is a trial comparing immediate surgery for benign prostatic hyperplasia with surveillance for symptoms before scheduling the procedure [15]. In this study, 89% of the surgery group underwent transurethral resection of the prostate within two weeks of randomization, while 24% had surgery over approximately 3 years.

References

1. Kaplan EL, Meier P. Nonparametric estimation from incomplete observations. J Am Stat Assoc. 1958;53:457–81.
2. Peto R, Peto J. Asymptotically efficient rank invariant test procedures (with discussion). J R Stat Soc Ser A. 1972;135:195–206.
3. Schoenfeld DA, Tsiatis AA. A modified log rank test for highly stratified data. Biometrika 1987;74:167–75.
4. Cox DR. Regression models and lifetables. J R Stat Soc. 1972;34:187–220.
5. Atroshi I, Larsson GU, Ornstein E, Hofer M, Johnsson R, Ranstam J. Outcomes of endoscopic surgery compared with open surgery for carpal tunnel syndrome among employed patients: randomised controlled trial. BMJ. 2006;332(7556):1473.
6. Grant AM, Cotton SC, Boachie C, Ramsay CR, Krukowski ZH, Heading RC, Campbell K. REFLUX trial group. Minimal access surgery compared with medical management for gastro-oesophageal reflux disease: five year follow-up of a randomized controlled trial (REFLUX). BMJ. 2013;346:f1908.

7. Putter H, Sasako M, Hartgrink HH, van de Velde CJ, van Houwelingen JC. Long-term survival with non-proportional hazards: results from the Dutch Gastric Cancer Trial. Stat Med. 2005;24(18):2807–21.
8. Bonenkamp JJ, Hermans J, Sasako M, van de Velde CJ, Welvaart K, Songun I, Meyer S, Plukker JT, Van Elk P, Obertop H, Gouma DJ, van Lanschot JJ, Taat CW, de Graaf PW, von Meyenfeldt MF, Tilanus H; Dutch Gastric Cancer Group. Extended lymph-node dissection for gastric cancer. N Engl J Med. 1999;340(12):908–14.
9. Songun I, Putter H, Kranenbarg EM, Sasako M, van de Velde CJ. Surgical treatment of gastric cancer: 15-year follow-up results of the randomised nationwide Dutch D1D2 trial. Lancet Oncol. 2010;11(5):439–49.
10. Cook JA, Ramsay CR, Fayers P. Statistical evaluation of learning curve effects in surgical trials. Clin Trials. 2004;1:421–7.
11. PREVENT IV Investigators. Efficacy and safety of edifoligide, an E2F transcription factor decoy, for prevention of vein graft failure following coronary artery bypass graft surgery PREVENT IV: a randomized controlled trial. JAMA. 2005;294(19):2446–54.
12. Lederle FA, Wilson SE, Johnson GR, Littooy FN, Acher C, Messina LM, Reinke DB, Ballard DJ. Design of the abdominal aortic Aneurysm Detection and Management Study. ADAM VA Cooperative Study Group. J Vasc Surg. 1994;20(2):296–303.
13. Boden WE, O'Rourke RA, Teo KK, Hartigan PM, Maron DJ, Kostuk WJ, Knudtson M, Dada M, Casperson P, Harris CL, Chaitman BR, Shaw L, Gosselin G, Nawaz S, Title LM, Gau G, Blaustein AS, Booth DC, Bates ER, Spertus JA, Berman DS, Mancini GB, Weintraub WS, COURAGE Trial Research Group. Optimal medical therapy with or without PCI for stable coronary disease. N Engl J Med. 2007;356(15):1503–16.
14. Lederle FA, Wilson SE, Johnson GR, Reinke DB, Littooy FN, Acher CW, Ballard DJ, Messina LM, Gordon IL, Chute EP, Krupski WC, Busuttil SJ, Barone GW, Sparks S, Graham LM, Rapp JH, Makaroun MS, Moneta GL, Cambria RA, Makhoul RG, Eton D, Ansel HJ, Freischlag JA, Bandyk D. Aneurysm Detection and Management Veterans Affairs Cooperative Study Group. Immediate repair compared with surveillance of small abdominal aortic aneurysms. N Engl J Med. 2002;346(19):1437–44.
15. Wasson JH, Reda DJ, Bruskewitz RC, Elinson J, Keller AM, Henderson WG. Acomparison of transurethral surgery with watchful waiting for moderate symptoms of benign prostatic hyperplasia. The Veterans Affairs Cooperative Study Group on Transurethral Resection of the Prostate. N Engl J Med. 1995;332(2):75–9.

Chapter 18
Advanced Statistical Methods

Hui Wang, Ilana Belitskaya-Lévy, Mei-Chiung Shih and Ying Lu

Introduction

With the development of medicine and data technologies, modern clinical trials are often situated to address sophisticated therapeutic questions that require advanced statistical techniques. This chapter introduces readers to several advanced statistical topics one may likely encounter in today's clinical trials. These topics include multiple endpoints, subgroup analysis, site and operator heterogeneity, and time-to-event outcomes. The chapter provides an intuitive overview and references for these methods and serves as a complement to the other chapters in section of *Statistical Considerations*.

Each topic is covered in a separate subsection. The subsection on multiple endpoints, which are used to measure multiple aspects of a disease, includes a discussion of advanced multiplicity adjustment and composite endpoints construction. Subgroup analysis introduces methods to evaluate efficacy and conduct hypothesis testing in multiple subpopulations in addition to the overall population. Site and operator heterogeneity can be considered a case of subgroup analysis of special importance for surgical procedures. Meta-analysis methods and mixed

H. Wang · I. Belitskaya-Lévy · M.-C. Shih · Y. Lu
Cooperative Studies Program Coordinating Center, VA Palo Alto Health
Care System, 701 North Shoreline Blvd, Mountain View, CA, USA
e-mail: Hui.Wang@va.gov

I. Belitskaya-Lévy
e-mail: ilana.belitskaya-levy@va.gov

M.-C. Shih
e-mail: Mei-Chiung.Shih@va.gov

Y. Lu (✉)
Department of Biomedical Data Science, Stanford University School of Medicine,
150 Governor's Lane T101B, Stanford, CA 94305-5405, USA
e-mail: ylu1@stanford.edu

© Springer International Publishing AG 2017
K.M.F. Itani and D.J. Reda (eds.), *Clinical Trials Design in Operative
and Non Operative Invasive Procedures*, DOI 10.1007/978-3-319-53877-8_18

163

models are also discussed. The time-to-event subsection introduces basic concepts of time-to-event derivation, censoring, and common analysis techniques such as Kaplan–Meier curve, proportional hazards regression, and restricted mean survival.

Multiple Endpoints

A clinical study may use multiple primary endpoints for claiming efficacy, especially for complex diseases when a single endpoint cannot fully characterize the outcomes of a disease. For example, patients with migraine experience severe headache, typically associated with photophobia, phonophobia, and nausea/vomiting. If a migraine trial shows evidence of treatment benefit only for the endpoint of "headache" and not for the other endpoints, then it may earn a claim of treatment benefit for headache, but it may fail to earn a claim of treatment benefit for "migraine." When the primary endpoint is a laboratory measurement, the regulatory agency may require a functional outcome to be added as a co-primary endpoint to show meaningful clinical benefit of treatment for patients. A detailed coverage of multiple endpoints is provided in Dmitrienko et al. [15].

If a treatment requires rejecting null hypotheses of no difference for all endpoints in order to be considered as acceptable, as in the examples above, there should be a concern of increased type II errors and joint statistical power should be evaluated in addition to the marginal power for each endpoint.

More often, however, a treatment is considered efficacious if it rejects at least one of the null hypotheses of no difference. For example, a cardiovascular trial may achieve its primary objective for a clinical benefit, if it establishes the efficacy for the study treatment either for all-cause mortality or for myocardial infarction or for stroke. In a special case like this, there is a greater chance for an endpoint to hit the usual line of type I error (for example, 0.05) even if treatment is not overall effective at 0.05 significant level. For example, in a trial with two primary endpoints, if we test each endpoint at a type I error level of 0.05, the likelihood that at least one endpoint is statistically significant will be $0.0975 = 1 - (1 - 0.05)(1 - 0.05)$ under the null hypothesis that treatment is not effective—much higher than the intended type I error of 0.05. This is known as a multiplicity issue in clinical trials.

A common approach to adjust for multiplicity is to control for the family-wise error rate (FWER). FWER is defined as the probability of rejecting the null hypothesis of no treatment effect for at least one of the endpoints when the null hypothesis is true. There are a number of statistical procedures to control for FWER. One strategy is to use classic multiple testing correction methods, such as Bonferroni [17, 18], Holm's step-down procedure [26] or Hochberg's step-up procedure [25]. The other strategy involves using sequential testing procedures based on the closed testing principle, such as the gatekeeping procedures [14] and the fallback procedures [40, 51] both falling into a more general class of approach —the chain procedures [31].

Classic Multiple Testing Correction Methods

Suppose that we have m primary endpoints to compare, at least one of which needs to be statistically significant for the study treatment to be considered efficacious. The Bonferroni correction rejects the null hypotheses for each of the endpoint at a significance level α/m in order to maintain FWER at α level. For example, if the overall significance level is 0.05 and there are two primary endpoints, we reject each one at 0.025 significance level in order to maintain the overall 0.05 FWER. This method does not require any distribution assumptions about dependence among the p-values. The disadvantage of Bonferroni correction is that it can be too conservative (the overall alpha level required to reject the null hypothesis is smaller than 0.05), particularly for a large number of co-primary endpoints. Thus, Bonferroni correction may result in not rejecting the null hypothesis when more accurate methods would reject.

Holm's step-down procedure offers a simple yet uniformly more powerful control for FWER than Bonferroni correction. In this approach, we first sort p-values for the primary endpoints from the smallest to the largest. From the smallest p-value and up, if the kth p-value $< \alpha/(m + 1 - k)$, reject the corresponding null hypothesis and continue to test the next higher p-value. Once kth p-value $\geq \alpha/(m + 1 - k)$, accept the corresponding null hypothesis and all hypotheses with p-value larger than the kth. Hochberg's step-up procedure starts in the opposite direction of Holm's step-down procedure by comparing the largest p-value against α. If it is smaller than α, reject all null hypotheses. Otherwise, continue to compare the next one against $\alpha/2$, and so on. When the first kth p-value is below $\alpha/(m + 1 - k)$, reject the corresponding hypothesis and all hypotheses with p-values below the kth.

Sequential Testing Procedures

Sequential testing procedures require endpoints to be ordered. These procedures include the gatekeeping procedure [2, 12, 13, 50], fallback procedure [40, 51], and the more general class of chain procedures [31]. The gatekeeping procedure is most suitable when hypothesis tests have a clear hierarchical tree structure. The endpoint in the higher hierarchy is tested at 0.05 level and, if significant, the procedure continues to the endpoint with lower hierarchy down the tree; otherwise, the procedure stops. For example, in diabetes trials, when HbA1c, fasting plasma glucose (FPG), and post-prandial glucose (PPG) are statistically tested, HbA1c is typically tested at 0.05 as the first gatekeeper. If HbA1c does not hit the 0.05 line, the gatekeeping procedure stops and the trial fails; if HbA1c is significant, FPG will be tested as the second gatekeeper and so on (Fig. 18.1). When a gatekeeping procedure stops in the middle, further discussion may be needed to claim complete efficacy. The advantage of a gatekeeping procedure is that one does not have to split

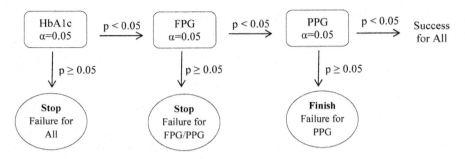

Fig. 18.1 Graphic illustration of gatekeeping procedure in diabetes trials

type I error and the most important endpoint is tested with full power. However, when the hierarchical ordering is not clear, a gatekeeping procedure can prevent endpoints down in the tree from being tested even if their p-values can be much less than 0.05. This leads to a fallback procedure that allows opportunities for all endpoints to be tested. Nevertheless, the gatekeeping procedure has gained much popularity due to its simplicity and has been widely used in the past few years. A detailed overview of the gatekeeping procedures for testing hierarchically ordered hypotheses is provided in Dmitrienko and Tamhane [14].

The fallback procedure [40, 51] tests the treatment effect for the (expected) least significant endpoint at a reduced level of α_0; if significant, the procedure stops and efficacy is claimed for both endpoints; otherwise, the treatment effect is tested for the (expected) more significant endpoint at α_+, where $\alpha_0 + \alpha_+ = \alpha$. The fallback procedure is further described in Section "Subgroup Analysis".

The fallback procedure belongs to a more general class of multiple testing procedures called the chain procedures [31]. The procedure is governed by an α allocation rule described by the proportions of α allocated to each hypothesis up-front and an α propagation rule described by the proportions of transferrable α among hypotheses upon rejection. For example, when two endpoints A and B are of equal interest, the allocation and propagation rule can be specified as $\omega_A = \omega_B = 0.5$ and $g_A = g_B = 1$. The treatment effect is tested for endpoint A with $\omega_A \, \alpha$. If test A is significant, the allocated α to test A is transferred to the test for endpoint B, and endpoint B is tested at level $(\omega_A g_A + \omega_B)\alpha = \alpha$; if not significant, the treatment effect is tested for endpoint B at $\omega_B \, \alpha$ and, if significant, endpoint A is tested again at level $(\omega_A + g_B \omega_B)\alpha = \alpha$.

Composite Endpoints

Composite endpoints combine multiple endpoints into one endpoint providing a single measure of effect based on a combination of individual endpoints. There are two classes of composite endpoints and the analysis methods for them can be quite different. One is time-to-event composite endpoints. A typical example is "MACE" (major adverse cardiac events) which might include cardiovascular death, nonfatal myocardial infraction, and nonfatal stroke. Time-to-event composite endpoints often use the time to the first component event as the outcome and are analyzed using regular survival analysis techniques.

The other class of composite endpoint involves combining continuous outcomes into one single endpoint. An established example is multiple sclerosis functional composite (MSFC) scale, which consists of a timed 25-foot walk, nine-hole peg test, and a paced auditory serial addition test. Combining continuous outcomes typically require techniques to standardize individual components and a reasonable weighting scheme. In the MS example, a Z-score approach is adopted to create a single MSFC score that involves comparing each component outcome with the mean and standard deviation found in a reference population. Choices of a reference population include a common population or baseline data within the study and should be evaluated carefully based on study objectives. The Z-scores are then summed up with equal weights to create the MSFC score. Another widely used approach is the O'Brien rank sum procedure [32], where ranks of each component are combined instead of standardized scores. Once the composite endpoint is created, analysis proceeds as usual.

Composite endpoints are particularly useful for evaluating treatments that can benefit patients in multiple domains or if component events are infrequent. Additionally, using composite endpoints helps avoid the multiplicity issues discussed earlier. Each component in a composite endpoint should itself be clinically meaningful, and, ideally, all components should be approximately equally meaningful and independent to support equal weighting. Efficacy should not be claimed for a composite endpoint, if it is driven by a less meaningful component, if there is evidence of a therapeutic disadvantage on a more meaningful component. As a result, each component in a composite endpoint needs to be analyzed separately to support the composite endpoint analysis.

Subgroup Analysis

Confirmatory (Phase 3) clinical trials aim to provide conclusive evidence on the efficacy and safety of new treatments, usually as compared to standard treatments. The conclusions from such studies are typically considered applicable to the whole study population. However, in light of growing biological and pharmacological knowledge leading to more personalized medicine and targeted therapies, it is well recognized that the treatment effect of a new drug might not be homogeneous across the study population [47]. For example, pharmacogenomic predictors that have been developed prior to a phase 3 trial may be used to identify patients with certain attributes that might be particularly sensitive to a given molecularly targeted therapy [42, 43]. For example, Herceptin is particularly effective for metastatic breast cancer patients with an HER2 protein overexpression [6]. In the surgical setting, the severity of injury at the surgical site may have an effect on recovery times or rates of infection following a surgical procedure [44]. When in addition to evaluating treatment effects overall, the researchers are interested in evaluating treatment effects in a subgroup of patients defined by a clinical or biological characteristic, this additional analysis is referred to as subgroup analysis.

Subgroup analyses can be classified into two main types: confirmatory and exploratory [33]. In the confirmatory setting, a small number of prospectively defined subgroups are investigated (usually in addition to the overall analysis) while controlling the number of false-positive results explicitly. In the exploratory setting, multiple subgroups may be considered, either post hoc or pre-specified in advance, and error rate control may not be addressed.

Exploratory subgroup analyses are routinely performed in observational studies. It is also common practice to conduct exploratory subgroup analysis in clinical trials—for each of many baseline characteristics, for each of several endpoints, or both [49]. Pocock et al. [35] found that at least one subgroup analysis was performed in addition to the main analysis in over 50% of clinical trials reported in three leading medical journals.

The results of exploratory subgroup analyses have had major effects, sometimes harmful, on treatment recommendations [34, 36, 38]. For example, many patients with suspected myocardial infarction who could have benefited from thrombolytic therapy may not have received this treatment as a result of subgroup analyses based on the duration of symptoms before treatment and the conclusion that streptokinase was only effective in patients treated within 6 h after the onset of pain [29]. A later, larger trial showed that streptokinase was effective up to 24 h after the onset of symptoms [34].

Conclusions based on exploratory subgroup analyses can have adverse consequences both when a particular category of patients is denied effective treatment (a "false-negative" conclusion), as in the above example, and when ineffective or even harmful treatment is given to a subgroup of patients (a "false-positive" conclusion). False-negative conclusions arise in subgroup analysis due to low power to detect treatment effects, especially in subgroups with low prevalence. False-positive conclusions arise in subgroup analysis due to multiple testing. When multiple subgroup analyses are performed, the probability of a false-positive finding can be substantial [28]. For example, if 10 independent subgroup analysis tests are performed at the 0.05 significance level, the chance of at least one false-positive result exceeds 40%. Thus, one must be cautious in interpretation of such results.

Exploratory subgroup analysis can be prespecified or performed post hoc [49]. A prespecified subgroup analysis is one that is planned and documented in the trial protocol before any examination of the data. Post hoc analyses refer to those in which the hypotheses being tested are not specified before any examination of the data. Such analyses are of particular concern because it is often unclear how many were undertaken and whether some were motivated by inspection of the data. However, both prespecified and post hoc analyses are subject to inflated false-positive rates arising from multiple testing.

Subgroup analyses are known to be prone to statistical and methodological issues such as inflation of false-positive rate due to multiple testing, low power, inappropriate statistical analyses, or lack of pre-specification. To deal with these issues, guidelines for the design, analysis, interpretation, and reporting of subgroup analyses have been proposed [11, 44–46]. They generally share the same main points: subgroup analysis should only be performed if the primary hypothesis is rejected, the number of subgroups to be tested should be small, subgroups of interest should be prespecified and based on a strong biological reasoning or based on observed effects in the subgroup in previous studies, adjustment for multiple testing should be included, subgroup-treatment interaction tests should be preferred to subgroup-specific tests, all subgroups tested should be reported including whether they are preplanned or post hoc.

If prior clinical or biological reasons exist why a certain subgroup may particularly benefit from a given treatment, then subgroup analyses are essential to interpret the results of clinical trials. For example, the estrogen receptor positive breast cancer appears to be more sensitive to endocrine therapy than the estrogen receptor negative breast cancer [43]. In recent years, an impressive amount of methodological research has been conducted to derive efficient trial designs and analysis strategies for confirmatory subgroup analysis to obtain evidence on the heterogeneity of treatment effects across subgroups.

Confirmatory phase III trials involving biomarkers often evaluate treatment effect in the overall population and a prespecified subgroup defined by a set of predictive biomarkers, based on prior clinical evidence that suggests that the biomarker-defined subgroups may respond differently to treatment. Patient subgroups are typically defined by genetic or proteomic biomarkers. A long-standing statistical problem is how to optimize the power for testing more than one population while controlling the false-positives rate.

An implicit assumption in the biomarker setting is that when the new treatment does not work in biomarker-positive patients, it also does not work in the biomarker-negative patients. If one is confident that the treatment will not benefit the biomarker-negative patients, then an enrichment phase III trial design, which randomizes only biomarker-positive patients, is appropriate [42]. However, there is often uncertainty about whether the treatment benefit, if any, extends to biomarker-negative patients. In this case, the phase III trial design should integrate treatment and biomarker evaluation [20–22, 41].

One strategy is to use a parallel subgroup-specific design (sometimes referred to as a biomarker-stratified design) [22]. This approach is used when strong belief exists that the positive subgroup will benefit from the treatment more than the negative subgroup. In this design, the treatment effect is tested separately in the biomarker-positive and biomarker-negative populations and a Bonferroni correction is typically used to control for multiple testing. However, the subgroup-specific design has less power than the traditional overall test of the entire population for detecting treatment benefit when the treatment effect is homogeneous across the biomarker subgroups.

A commonly used alternative design tests the treatment effect in the overall patient population and the biomarker-positive subgroup, but not in the biomarker-negative patients. This design may be useful when the rationale for the biomarker is weak (i.e., the treatment is expected to be broadly effective). Multiple versions of this overall/biomarker-positive approach have been developed [7, 40]. A well-known approach is the fallback analysis [40]: the treatment effect is tested in the overall population first and, if not significant, retested in the marker-positive group. The fallback approach was designed to cover a less likely scenario that the benefit is limited to a relatively small biomarker subgroup or when the biomarker is developed only if the overall test is not significant [23]. The problem with the overall/biomarker-positive designs is that when the treatment only works in the biomarker-positive patients, the probability of erroneously recommending the new treatment for biomarker-negative patients can be very large (i.e., when the treatment effect in the overall population is dominated by the marker-positive population) [20].

The more recent developments include the marker sequential test (MaST) design [21] that involves all three groups (overall, marker positive and marker negative) and the chain procedure—a general class of multiple testing procedures that can be applied to subgroup analysis [16, 31]. Song and Chi [43] used a similar concept and proposed a sequential test taking into account the correlations between the test statistics derived from the overall population and the subgroup. MaST prioritizes the testing in a subgroup, while the fallback procedure and Song and Chi's approach prioritize on the overall treatment effect.

Most of the methods described above are carried out in a sequential manner. Although simple to implement, sequential tests are multistep and the decision in each step is binary, regardless of the number of hypotheses. As a result, sequential tests are typically laid out in a framework of rejecting the null hypothesis of no treatment effect either in the overall population or the subgroup regardless of the specific components of composite alternatives, which may lead to a loss of power and less accurate decisions. Rosenblum et al. [37] used the Bayesian framework and proposed a simultaneous subgroup test based on the distribution of treatment effects in the marker-positive and negative subgroups. Most recently, Belitskaya-Levy and Wang, proposed the frequentist version of the simultaneous test for testing the treatment effect in the overall population and a prespecified target subgroup [3]. This test has higher power to detect treatment effects in the overall population and the biomarker-positive subgroup than most sequential procedures while controlling the false positive rate. This test also imposes a safety boundary for the test statistic in the marker-negative subgroup addressing the concern that a harmful effect in a subgroup may be masked when using an overall test statistic, in response to the request of considering safety in subgroup analysis from the European Medicines Agency [19].

Site and Operator Heterogeneity

Today, trials are routinely conducted in multiple centers (with multiple investigators). On one hand, multicenter trials provide a basis for subsequent generalization of clinical findings; on the other hand, for some conditions, having multiple sites may be the only means to achieve research goals in a given time frame. It is often of research interest to investigate the consistency of efficacy across sites for multi-center trials, particularly true for invasive procedures as the outcome of such procedures can be largely affected by the care level of a hospital and the experience level of an operator, causing heterogeneity in effect estimates. As a result, the consistency of effect estimates of an invasive treatment across sites and operators has become a subject of scrutiny for regulatory agencies, sometimes referred to as poolability examination. At minimum, one wants to make certain that the effectiveness and safety of a treatment cannot be attributed to site and operator differences. Some studies have a few sites each with a large number of enrollments; others have a large number of sites with few enrollments per site. The latter may be less relevant here as typically one does not expect site, in this case, to have a meaningful impact on results.

Trial conductors should address site heterogeneity as much as possible at the design stage of a trial. First of all, for a multicenter trial to be meaningful and interpretable, the protocol should be implemented in a similar fashion across sites and operators. For instance, it is good practice to ensure comparable enrollments at each site to avoid excessive or insufficient weight to an individual site in subsequent analyses. For randomized parallel arm trials, inclusion of various levels of hospital sites and operators can make results more credible and generalizable, and randomization is commonly stratified by site, and sometimes by operator. Meanwhile, for single-arm studies, one may want to choose similar sites and operators to reduce confounding. When a new surgical procedure is tested against a more mature one, a lead-in period is often built into a trial in which the first several procedures will be considered as "learning" cases and excluded from analysis.

In the analysis stage of a trial, statistical techniques are available to assess the heterogeneity of treatment effect across sites and operators. There are two major classes of methods: one class is stratum-based analysis; the other class assesses treatment by site-interaction effect (often in a regression model). The interaction-based method is less used than stratified analysis due to lack of power. A popular stratified analysis is the Breslow–Day (BD) [5] test often used in conjunction with the Cochran–Mantel–Haenszel (CMH) [8, 30] estimates for contingency tables. The BD statistic tests for the equivalence of conditional odds ratios computed from a series of contingency tables given a stratum variable. In our context, the BD test tests the null hypothesis that the odds ratios of a treatment for different sites (or operators) are equal. The BD test is sometimes criticized for lack of power to detect heterogeneity when the number of sites is large [1].

A more general approach, with the potential to handle multiple types of outcomes and single-arm studies, is the random effect model in meta-analysis. As an illustration, suppose that there are k sites ($i = 1, 2, \ldots, k$) in a study and each has an effect estimate T_i. We acknowledge the differences among sites and assume that each site has a different treatment effect θ_i which is a random draw from a normal distribution $N(\mu, \tau^2)$. We can then write θ_i as:

$$\theta_i = \mu + \alpha_i,$$

where α_i is a random error from $N(0, \tau^2)$. Similarly T_i can be written as

$$T_i = \mu + \alpha_i + e_i,$$

where e_i is a random error from $N(0, \sigma_i^2)$. The α_i and e_i represent the two sources of variability in T_i: α_i is the between-site variability and e_i is the within-site variability. The within-site variability is typically attributed to sampling error. The between-site variability is due to capacity and care practice differences among study sites and represents truly the heterogeneity we are studying here. Hence the null hypothesis of no heterogeneity is equivalent to $\tau^2 = 0$.

Three metrics that can be used to assess heterogeneity from a random effect model are referenced here. A usual quantity is the Cochran's Q-statistic [9]. The Q-statistic can be underpowered when there are few sites and overpowered when there are many. As an alternative, Higgins and Thompson [24] proposed an I^2 index to quantify the between-group heterogeneity instead of testing for it. The I^2 index compares the Q-statistic with its expected value. It can be interpreted as the percentage of total variances among treatment estimates that can be attributed to heterogeneity. I^2 index has gained popularity due to its simple calculation and easy interpretation [27]. Finally, the between-site variance estimate can also serve as a measurement for heterogeneity.

Analysis of site heterogeneity can be considered a special case of subgroup analysis. Virtually, any subgroup analysis method has a potential to apply to site analysis. What we have discussed are the most standard approaches. Graphic methods such as the forest plot are also quite popular to visualize site heterogeneity. There is a wide array of statistical techniques to handle site heterogeneity, and the soundest one will depend on the specific research question to be answered.

To conclude this section, we present a case study from a panel meeting for the Premarket Approval Application for NaviStar ThermoCool Radio Frequency (RF) Ablation Catheters [4]. In this application, the RF ablation is compared to anti-arrhythmic drugs (AAD) for freedom from recurrent symptomatic atrial fibrillation (AF) during a 9 month evaluation period. At 9 months, the overall rate for freedom of AF was 63% for RF ablation and 16% for AAD control, in agreement with general beliefs for RF ablation and AAD. However, when effectiveness of RF ablation was examined within each site, it was discovered that one large site OUS-1 had achieved an exceptional 100% rate of freedom of AF at 9 months and relatively lower-than-average performance for AAD. Meanwhile, the remaining sites combined achieved a disappointing 47% rate of AF freedom. Hence, the satisfactory result of 63% for RF ablation in the overall population can be driven by this outlying site alone. Results of this study are summarized in Table 18.1 and Fig. 18.2. Such site heterogeneity often warrants a panel discussion and requires further investigations.

Table 18.1 Summary of result for the study of ThermoCool RF ablation versus ADD

Site	Total number of subjects	Freedom from AF at 9-month		Relative risk
		RF ablation (%)	AAD (%)	
OUS-1	49	100	11	9.0
Non OUS-1	110	47	18	2.6
All Sites	159	63	16	4.0

Fig. 18.2 Forest plot for the study result of ThermoCool RF Ablation versus ADD. Relative risks of RF ablation to ADD and their 95% confidence intervals are presented. The size of the *square* represents the magnitude of relative risk

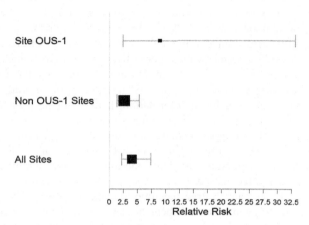

Time-to-Event Endpoints

Many clinical trials evaluate the treatment efficacy by measuring the time to a clinically significant event as the primary endpoint or one of the secondary endpoints. Examples are the recurrence-free survival time in cancer trials and the time to major adverse cardiac events (MACE) in cardiology trials, etc. The event to be evaluated does not have to be fatal, or undesirable, for example, the length of hospital stay after surgery. In the statistical literature, the statistical method analyzing time-to-event data is called survival analysis, and the time-to-event is called survival time.

To select a time-to-event endpoint in a clinical trial, one needs to consider the following important aspects. First, the event has to be critically and clinically relevant to the scientific inquiry such that the time difference between two treatments can change clinical practice. Second, there should be a well-defined beginning point of time. Many clinical trials use randomization time as an anchor point to start the calculation. In surgical trials, however, the date of intervention, i.e., surgeries, may be a better origin for the calculation of time-to-event. Third, time-to-event should be defined without ambiguity. For instance, time to death is considered one of the most objective measurements. That said, some events can be hard to determine. As an example, the determination of time to cardiovascular death, often used as a primary endpoint in trials for cardiovascular conditions, needs information on cause of death which may not be obvious from death report; some MACE need careful examination of medical records and chart review; time to tumor progression is determined based on radiological images and requires sophisticated algorithms. For many trials, a clinical endpoint evaluation committee is required to adjudicate the nature of the clinical events and determine the time when they actually occur. When the appropriate event is selected, the beginning is determined, and method to assess the event occurrence is established, one can use time-to-event (or survival time) to measure treatment effectiveness (or safety).

In Statistics 101, data are grouped into four types: the nominal categorical data, ordinal categorical data, discrete data, and continuous data. Survival time is typically measured continuously, but can also be discrete (for example, number of days). Sometimes we are interested in the survival time at a fixed interval, such as a 5-year disease free survival. In this case, we make the continuous survival time into a binary variable, i.e., survived by 5 years or beyond. While continuous survival time carries a lot of information, it may not be necessarily relevant to a clinical research question. For example, to compare the time to target vessel failure due to two different types of stents in a clinical trial, the primary interest of the study is the failure rate within a year, because there are other factors likely to contribute to failures beyond a year. Thus, the time to failure within a year is more relevant than events after one year.

If we can observe the time-to-event for every trial participant, the analysis of time-to-event data will bear no special challenge as conventional statistics can be used. With increasing use of various data sources, such as cooperative data warehouses from healthcare systems and informatics, it is possible in the future that we will get most if not all survival information for our study participants.

The main challenge in survival analysis is that time-to-event data may not be observed before the trial ends. Participants who do not develop the clinical event of interest before trial termination or who prematurely withdraw from the trial will have no information about when they will have the event. This is called right censoring as the true event time will be after the time of last contact. Another case is the evaluation of new lesions in cancer studies that may occur between two MRI scans. Thus, we know that the time-to-event is between two scans but do not know the exact time for progression. We call this interval censored data. Most survival analysis methods require the censoring time to be non-informative or independent of the survival time, i.e., we cannot tell the differences between time-to-event for any two patients based on when they leave (or remain in) the trial.

Because time is one dimensionally directional and always increases, the censored participants provide partial information about time-to-event, i.e., the survival time is longer than withdrawal time for right censored data or the survival time is in between two examinations for interval censored data.

The Kaplan–Meier survival curve is a commonly used graphic presentation of survival data. Figure 18.3 presents an example of a Kaplan–Meier curve for a token example presented in Table 18.2. The x-axis of a Kaplan–Meier survival curve is the time since the origin. The y-axis is the probability of survival to time x. At the beginning of the study, everyone is alive, and thus the survival probability is 1.

Whenever we observe one or multiple deaths, at day 7 and day 18 in Table 18.1, we calculate the number of subjects still alive right before that time (thus exclude all participants who died or were censored before). This number is usually referred to as the number of subjects at risk. The ratio of the number of participants who have events at time days 7 and 18 over the number of subjects at risk is the conditional probability of having the event for participants who have survived to day 7 and day 18 respectively, often referred to as the hazard function. Subtracting the hazard function from 1 will lead to the conditional survival probability beyond time x for those still alive before time x. Multiplying this conditional survival probability with the overall probability prior to the time x results in the overall survival probability at time x (i.e., the y-axis value). The higher the value on y-axis, the less likely an event will occur. In the presence of right censoring, the correct estimation of the event rate at a fixed time x should be the y-value of the Kaplan–Meier curve at x. The ratio of deaths before time x over all patients or over all patients who are followed to time x can be biased because they will incorrectly handle the censored observations.

In the presence of censoring, the last patients may be censored. In such case, the Kaplan–Meier survival curve will not hit zero, and the mean survival time, a commonly used descriptive statistics for distribution location, is not estimable. More often than not (although not always) we can observe the time when the Kaplan–Meier curve passes the 50% threshold on the y-axis. When the y-value is equal to 0.5, the corresponding x-value is the median survival time, a common alternative description of survival data. When the survival probability of the last observation is above 50%, i.e., the curve does not hit the $y = 50\%$ line as shown in Fig. 18.3, the median survival time is also not estimable. A model-based approach or other summary statistics, such as the probability of survival given a fixed time point or the restricted mean survival time (to be discussed later) can be used to describe the data.

Fig. 18.3 Kaplan–Meier survival curve for the token example

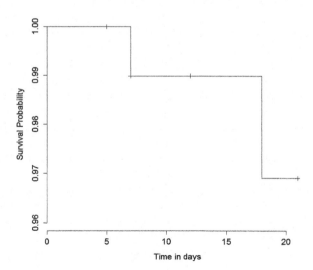

Table 18.2 A token example for calculation of Kaplan–Meier survival curve

x-axis: time (days)	0	5	7	12	18	21
# of participants prior to x	100	100	99	97	95	93
# of deaths	0	0	1	0	2	0
# of right censored	0	1	1	2	0	93
Hazard function	0%	0%	1/99 = 1.01%	0%	2/95 = 2.11%	0%
y-axis: survival function	100%	100%	98.99%	98.99%	96.91%	96.91%

A hazard function on an instantaneously continuous time scale is defined as the hazard rate—the speed of probability of death at time of x among those alive prior to x. The higher the hazard rate, the more likely an event occurs in the next instantaneous moment. Thus, we can use the ratio of two hazard rates from treatment A and treatment B to describe the survival difference between two treatments. The well-known Cox regression model assumes that the log of the hazard ratio is a function of covariates independent of time [10]. The Cox regression, also called proportional hazards regression, and Kaplan–Meier survival curves are the most commonly used methods in clinical trials to analyze survival data. A standard statistical test to determine the significance of the differences between two Kaplan–Meier survival curves or the significance of a covariate in a Cox regression is the log-rank test.

While the Cox proportional hazard model is flexible and powerful, it has an assumption that the hazards from different covariates values including treatments are proportional over time. Also, the effect of the hazard ratio to the actual clinical concern on survival probability may be counter intuitive. For example, a hazard ratio of 0.5 for treatment A versus B is commonly interpreted as that treatment B reduces the hazard of treatment A by 50%. However, to translate the reduction into survival probabilities at different time points is not 50% and not even constant. For example, if the survival probability of A is 90%, then that of B should be 95%; Similar relationships are 70% versus 84%; 50% versus 71%; 30% versus 55%, and 10% versus 32%. Thus depending on the survival probability of A, the relative impact on survival probability can be different under the same hazard ratio.

The proportional hazards assumption can be examined visually in the Kaplan–Meier curve: when two survival curves cross, the proportional hazards assumption is violated. Alternatively, one can plot the negative log of survival functions of two groups to examine whether they are parallel. Another approach is to examine and test whether the Schoenfield residuals from Cox regression model [39] are independent of time. If independent, the proportional hazards assumption is acceptable. Otherwise, the assumption is violated and the hazard ratio is not the best statistic of the treatment difference because the benefit and harm can change over time.

Recently, there was a call to move beyond the use of hazard ratio in quantifying the between-group difference in survival analysis [48]. The restricted mean survival time (RSMT) has been proposed as one of the alternatives. A RMST measures the mean survival time up to a clinically relevant time point, such as the mean survival time up to 5 years. The interpretation is the mean survival time if we follow the participants to 5 years in this case. Mathematically, a 5-year RMST is the area under the Kaplan–Meier survival curve up to 5 years. The choice of the time window depends on clinical relevance. The difference of two RMSTs measures the difference of two areas under the two survival curves. The main advantages of RMST are the following: (1) it is easier to communicate the meaning among clinicians, patients, and statisticians; (2) It is estimable even for rare events where the median survival time cannot be achieved; (3) It is nonparametric and free from assumptions such as the proportional hazards; (4) comparison of survival difference via RMSTs can be more powerful than the log-rank test when the proportional hazards assumption is not true; (5) comparison of survival difference via RMSTs integrates difference in survival probabilities from the beginning to the end of the follow-up time, thus a more meaningful difference.

In summary, survival analysis is an important area in clinical trials. Due to the various censoring mechanisms for time-to-event data in clinical studies, it is worth a special consideration. Kaplan–Meier survival curve is a standard graphic presentation of time-to-event data. Median survival time, survival probability at a fixed time, and restricted mean survival time in a clinically meaningful time window are commonly used summary statistics. Additional advanced topics for survival analysis include but are not limited to multiple times to events (such as individual time for each event in the composite MACE endpoint), recurrent events, interval censoring, informative censoring that the censoring time is related to the time-to-event, time dependent Cox regression model, and stochastic modeling, etc. It is recommended to consult professional statisticians for any major projects that involve survival endpoints.

References

1. Bagheri Z, Ayatollahi SMT, Jafari P. Comparison of three tests of homogeneity of odds ratios in multicenter trials with unequal sample sizes within and among centers. BMC Med Res Methodol. 2011;11:58.
2. Bauer P, Röhmel J, Maurer W, Hothorn L. Testing strategies in multi-dose experiments including active control. Stat Med. 1998;17:2133–46.
3. Belitskaya-Levy I, Wang H, Shih MC, Tian L, Doros G, Lew RA, Lu Y. A new overall-subgroup simultaneous test for optimal inference in biomarker-targeted confirmatory trials. Stat. Biosci. doi:10.1007/s12561-016-9174-8.
4. Biosense Webster Inc. FDA executive summary prepared for the November 20, 2008 meeting of the Circulatory System Devices Panel P030031/S011 NaviStar ThermoCool RF Ablation Catheters. 2008. http://www.fda.gov/ohrms/dockets/ac/08/briefing/2008-4393b1-01%20%20FDA%20executive%20summary%20FINAL.pdf.
5. Breslow NE, Day NE. Statistical methods in cancer research: volume 1—the analysis of case-control studies. Lyon, France: IARC Scientific Publications; 1980.
6. Burstein HJ. The distinctive nature of HER2-positive breast cancers. N Engl J Med. 2005; 353(16):1652–4.

7. Cappuzzo F, Ciuleanu T, Stelmakh L, et al. Erlotinib as maintenance treatment in advanced non-small-cell lung cancer: a multicentre, randomised, placebo-controlled phase 3 study. Lancet Oncol. 2010;11:521–9.
8. Cochran WG. The combination of estimates from different experiments. Biometrics. 1954;10:101–29.
9. Cochran WG. Some methods for strengthening the common χ^2 tests. Biometrics. 1954;10(4): 417–51.
10. Cox DR. Regression models and life-tables. J R Stat Soc. 1972;34:187–220.
11. Dijkman B, Kooistra B, Bhandari M. How to work with a subgroup analysis. Can J Surg. 2009;52:515–22.
12. Dmitrienko A, Offen WW, Westfall PH. Gatekeeping strategies for clinical trials that do not require all primary effects to be significant. Stat Med. 2003;22:2387–400.
13. Dmitrienko A, Tamhane AC, Wang X, Chen X. Stepwise gatekeeping procedures in clinical trial applications. Biometrical J. 2006;48(6):984–91.
14. Dmitrienko A, Tamhane AC. Gatekeeping procedures with clinical trial applications. Pharm Statistics. 2007;6:171–80.
15. Dmitrienko A, Tamhane AC, Bretz F. Multiple testing problems in pharmaceutical statistics. 1st ed. Boca Raton: Chapman and Hall, CRC Biostatistics Series; 2009.
16. Dmitrienko A, D'Agostino RB. Tutorial in biostatistics: traditional multiplicity adjustment methods in clinical trials. Stat Med. 2013;32:5172–218.
17. Dunn OJ. Estimation of the medians for dependent variables. Ann Math Stat. 1959;30(1): 192–7. doi:10.1214/aoms/1177706374.JSTOR2237135.
18. Dunn OJ. Multiple comparisons among means. J Am Stat Assoc. 1961;56(293):52–64. doi:10.1080/01621459.1961.10482090.
19. European Medicines Agency, Committee for Medicinal Products for Human Use. Concept paper on the need for a guideline on the use of subgroup analyses in randomized controlled trials. 2010. http://www.ema.europa.eu/docs/en_GB/document_library/Scientific_guideline/2010/05/WC500090116.pdf. Accessed January 14, 2016.
20. Freidlin B, Korn EL. Biomarker enrichment strategies: matching trial design to biomarker credentials. Nat Rev Clin Oncol. 2014;11(2):81–90.
21. Freidlin B, Korn EL, Gray R. Marker sequential test (MaST) design. Clin Trials. 2014;11(1): 19–27.
22. Freidlin B, McShane LM, Korn EL. Randomized clinical trials with biomarkers: design issues. J Natl Cancer Inst. 2010;102:152.
23. Freidlin B, Simon R. Adaptive signature design: an adaptive clinical trial design for generating and prospectively testing a gene expression signature for sensitive patients. Clin Cancer Res. 2005;11:7872–78.
24. Higgins JPT, Thompson SG. Quantifying heterogeneity in a meta-analysis. Stat Med. 2002;21:1539–58.
25. Hochberg Y. A sharper Bonferroni procedure for multiple tests of significance. Biometrika. 1988;75:800–2.
26. Holm S. A simple sequentially rejective multiple test procedure. Scand J Stat. 1979;6(2): 65–70.
27. Huedo-Medina, TB, Sánchez-Meca J, Marín-Martínez F, Botella J. Assessing heterogeneity in meta-analysis: Q statistics or I2 index. Psychol Methods. 2006;11(2):193–206.
28. Lagakos SW. The challenge of subgroup analyses—reporting without distorting. N Engl J Med. 2006;354:1667–9.
29. Lee TH, Weisberg MC, Brand DA, Rouan GW, Goldman L. Candidates for thrombolysis among emergency room patients with acute chest pain. Ann Intern Med. 1989;110:957–62.
30. Mantel N, William Haenszel W. Statistical aspects of the analysis of data from retrospective studies of disease. J Natl Cancer Inst. 1959;22(4):719–48.
31. Millen BA, Dmitrienko A. Chain procedures: a class of flexible closed testing procedures with clinical trial applications. Stat Biopharm Res. 2011;3:14–30.

32. O'Brien PC. Procedures for comparing samples with multiple endpoints. Biometrics. 1984;40 (4):1079–87.
33. Ondra T, Dmitrenko A, Friede T, Gra A, Miller F, Stallard N, Rosch M. Methods for identification and confirmation of targeted subgroups in clinical trials: a systematic review. J Biopharm Stat. 2016;26(1):99–119.
34. Oxman AD, Guyatt GH. A consumer's guide to subgroup analyses. Ann Intern Med. 1992;116:78–84.
35. Pocock SJ, Hughes MD, Lee RJ. Statistical problems in the reporting of clinical trials. NEJM. 1987;317:426–32.
36. Pocock SJ, Assmann SF, Enos LE, Kasten LE. Subgroup analysis, covariate adjustment and baseline comparisons in clinical trial reporting: current practice and problems. Stat Med. 2002;21:2917–30.
37. Rosenblum M, Liu H, Yen E-H. Optimal tests of treatment effects for the overall population and two subpopulations in randomized trials, using sparse linear programming. J Am Stat Assoc. 2014;109(507):1216–28.
38. Rothwell PM. Subgroup Analysis in randomized controlled trials: importance, indications, and interpretation. Lancet. 2005;2005(365):176–86.
39. Schoenfeld D. Partial residuals for the proportional hazards regression model. Biometrika. 1982;69:239–41.
40. Simon R. The use of genomics in clinical trial design. Clin Cancer Res. 2008;14:5984–93.
41. Simon R. Clinical trials for predictive medicine. Stat Med. 2012;31:3031–40.
42. Simon RM, Maitournam A. Evaluating the efficiency of targeted designs for randomized clinical trials. Clin Cancer Res. 2004;10:6759–63.
43. Song Y, Chi GYH. A method for testing a prespecified subgroup in clinical trials. Stat Med. 2007;26:3535–49.
44. Sun X, Heels-Ansdell D, Walter SD, Guyatt G, Sprague S, Bhandari M, Sanders D, Schemitsch E, Tornetta P, Swiontkowski M. Is a subgroup claim believable? A user's guide to subgroup analyses in the surgical literature. J Bone Joint Surg Am. 2011;93:e8.
45. Sun X, Briel M, Busse JW, You JJ, Akl EA, Mejza F, Bala MM, Bassler D, Mertz D, Diaz-Granados N, Vandvik PO, Malaga G, Srinathan SK, Dahm P, Johnston BC, Alonso-Coello P, Hassouneh B, Walter SD, Heels-Ansdell D, Bhatnagar N, Altman DG, Guyatt GH. Credibility of claims of subgroup effects in randomised controlled trials: systematic review. BMJ. 2012;344:e1553.
46. Sun X, Ioannidis JP, Agoritsas T, Alba AC, Guyatt G. How to use a subgroup analysis: users' guide to the medical literature. JAMA. 2014;311:405–11.
47. Tanniou J, van der Tweel I, Teerenstra S, Roes KCB. Subgroup analysis in confirmatory clinical trials: time to be specific about their purposes. BMC Med Res Methodol. 2016;16:20.
48. Uno H, Claggett B, Tian L, Inoue E, Gallo P, Miyata T, Schrag D, Takeuchi M, Uyama Y, Zhao L, Skali H, Solomon S, Jacobus S, Hughes M, Packer M, Wei LJ. Moving beyond the hazard ratio in quantifying between-group difference in survival analysis. J Clin Oncol. 2014;32(22):2380–5.
49. Wang R, Lagakos SW, Ware JH, Hunter DJ, Drazen JM. Statistics in medicine—reporting of subgroup analyses in clinical trials. NEJM. 2007;357(21):2189–94.
50. Westfall PH, Krishen A. Optimally weighted, fixed sequence and gatekeeper multiple testing procedures. J Stat Plan Infer. 2001;99:25–41.
51. Wiens BL, Dmitrienko A. The fallback procedure for evaluating a single family of hypotheses. J Biopharm Stat. 2005;15(6):929–42.

Chapter 19
Missing Data

Kousick Biswas

Introduction

The validity of primary findings from a RCT is critically dependent on the completeness and accuracy of collected data. Complete and accurate data ensure that the designed power is achieved and the analysis bias is minimized. Presence of missing data in a RCT, if ignored, makes the interpretation of the trial results problematic as it not only reduces the power but also introduces response bias, reducing the robustness of findings that result from randomization. Data, in a RCT, can be missing for a multitude of reasons (e.g., participants' refusal to continue the study intervention, participants' decision to dropout due to either no perceived efficacy or perceived efficacy, or due to adverse reactions experienced during participation, participants moving out from the area, etc.) at various time points, e.g., baseline, one, several or all follow-ups etc., which provide the foundations of various missing data mechanisms. The mechanisms along with missing data should be taken into account while deciding on strategies to deal with missing data. It is always desirable that the intended strategies to deal with missing data based on anticipated missing data mechanism(s) are taken into account during the design phase of a RCT. There is no universally accepted method to deal with missing data as it is difficult to test the hypothetical missing mechanism [1]. A more commonly accepted practice is to conduct a sensitivity analysis by utilizing various methods that deal with missing data with respective assumptions to demonstrate the robustness of the findings. As a bottom line, prevention and the strategies to deal with missing data are the two most important issues that must be dealt with during planning of RCTs irrespective of disease areas to ensure valid inferences based on anticipated missing data mechanism.

K. Biswas (✉)
US Department of Veteran Affairs, Cooperative Studies Program Coordinating Center,
Office of Research and Development, VA Medical Center, 5th Boiler Street,
Perry Point, MD 21902, USA
e-mail: Kousick.Biswas@va.gov

© Springer International Publishing AG 2017   181
K.M.F. Itani and D.J. Reda (eds.), *Clinical Trials Design in Operative
and Non Operative Invasive Procedures*, DOI 10.1007/978-3-319-53877-8_19

Background

Notations

In general, a dataset is organized as a rectangular matrix Y with m rows and n columns where rows correspond to the units (or participants) and the columns correspond to the variables (age, gender, outcome measures, such as, CAPS scores, etc.) at different time points, as per the design (e.g., Baseline, 3, 6, 9 months follow up visits, etc.). So, y_{ijk} is the value of a variable j (j can take a value between 1 and n) for participant i (i can take a value between 1 and m) at k time point (k can take a value between 1 and total number of time points in a trial) and it could be either a value(s) of a single outcome or a set of outcomes or values of covariates. M is the missing data indicator matrix where each entry M_{ijk} can take a value of 1 (if y_{ijk} is observed) or 0 (if y_{ijk} is missing).

Missing Data Patterns

The following missing data patterns are common in RCTs [2]:

(a) *Univariate*—For this pattern all the covariates are collected but the outcome values were missed. The outcome values can be of a single outcome or a group of outcomes which, in this case, are either completely observed or completely missed. (y_{ijk} are missing, either for a single outcome or for a set of outcomes)
(b) *Monotone*—This pattern is very common in longitudinal studies where all repeating observations at future time points are missing once a participant is dropped out of the trial. (all y_{ijk} are missing irrespective of types—outcome or covariates—after the dropout time point)
(c) *Arbitrary*—In the rectangular data grid ($Y_{m \times n}$) any data items can be missing for any participants without following any particular pattern. Occasional missed visits by the participants (but not completely dropping out) or mistakenly omitted forms can produce this pattern of missing data (any y_{ijk} can be missing).

Missing Data Mechanism

Missing data mechanism or dropout mechanism (denoted by $P(M|Y, \theta)$ where θ is a parameter of interest) governs the relationship between the missing information and its underlying dependencies on the observed or unobserved data. Mechanisms of missing data in RCTs were suggested and described by Rubin [3] and Little and Rubin [4] in detail and are briefly described below:

(a) *Missing-Completely-at-Random (MCAR)*—The probability of missing is unrelated to the values of any data, observed, or missing. These missing values do not introduce bias but do impact the power of analysis when removed from the analysis, if the proportion of missing is high. For MCAR, any standard analysis approach will produce valid results in a dataset with limited missing information. The MCAR assumption is a very rare possibility in RCTs.

$$P(M|Y, \theta) = P(M|\theta)$$

Examples: Data is missing due to incarceration of a participant or the person is leaving the area due to a job change.

(b) *Missing-at-Random (MAR)*—The probability of missing is related to the observed data but not to the unobserved data. The missing data with MAR assumption is ignorable. In other words, a missing observation will satisfy this assumption if it is in itself not informative about the treatment effect.

$$P(M|Y, \theta) = P(M|Y_{\text{obs}}, \theta)$$

Example: Participant termination as a result of reaching a threshold on a certain measure, such as the systolic blood pressure rising above a predefined safety limit.

(c) *Missing-not-at-Random (MNAR)*—The probability of missing is related to unobserved future data. In other words, if the missing data is neither MCAR nor MAR, then they are MNAR. The MNAR data is non-ignorable and thus needs to be taken into the analysis.

$$P(M|Y, \theta) = P(M|Y_{\text{miss}}, \theta)$$

Example: Participant drops out because their symptoms have worsened since the last study visit but they do not report that to the study investigator.

Impact of Missing Data

It is very important to have an appreciation about the impacts of missing data on primary findings of RCTs if the missing data and the underlying missing mechanism are not taken into account during the analysis [5].

Statistical Power and Variability—In RCTs, the statistical power, for a specific outcome analysis, is directly proportional to the number of observations and inversely proportional to the variability in the outcome of interest. So, if participants with missing data are removed then the number of observations available for a given analysis is reduced and thus weakens the power of the analysis. On the other hand, most often the participants who drop out are likely to have more extreme outcomes. So, analysis excluding these non-completers yields reduced variability and narrower confidence intervals which falsely indicate more precise treatment effect.

Analysis Bias—Analysis of RCT data with missing information can be biased in two ways:

(i) Differential missing proportions in treatment arms—If only complete cases are included in the analysis and proportions of missing data are not balanced across the treatment arms then the analysis will be biased toward the treatment arm that has the least amount of missing information.

(ii) Relationship between missing data and underlying mechanism—The analysis will be biased if the anticipated missing mechanism is not a good fit for the type of missing information and as a result inappropriate statistical methods are used for inferences.

Strategy to Deal with Missing Data

Strategy to deal with missing data in RCTs is a two-step process. First, a smart and patient-centric trial design/implementation plan is utilized to minimize or to prevent missing data. Second, based on the anticipated type of missing data (e.g., MAR), suitable analytic methods are chosen to ensure unbiased and robust findings.

Prevention of Missing Data

During the conduct of RCTs, missing data occurs in a variety of trial design and implementation scenarios. Majority of these missing data either can be avoided or minimized by implementing simple changes in the study design and implementation [1, 6]. The drivers for these missing data can be categorized in three broad categories [6]—(a) Data missed because of participants' action or inaction, (b) Data missed because of investigator's or study personnel's action or inaction and (c) Data missed because of inefficient study design. Recommendations for improving (a) study design and implementation, (b) design of data collection instruments, and (c) the role of study personnel during trial implementation so that missing information can be prevented from occurring during the study conduct as much as possible are discussed in detail in Biswas [6].

Statistical Treatment of Missing Data

Even with careful trial design and smart implementation of trials it is practically impossible to eliminate missing data completely. The only way to deal with a data set with missing information is to utilize statistical methods that are appropriate for underlying missing mechanisms [1]. It is important to prespecify the anticipated proportion of participants who are likely to be dropped out along with the anticipated missing mechanism (e.g., MCAR or MAR) based on past RCT experiences with similar population or disease areas. Prespecification of anticipated missing data proportion allows the inflation of the sample size during the design phase so that the designed power can be achieved and the specification of the anticipated missing data mechanism helps to choose the appropriate analytical methods for data analysis. A sensitivity analysis (by utilizing a variety of methods under different missing data mechanism assumptions) provides the robustness of the analysis in case of a departure from the anticipated missing data mechanism(s) as testing of assumed missing data mechanism is often impossible [1].

Statistical Methods for Ignorable Missing Data (MCAR and MAR)

Complete Case (CC) Analysis (listwise deletion)—Only cases with complete data are retained for analysis with the assumption that missing data are completely at random (MCAR). In the instance where MCAR assumption holds, CC provides valid parameter estimates but with reduced power [7].

Available Case (AC) Analysis (pairwise deletion)—Different sets of values are used to estimate different parameters of interest. AC yields consistent estimates if the variables are moderately to weakly correlated [6] but it can produce an erroneous covariance matrix based on estimated correlations outside the range of -1.0 to 1.0. AC fails to adequately address the missing values even under MCAR assumption [7].

Single Value Imputation—Missing values are imputed with a single probable value, e.g., the mean calculated from the observed values [8]. This imputation technique retains all the observations as per the design of the trial (i.e., no listwise or pairwise deletion) but as the missing values are replaced by a single value, such as the mean of the observations in the rest of the dataset, the distribution of the variable changes because of reduced variability. Smaller standard error, as a result of the retained sample size and reduced variability, provides a false impression of reduced uncertainties in the data. Some of the commonly used single value imputations are [9] (i) Mean substitution—mean of the observed values replaces the missing values, (ii) Hot Deck imputation—missing values are replaced with observed values from participants with similar attributes, (iii) Conditional Mean Substitution—missing values (as response variables) are predicted from observed variables (as predictors), and (iv) Conditional Distribution Imputation—missing values are replaced with random picks from conditional distribution of the variable (that is missing) on the other variables (that are observed).

Model Based Methods

The model based methods work under two main assumptions—(a) the joint distribution of the data is multivariate normal, and (b) the missing data mechanism is ignorable (MAR).

Maximum Likelihood (ML) using Expectation-Maximization (EM) algorithm—The ML method yields estimates of parameters of interest (e.g., *mean*) which would maximize the probability of observed data (y_{ijk}). A log likelihood (LL) function, the probability of the data as a function of the data and the unknown parameter, is maximized with a value of *mean* using an iterative process.

EM algorithm can be used, as suggested by Little and Rubin [4] and Schafer [2] to obtain ML estimates with missing data with the assumption that the data is multivariate normal. This is a two-step process—first, the expected value of the LL function is obtained for the observed data based on the current parameter values (the E step), then second, the expected LL is maximized to obtain new parameter values (the M step). These two steps are repeated until convergence criterion is met [8]. For multivariate normal data, the parameters of interest are means, variances, and covariances. The ML method with EM algorithm does not generate estimates of missing values but provides estimates for means and variance-covariance matrix of the variables with missing values which are then used to obtain estimates for the model parameters, e.g., coefficients of a regression model [8].

Multiple Imputation (MI)—Missing values are imputed using random draws from the distribution of the missing values given the observed values to generate a complete data set. This process is repeated multiple times (at least 5 completed data sets are generated). Each of these completed datasets is analyzed using standard statistical methods and the parameter estimates from each of these analyses are then pooled, using rules suggested by Rubin [7], to obtain the final estimates.

Statistical Methods for Non-ignorable Missing Data (MNAR)

If missing data are non-ignorable then the missingness needs to be modeled along with the modeling of the complete data. The following methods can be used to accomplish that:

Pattern Mixture—The participants are classified according to the pattern of their missingness with the available data in each pattern. The parameters are estimated in each pattern using the complete data model and the final estimates are obtained by averaging across the missing data patterns [10].

Selection Models—The distribution of the complete data is specified first and then how the missingness is dependent on the data is specified [1]. Based on a marginal distribution of the complete data and a conditional distribution of missing given the complete data, a selection model establishes the joint distribution of the complete data and the missingness. A detailed review of selection models for longitudinal data with missing observations can be found in Little [11] and Verbeke and Molenbergs [12].

Sensitivity Analysis

It is very important that the trial designers identify the basic assumptions about the missing data mechanisms during the design stage of the study. These assumptions can then provide the basis of sensitivity analysis. In general, a MAR assumption can be a reasonable starting point and the assumptions should be made in consultations with the clinicians depending on the disease areas. The main idea of conducting a sensitivity analysis is to capture the robustness of the analysis. If the basic assumption of missing data mechanism holds then the variations in the parameter estimates and the standard errors would be minimal [1]. A commonly used method for sensitivity analysis that can be easily implemented in SAS is called "Tipping Point Approach". In this method a progressive stress-testing is employed, using multiple imputation (MI) under a suspected missing mechanism of MNAR, to identify the "Tipping Point" that reverses the analysis conclusion (e.g., the statistical significance $(P < 0.05)$ changes to nonsignificance $(P > 0.05)$ when the analysis is done using MI under the assumption of MAR). The stress-test is implemented by using shift parameters to adjust the imputed values in steps, commonly in the active arm only. If the change needed (the magnitude of the shift parameter) to reverse the original analysis conclusion is implausible (according to the subject matter experts) then the MAR assumption holds for the missing values. This method can be implemented using PROC MI and PROC MIANALYZE in SAS [13].

References

1. National Research Council of the National Academies. The prevention and treatment of missing data in clinical trials. Washington DC: National Academies Press; 2010.
2. Schafer JL. Analysis of incomplete multivariate data. New York: Chapman & Hall; 1997.
3. Rubin DB. Inference and missing data. Biometrika. 1976;63:581–92.
4. Little RJA, Rubin DB. Statistical analysis with missing data. 2nd ed. Wiley: New York; 2002.
5. European Medicines Agency. Guideline on missing data in confirmatory clinical trials. 2009. EMA/CPMP/EWP/1776/99 rev. 1, Committee for Medicinal Products for Human Use (July). Available from http://www.ema.europa.eu/docs/en_GB/document_library/Scientific_guideline/2010/09/WC500096793.pdf.

6. Biswas K. Prevention and management of missing data during conduct of a clinical study. Biostatistics Psychiatry. 2012;24(4):235–7.
7. Rubin DB. Multiple imputation for non-response in surveys. New York: Wiley; 1987.
8. Pigott TD. A review of Methods for Missing Data. Educ Res Eval. 2001;7(4):353–83.
9. Schafer JL, Graham JW. Missing data: our view of the state of the art. Psychol Methods. 2002;7(2):147–77.
10. Ratitch B, O'Kelly M. Implementation of pattern-mixture models using standard SAS/STAT procedures. 2011. PharmaSug2011—Paper SP04. Available: http://pharmasug.org/proceedings/2011/SP/PharmaSUG-2011-SP04.pdf.
11. Little RJA. Modeling the dropout mechanism in repeated-measures studies. J Am Stat Assoc. 1995;90:1112–21.
12. Verbeke G, Molenbergs G. Linear mixed models for longitudinal data. New York: Springer; 2000.
13. SAS/STAT(R) 13.1 User's guide, the MIANALYZE procedure. SAS Institute; Available from http://support.sas.com/documentation/cdl/en/statug/66859/HTML/default/viewer.htm#statug_mianalyze_examples13.htm.

Chapter 20
Interim Monitoring

Joseph F. Collins

Interim Monitoring

In any clinical trial, the primary concern is patient safety. While study design, data integrity, study methods and so forth are all extremely important, patient safety is of the utmost importance and requires that studies be reviewed in a routine fashion to ensure that no harm is being done to study participants. In addition, clinical trials have become time consuming, labor intensive, and costly endeavors that need to be monitored regularly to ensure that study progress is going as expected and that study results are not already conclusive (positively or negatively).

Interim monitoring is a way of ensuring that patient safety, study progress, protocol adherence, and study outcomes (when possible) are routinely reviewed. It is an ongoing review of outcomes data for groups of patients that determines if a clinical trial needs modification or early stopping for reasons of efficacy or safety. Trials that require outcomes monitoring are any trials in which the treatments have the potential for producing an adverse or beneficial treatment effect and where it is possible to detect and act upon such effects during the course of the trial. While most randomized clinical trials can be monitored for recruitment, protocol adherence, and patient safety, some cannot be monitored meaningfully for study outcomes. For example, a surgery study with a one-year recruitment period and a one-year or more follow-up to reach the primary outcome would not benefit greatly from outcome monitoring since all of the treatments would have been delivered before it was possible to determine outcomes.

Plans for interim monitoring need to be prepared prior to study start-up, and should identify who will do the monitoring. The National Institutes of Health (NIH) recommends that every clinical trial should have provisions for data and

J.F. Collins (✉)
Department of Veteran Affairs, Cooperative Studies Program Coordinating Center,
VA Medical Center, Building 362T, Perry Point, MD 21902, USA
e-mail: joseph.collins2@va.gov

© Springer International Publishing AG 2017   189
K.M.F. Itani and D.J. Reda (eds.), *Clinical Trials Design in Operative
and Non Operative Invasive Procedures*, DOI 10.1007/978-3-319-53877-8_20

safety monitoring, that the provisions should be approved by an Institutional Review Board (IRB), and that multicenter trials should have an independent Data and Safety Monitoring Board (DSMB). For phase I and II clinical trials, NIH requires that investigators submit a general description of the data and safety monitoring plans as part of research applications. At a minimum, plans should describe reporting mechanisms of adverse events to the IRB, the Food and Drug Administration (FDA), and NIH. For multisite trials, NIH requires a central reporting entity to prepare summary reports of adverse events for distribution to sites and IRB's as well as to FDA and NIH.

The plans for interim monitoring should also be included in the study proposal. The plans at a minimum should include what variables will be considered, how often these variables will be presented, to whom these data will be presented, how they will be presented, and what statistical methods, if any, will be used. The variables to be considered should include recruitment and safety variables at a minimum. Recruitment needs to be reviewed regularly to ensure that the trial is on track to reach its planned goal. If it is not on track, then this will allow the investigator to consider making changes to the study, such as expanding entry criteria or asking for an extension, or to consider terminating the study. Safety variables need to be considered on a routine basis also. While serious adverse events (SAE's) should be reported to IRB's and funding agencies (if appropriate) when they are detected, summaries of adverse events should be considered regularly to ensure that there are no unexpected or greater than expected risks to the patients. In addition to recruitment and safety, outcome measures should also be considered for inclusion in the interim monitoring plan when appropriate. At a minimum, these should include the primary outcome measure(s). In some instances, any major secondary outcomes that might influence any decisions based on the primary outcomes should be included. The inclusion of secondary outcome measures should be limited to the important ones to guard against chance findings.

The number of proposed looks at the variables during the course of the study, especially for the primary and any secondary outcome measures, needs to be presented in the monitoring plan also. While the recruitment and safety data can be routinely presented (e.g., every month), outcome data cannot be presented meaningfully until sufficient data has been collected. Then, since statistics would be calculated, a reasonable time frame between looks at the data needs to be determined to ensure that obtaining any meaningful results will not be delayed, but that too many looks at the data are not performed so that chance findings are obtained.

Who does the monitoring depends on the level of risks, phase of the trial, and whether the trial is multicenter or single center research. For single center studies, the monitoring may be (1) an appointed monitor, (2) a committee comprised of study investigators/personnel, (3) a standing DSMB (at some institutions), or (4) an independent board such as an independent study or central DSMB. Multicenter trials, especially if funded by NIH, Department of Veteran Affairs (VA) or other federal agencies will use an independent or central DSMB. These trial monitors will be in addition to the safety reviews of the local or central IRB's.

When an independent board, especially for multicenter trials, is used to monitor a trial, the board should be a multidisciplinary review team with appropriate medical, biostatistical, and bioethical expertise. At least one team member should have first-hand clinical experience with the treatments under study and be familiar with the nuances of the treatment protocol. No voting member can be dependent on funding from the trial or stand to gain or lose financially from the recommendations concerning the trial results. The primary responsibilities of the DSMB are (1) to periodically review and evaluate accumulated data for participant safety, study conduct, and progress, and when appropriate, efficacy and (2) to make recommendations concerning continuation, modification, or termination of the trial. This board should also (1) monitor performances of sites and adherence to protocol, (2) monitor data quality, completeness, and timeliness, (3) consider factors external to the study, such as scientific or therapeutic developments that might impact equipoise, participant safety or willingness to continue, and (4) review and approve proposed changes to the protocol or any sub-protocols.

The plans for interim monitoring should include a description of exactly what data will be presented and how the data will be presented to the monitors. Table templates should be presented in the study protocol appendices and/or the statistical analysis plan. The templates should indicate exactly how the data is proposed to be given including whether the results will be given by specifically identifying the treatment groups or by coding the treatment groups, such as Treatment A and Treatment B. Some monitors/DSMBs want to know actual groups, while others prefer to be blinded. While it is hoped that exactly what data will be presented for monitoring can be given in the original study protocol/research application, this is not always possible as monitors/DSMBs might want to see additional information when they first review the trial or, during the trial, issues may be raised that require additional information. Thus, these plans for monitoring need to be flexible.

Many phase III clinical trials and some smaller trials will conduct interim analyses of outcome measures over the course of the trial. These interim analyses have potential biostatistical drawbacks that need to be addressed in the interim monitoring plan. The p-value or significance level of 0.05 is based on a single look, which, in effect states, that for a single look, there is a 5 in 100 chance that the significant difference seen might be a chance occurrence and that there really is no difference between the treatment groups. If more than one look is taken, then the p-value will increase above 5%. For example, Fleming et al. [1] reported that if interim analyses were conducted every three months for three years, the probability of at least one those analyses achieving a p-value of 0.05 could be as high as 26%. Thus, there is a need to develop a plan at the beginning of the study to guard against reporting chance findings and stopping the study too early.

There are a number of statistical designs that can be used to plan for the interim analyses to guard against reporting chance findings [e.g., 2–6]. These methods vary but are based on the principle that the interval analyses are conducted at a reduced level of significance with the final test corrected according to these prior analyses. For example, Pocock's [2] method consists of having the planned numbers of looks all at the same p-value including the final look (e.g., 4 looks each with a p-value of 0.0125). For Peto's [3] method, the interval tests have a very low p-value (e.g., $p = 0.001$), which has very little impact on the significance level of the final test. The O'Brien-Fleming method [4] is intermediate to the first two methods in that the first test is run with a very low p-value, the second is run with a slightly higher p-value, etc., until the final test, which has a p-value that is reduced by the amount of the previous p-values. Other methods [5, 6] use flexible levels of significance making it possible to use the amount of the p-value available for the final look and to vary the number of looks, for example, if the study is extended.

It is important to note that each of the methods discussed above, as well as others not discussed, will have their advantages and disadvantages. For instance, Pocock's method may discover important events sooner but could miss an overall significant result at the end such as a p-value < 0.05 but greater than 0.0125 for four looks. Also, the number of looks is fixed at the beginning. For Peto's method, important differences could be missed until the end due to the small p-value at interim looks. The O'Brien-Fleming method might delay finding an important difference and would miss declaring a significant difference at the end if a p-value is just under 0.05. It also requires a fixed number of looks. Some of the methods with flexible levels of significance such as Lan-DeMets [5] can have a flexible number of looks due to the small p-values at the interim looks, but they could also delay finding important differences until the end.

In addition to doing interim analyses to determine how a study is doing in achieving its primary purpose, it may also be necessary when reviewing outcome data, especially the primary outcome, to conduct futility analyses to determine whether it is worth continuing the study from both the point of view of patient safety and the use of valuable resources. For example, if in a study comparing an active drug to a placebo, the placebo was doing substantially better, a futility analysis would provide valuable information concerning the likelihood that the active drug could possibly do better by the projected end of the study. Conditional probability is one method of testing this [7].

When conducting interim monitoring during the course of a clinical trial, it is important that there is timely collection of the data and that the data is submitted for report generation in a timely fashion. This will ensure that the reports generated for monitoring will contain the latest data. It is also important that there is regular generation and review of the reports to ensure that the issues concerning the study are detected as soon as possible. It is also important that these interim reports are not made available to the study investigators or sponsors, especially any efficacy data. Knowing these interim data could (1) change accrual patterns as investigators might begin to limit the types of patients they enter because of these results, (2) cause biased consideration of changes in analytical approaches after one or more interim analyses have been conducted, and (3) cause early study termination that might not permit the study question to be answered conclusively.

When conducting interim monitoring, there is an ethical dilemma faced by the monitors or DSMBs. These are the individual ethics concerning the needs of the next eligible study participant. You never want to randomize a participant to an established inferior treatment. On the other hand, there are the collective ethics concerning the correct policy for future patients. There needs to be sufficient evidence to change clinical practice for the better and to keep future patients from being denied the superior treatment. Failure to achieve a clear convincing result could be unethical as could be enrolling study patients in an inferior treatment unnecessarily. Monitors/DSMBs need to balance these two concerns when reviewing interim reports.

The following are examples of the importance of interim monitoring and the need for having a monitor/DSMB to review study progress. The first study was a VA Cooperative Study entitled "Oxandrolone for Healing Pressure Ulcers in Spinal Cord Injured Patients" [8]. This was planned as a 400 subject, parallel-group, placebo-controlled multisite randomized trial to determine whether oxandrolone increases the percentage of healed target pressure ulcers within 24 weeks compared to placebo. The DSMB had requested that they be blinded to the treatment groups. After 164 patients had full data, the results were, Drug A had a healing rate of 25% and Drug B a rate of 31%. The DSMB was ok with continuing the study if Drug A was placebo and Drug B was oxandrolone but if the reverse was true, they wanted a futility analysis performed. The reverse was true and a futility analysis was performed. This analysis indicated that for the remaining 236 patients to be recruited, the active drug would need to increase from the current 25% healing to over 50%, to achieve the originally estimated 40% healing and the placebo group would need to drop from its current 31% healing rate to 20% to achieve the originally estimated 25%. The conditional probability {7} of this occurring was $p = 0.000005$. The DSMB recommended terminating the study and the study was terminated within 2 months. Thus, the result of this study's interim monitoring was that subjects were not treated with a drug that was of no benefit to them and the VA saved valuable resources.

The second study is also a VA Cooperative Study and indicates the importance of monitoring recruitment, safety, and not stopping a study early. A Comparison of Four Treatments for Generalized Convulsive Status Epilepticus [9] was a randomized, multicenter, double-blind clinical trial testing four intravenous drug regimens (lorazepam, phenobarbital, phenytoin, diazepam followed by phenytoin) to treat two types of generalized convulsive status epilepticus: overt and subtle. During the course of the study, two problems emerged that needed to be addressed: poor recruitment and unexpected 30-day mortality differences between treatment groups [10]. The study's DSMB met yearly with reports given in between. The recruitment issue was noted at the first yearly meeting with 78 patients entered and 305 expected (25.6% of expected). The DSMB recommended (1) where possible, recruit from universities affiliated with the VA Medical Center, (2) the Study Chair visit each participating site, and (3) replace poor performing sites. At the second annual meeting, recruitment had only improved marginally to 30% of expected. Study leadership submitted a plan to increase the recruitment period from 3 to 5 years and to reduce sample size in the overt status arm from 512 to 436 and in the subtle status arm from 640 to 348. The DSMB agreed to the plan contingent on eliminating nonproductive sites. Four sites were immediately terminated and one was placed on probation. With the DSMB's recommendation, VA Central Office approved the plan. By the third annual meeting, the overt status arm was basically on target to achieve the new sample size, but the subtle status arm was still badly lagging. The DSMB recommended to continue both study arms because, since recruitment relied on subjects being referred for this emergency condition, they were afraid the referrals to the overt status arm might be reduced if the study started rejecting the subtle status patients. They also believed that some useful information could still be obtained for subtle status patients. At the end of 5 years, 395 overt status patients (91% of expected) and 175 subtle status patients (50% of expected) were recruited. Thus, monitoring recruitment helped this study to be successful.

The second issue raised in the monitoring of this study was a safety issue. At the second yearly meeting, it was seen that one of the study drugs had a much higher 30-day mortality rate than the other drugs (34.2% vs. 15.8, 17.1, and 27.6%). While the differences were not statistically significant ($p = 0.193$ overall), the fact that it was the death variable and one drug had a doubling of deaths over two of the other drugs raised serious concerns. Since the difference was not statistically significant, the DSMB decided to continue the study but wanted increased monitoring and wanted to see monthly death reports. These monthly reports continued to show large differences between the drugs with the significance level dropping to $p = 0.056$. Also, instead of one drug having a doubling of deaths over the others, there were now two drugs doubling the deaths over the other two drugs and these two drugs were of the same class, diazepam, and lorazepam. While the doubling of deaths continued for a 10-month period, the DSMB, after the first couple of months, requested analyses comparing the treatment groups on demographics, primary and secondary causes of death, the use of Do Not Resuscitate (DNR) orders, and times of death to explore potential causes of the imbalances in deaths. These analyses indicated that patients on one drug with a high death rate were 4–6 years older than patients on the other three drugs, that patients on the other drug with a high-death rate had more preexisting medical conditions than either of the two drug group patients with the lower death rates, and that patients on the two drugs with the higher death rates had more DNR orders than the other two groups. These findings convinced the DSMB to continue with the study even with the lowering significance values. After reaching the low p-value of 0.056 at 10 months of observation, things started to improve to the point that at the end of the study, the p-value for 30-day mortality was 0.862 with death rates of 23.9, 27.0, 29.3, and 27.9%. Also, what was seen was that the differences found when looking for potential causes of deaths also disappeared over time. Thus, while the monitoring for safety found a potential major problem, working with the DSMB to explore the reasons for the cause of the increased deaths in two of the drug groups, allowed the study to continue and to be completed successfully.

A third trial where the DSMB faced a difficult decision at one of its interim reviews was a surgical VA study comparing open Chevrel and laparoscopic repair of ventral incisional hernia [11]. The primary outcome for this trial was the complication rate 8 weeks after surgery and the target sample size of 310 was determined to provide 80% power to detect a difference of 32% versus 17% in the primary outcome. The study faced considerable recruitment challenges and the DSMB was asked to consider an unfunded extension of recruitment. At the time funding ended, 162 patients had been randomized into the trial. The DSMB asked to review the primary outcome and determined that a statistically significant difference was evident (laparoscopic repair [31.5%], open repair [47.9%], $p = 0.03$). Typically, a DSMB would want to see at least two consecutive looks at the data to determine whether the difference observed would remain after additional patients were recruited. However, that would have required approving the unfunded extension. In order to assess whether this observed difference was reliable, the DSMB requested additional analyses. The DSMB voted not to extend the recruitment period because the statistically significant difference in the primary outcome measure showed consistency by calendar time in the study and across the four study sites. While it is possible that that the results could have changed if the study was allowed to continue, it is likely that the DSMB review at this interim monitoring visit saved VA resources and prevented the additional participants from being exposed to an inferior treatment.

In summary, interim monitoring is an important tool for the conduct of clinical trials. It ensures patient safety and that study progress and conduct are appropriate, and it allows the study early determination of efficacy/effectiveness. An essential component of interim monitoring is the use of independent monitors or DSMBs. Monitors and DSMBs can provide investigators with appropriate advice on conducting the study and help them with any ethical concerns such as individual verses collective ethics that may arise. Interim monitoring plans should be included in study proposals and/or statistical analysis plans.

References

1. Fleming TR, Green SJ, Harrington DP. Considerations for monitoring and evaluating effects in clinical trials. Control Clin Trials. 1984;5:55–66.
2. Pocock SJ. Interim analyses for randomized clinical trials: the group sequential approach. Biometrics. 1982;38:153–62.
3. Peto R, Pike MC, Armitase P, et al. Design and analysis of randomized clinical trials requiring prolonged observation of each patient. I. Introduction and design. Br J Cancer. 1976;34:585–612.
4. O'Brien PC, Fleming TR. A multiple testing procedure for clinical trials. Biometrics. 1979;35:549–56.
5. Lan KKG, Demets DL. Discrete sequential boundaries for clinical trials. Biometrika. 1983;70:659–63.
6. Kim K, DeMets DL. Designs and analysis of group sequential tests based on Type I error spending rate Function. Biometrika. 1987;74:149–54.
7. Lan KK, Wittes J. The B-value: a tool for monitoring Data. Biometrics. 1988;44:579–85.
8. Bauman WA, Spungen AM, Collins JF, Raisch DW, Ho C, Dietrick GA, et al. The effect of oxandrolone on the healing of chronic pressure ulcers in persons with spinal cord injury. Ann Int Med. 2013;158:718–26.
9. Treiman DM, Meyers PD, Walton NY, Collins JF, Colling C, Rowan J, et al. A comparison of four treatments for generalized convulsive status epilepticus. NEJM. 1998;339:792–8.

10. Collins JF. Data and safety monitoring board issues raised in the VA status epilepticus study. Control Clin Trials. 2003;24: 71–7.
11. Itani KMF, Hur K, Kim LT, et al. Comparison of laparoscopic and open repair with mesh for the treatment of ventral incisional hernia. Arch Surg. 2010;145:322–8.

Part IV
Ethical Considerations

Chapter 21
Ethical Considerations in Clinical Trials

Jennifer Tseng and Peter Angelos

Clinical trials are crucial to answering important questions in surgery, but they do raise ethical issues. After the historical atrocities of the experiments conducted by Nazi physician researchers on prisoners in concentration camps during World War II, the current standards of ethical conduct are based on protecting human subjects. Several key issues arise when determining the ethicality of human experimentation. When does medical practice cross the line to biomedical research? When do risks outweigh the benefits? What constitutes informed consent in clinical research?

The Nuremberg Code, Declaration of Helsinki, Belmont Report, and the International Ethical Guidelines for Biomedical Research Involving Human Subjects form the present basis for ethical conduct of clinical research. The Nuremberg Code of 1947, considered to be the first time it was outlined that human experimentation should be rooted in informed consent, emphasized the need for consent and favorable risk–benefit ratio [1]. The Declaration of Helsinki highlighted the necessity of independent review, distinguishing between therapeutic and nontherapeutic research [2]. The Belmont Report was written to protect vulnerable populations after the Tuskegee and Willowbrook scandals [3–6]. Beauchamp and Childress proposed four classic principles of biomedical ethics: autonomy, nonmaleficence, beneficence, and justice [7]. Nonmaleficence is defined as inflicting the least harm possible to reach a beneficial result. Beneficence requires researchers keep the welfare of the human participant as the ultimate overall goal of the

J. Tseng (✉) · P. Angelos
Department of Surgery, The University of Chicago Medicine,
5841 S. Maryland Avenue, Chicago, IL 60637, USA
e-mail: jennifer.tseng@uchospitals.edu

P. Angelos
e-mail: pangelos@surgery.bsd.uchicago.edu

© Springer International Publishing AG 2017   199
K.M.F. Itani and D.J. Reda (eds.), *Clinical Trials Design in Operative and Non Operative Invasive Procedures*, DOI 10.1007/978-3-319-53877-8_21

experimentation. In his research, David Resnik proposed four slightly different "standards" or ethical principles for biomedical research [8]. The four ideals include truth telling or veracity, dialogue or free exchange, caution or prudence, and social responsibility or civic duty.

Truth telling is vital in research as scientists have a moral obligation to report accurate results and avoid all fabrication, falsification, and plagiarism of data [9]. Fabrication is the creation of data in the absence of experimental results. One of the more notorious cases of research fabrication was William T. Summerlin's misrepresentation of results relating to immunological rejection of transplanted tissues in a mouse model in 1974. This scandal highlighted some of the pressures clinical researchers face to publicize positive results [10]. Falsification relates to the manipulation or misrepresentation of experimental results and can occur during data collection, statistical analysis, or with omission of contradictory findings [9]. Plagiarism is defined as taking credit for another researcher's work. This includes taking ideas, methods, and techniques or not attributing appropriate credit for previous work. Dishonesty erodes confidence in research findings among the scientific community and the public at large. Unfortunately, scientific dishonesty can be ambiguous and difficult to prove.

Ideally, the scientific community promotes free exchange of ideas through the peer review process. However, researchers often compete for the same funding resources, academic promotions, and prestige that may lead to secrecy of ideas and techniques. Open dialogue promotes sharing of information, methods and data allowing for more efficient use of resources and potentially faster achievement of research objectives [9].

Caution or prudence is crucial to minimize errors. Errors can be categorized as practical errors (mistakes made by people using instruments, performing calculations, or recording data) or theoretical errors (bias in analysis). Resnik proposed informal rules of scientific methodology, including use of controlled experiments, repeating experiments to confirm findings, use of reliable instrumentation, necessity of using instrumentation correctly and reliably, careful recording and duplication of data records and regular engagement in informal peer review of experimental design and data interpretation [8]. Clinical researchers have a social responsibility to behave humanely and utilize scarce resources in a judicious manner when designing and performing experiments. In addition, they should strive to minimize harm and ensure the social utility and benefit of their research [9].

Building on Resnik's work, Emanuel et al. subsequently defined seven ethical requirements for clinical research. These requirements include social or scientific value, scientific validity, fair subject selection, favorable risk–benefit ratio, independent review, informed consent, and respect for potential and enrolled subjects. These requirements draw from the ethical principles of scarce resources and non-exploitation, justice, nonmaleficence, public accountability, and respect for subject autonomy (Table 21.1) [11].

In designing clinical trials, evaluating operative and nonoperative procedures, certain ethical issues arise. There is an ongoing ethical debate regarding "sham surgery." Beecher published the first paper on surgery as placebo in 1961 [12]. Since

Table 21.1 Seven requirements for determining whether a research trial is ethical

Requirement	Explanation	Justifying ethical values	Expertise for evaluation
Social or scientific value	Evaluation of a treatment, intervention, or theory that will improve health and well-being or increase knowledge	Scarce resources and nonexploitation	Scientific knowledge; citizen's understanding of social priorities
Scientific validity	Use of accepted scientific principles and methods, including statistical techniques, to produce reliable and valid data	Scarce resources and nonexploitation	Scientific and statistical knowledge; knowledge of condition and population to assess feasibility
Fair subject selection	Selection of subjects so that stigmatized and vulnerable individuals are not targeted for risky research and the rich and socially powerful not favored for potentially beneficial research	Justice	Scientific knowledge; ethical and legal knowledge
Favorable risk-benefit ratio	Minimization of risks; enhancement of potential benefits; risks to the subject are proportionate to the benefits to the subject and society	Nonmaleficence, beneficence, and nonexploitation	Scientific knowledge; citizen's understanding of social values
Independent review	Review of the design of the research trial, its proposed subject population, and risk-benefit ratio by individuals unaffiliated with the research	Public accountability; minimizing influence of potential conflicts of interest	Intellectual, financial and otherwise independent researchers; scientific and ethical knowledge
Informed consent	Provision of information to subjects about purpose of the research, its procedures, potential risks, benefits, and alternatives, so that the individual understands this information and can make a voluntary decision whether to enroll and continue to participate	Respect for subject autonomy	Scientific knowledge; ethical and legal knowledge
Respect of potential and enrolled subjects	Respect for subjects by 1. Permitting withdrawal form the research 2. Protecting privacy through confidentiality 3. Informing subjects of newly discovered risks/benefits 4. Informing subjects of results of clinical research 5. Maintaining welfare of subjects	Respect for subject autonomy and welfare	Scientific knowledge; ethical and legal knowledge; knowledge of particular subject population

Based on data from Ref. [11]

Table 21.2 Placebo-controlled trials

The research design addresses a valuable, clinically relevant question
The placebo control is methodologically necessary
The risk of placebo is minimized, does not exceed acceptable research risk and is justified by clinical knowledge to be gained
Deception used to blind the placebo arm is disclosed to and authorized by participants
There is an ability to cross over to the active intervention arm

Based on data from Refs. [16, 17]

that time, patients have infrequently been placed under anesthesia and had surgical incisions created for the placebo arms of surgical trials [13, 14]. Opponents argue that unlike a placebo medication (or sugar pill) that has no risk associated with it, research participants are necessarily put at some risk in a sham surgery trial, violating the principle of nonmaleficence. Conversely, those in favor of placebo-controlled surgical trials cite the existence of the placebo effect and thus the necessity of these trials to determine the true efficacy of treatment [15]. Proponents argue that in the realm of clinical research, there is no requirement to offer participants direct benefit. Participants in the placebo arm may actually be exposed to less risk, as they would not encounter the potentially adverse effects of the intervention.

Sham surgery mandates thorough informed consent. Researchers should be cautious of enrolling patients who do not have decision-making capacity. Placebo-controlled trials should optimally minimize risk, be justified in forwarding clinical knowledge, and fully disclose the deception used to blind the placebo arm (Table 21.2) [16, 17]. The research must be peer-reviewed to determine that the question being asked is important to clinical medicine and that the knowledge gained justifies a placebo arm to determine the true benefit of the intervention. The placebo arm should be disclosed to offer no direct therapeutic benefit and its risks should be minimized and not be considered unduly excessive. There may be a role for pre-research consultation with patient groups in potentially controversial clinical trials to ameliorate concerns and optimize patient educational materials. If possible, agreement should be sought in advance for the participation of non-surgeon clinicians (i.e., anesthesiologists) and support staff who will necessarily be participating in the research [15, 18, 19].

References

1. Nuremberg Military T. The Nuremberg code. JAMA. 1996;276(20):1691. PubMed PMID: 11644854.
2. World Medical Association declaration of Helsinki. Recommendations guiding physicians in biomedical research involving human subjects. JAMA. 1997;277(11):925–6.
3. United States. National Commission for the Protection of Human Subjects of Biomedical and Behavioral Research. The Belmont report: ethical principles and guidelines for the protection

of human subjects of research. Bethesda, Md. Washington: The Commission; for sale by the Supt. of Docs., U.S. Govt. Print. Off.;1978. 20 p.

4. Jones JH, Tuskegee Institute. Bad blood: the Tuskegee syphilis experiment. New York London: Free Press; Collier Macmillan Publishers; 1981. xii, 272 p., 8 leaves of plates p.

5. Rothman DJ, Rothman SM. The Willowbrook wars. 1st ed. New York: Harper & Row; 1984. viii, 405 p.

6. Krugman S. The Willowbrook hepatitis studies revisited: ethical aspects. Rev Infect Dis. 1986;8(1):157–62.

7. Beauchamp TL, Childress JF. Principles of biomedical ethics. 3rd ed. New York: Oxford University Press; 1989. x, 470 p.

8. Resnik DB. The ethics of science: an introduction. London; New York: Routledge; 1998. ix, 221 p.

9. Souba WW, Wilmore DW. Surgical research. San Diego, CA: Academic Press; 2001. xxxii, 1460 p.

10. Hixson JR. The patchwork mouse. 1st ed. Garden City, N.Y.: Anchor Press; 1976. x, 228 p.

11. Emanuel EJ, Wendler D, Grady C. What makes clinical research ethical? JAMA. 2000;283 (20):2701–11.

12. Hk B. Surgery as placebo: a quantitative study of bias. JAMA. 1961;176(13):1102–7.

13. Moseley JB, O'Malley K, Petersen NJ, Menke TJ, Brody BA, Kuykendall DH, Hollingsworth JC, Ashton CM, Wray NP. A controlled trial of arthroscopic surgery for osteoarthritis of the knee. N Engl J Med. 2002;347(2):81–8. doi:10.1056/NEJMoa013259.

14. Freeman TB, Vawter DE, Leaverton PE, Godbold JH, Hauser RA, Goetz CG, Olanow CW. Use of placebo surgery in controlled trials of a cellular-based therapy for Parkinson's disease. N Engl J Med. 1999;341(13):988–92. doi:10.1056/NEJM199909233411311.

15. Rogers W, Hutchison K, Skea ZC, Campbell MK. Strengthening the ethical assessment of placebo-controlled surgical trials: three proposals. BMC Med Ethics. 2014;15:78. doi:10. 1186/1472-6939-15-78. PubMed PMID: 25341496; PMCID: PMC4223753.

16. Horng S, Miller FG. Ethical framework for the use of sham procedures in clinical trials. Crit Care Med. 2003;31(3 Suppl):S126–30. doi:10.1097/01.CCM.0000054906.49187.67.

17. Horng SH, Miller FG. Placebo-controlled procedural trials for neurological conditions. Neurotherapeutics. 2007;4(3):531–6. doi:10.1016/j.nurt.2007.03.001. PubMed PMID: 17599718; PMCID: PMC2043150.

18. Marsden J, Bradburn J, Consumers' Advisory Group for Clinical T, Lynda Jackson Macmillan C. Patient and clinician collaboration in the design of a national randomized breast cancer trial. Health Expect. 2004;7(1):6–17. doi:10.1111/j.1369-7625.2004.00232.x. PubMed PMID: 14982495.

19. Koops L, Lindley RI. Thrombolysis for acute ischaemic stroke: consumer involvement in design of new randomised controlled trial. BMJ. 2002;325(7361):415. PubMed PMID: 12193356; PMCID: PMC119434.

Chapter 22
IRB and Review Process for Multisite Trials

Jennifer Tseng and Peter Angelos

The Common Rule is a federal policy regarding human subjects protection and dictates requirements for institutional review boards (IRB) membership, function, operations, review of research, and record keeping. IRBs are traditionally local bodies made up of peers at a medical institution. They play a legally mandated role in reviewing both the scientific validity and ethical basis of clinical research. Researchers must adhere to certain minimum requirements for conduct of human research (Table 22.1) [1, 2]. IRBs review the design and protocol of the study, the informed consent for participation in the study, and monitor the conduct of the research throughout the trial period. Investigators must ethically and legally report adverse events to the IRB. The IRB evaluates the extent of conflicts of interest and whether potential bias precludes the researcher from continuing the research. The IRB creates local research policy and determines standards for review of human subjects research as well as dealing with violations of institutional policies and conflicts of interest [1]. Independent review allows for social accountability. As clinical research poses risks to subjects, the IRB ensures ethical treatment for human subjects across various participating sites [3].

Despite the fact that IRBs have traditionally been at local institutions, the National Institutes of Health has promoted the use of a single IRB for large, multisite clinical trials since late 2014. As there is no evidence that multiple IRB reviews enhance human subject protection, a single IRB is thought to potentially increase protections by "eliminating the problem of distributed accountability [and] minimizing institutional conflicts of interest." [4]. However, concerns have been raised about the different definitions of "minimal risk" in ethical guidelines across

J. Tseng (✉) · P. Angelos
Department of Surgery, The University of Chicago Medicine,
5841 S. Maryland Avenue, Chicago, IL 60637, USA
e-mail: jennifer.tseng@uchospitals.edu

P. Angelos
e-mail: pangelos@surgery.bsd.uchicago.edu

© Springer International Publishing AG 2017   205
K.M.F. Itani and D.J. Reda (eds.), *Clinical Trials Design in Operative
and Non Operative Invasive Procedures*, DOI 10.1007/978-3-319-53877-8_22

Table 22.1 Minimum requirements for the conduct of human research

Study design and implementation
The research must be expected to yield significant benefits of the individual patient or society
The risk of research must be proportional to the expected benefit
The question addressed must justify the risk posed to participants
The study must be well designed
The planned experimental procedures must have been previously tested in animal models
The investigations must be conducted honestly
Rights of human subjects
Informed consent
Ability to deny or quit treatment
Privacy and confidentiality
Anonymity

Based on data from Refs. [1, 2]

institutions [5]. Therefore, even though the research community is striving to standardize the oversight of clinical trials, continued vigilance is warranted in protecting vulnerable populations at an individual institutional level in the midst of centralization.

With the emergence of global health foundations and the multinational presence of pharmaceutical companies, there are now additional international challenges with multisite clinical trials. There is concern that developing countries might be exploited by higher resourced countries. Definitions of autonomy and informed consent certainly vary across countries due to different cultural and societal factors. It is challenging to know what standard to apply when a trial spans several different countries. Language barriers between researchers and subjects create additional concerns. Participants may be less likely to ask questions of an interpreter seen to be in a higher position of power [6]. One must consider whether research subjects who are also patients are truly free to choose to participate in clinical trials when access to medications or procedures may be tied to research [7]. There may also be explicit or implicit pressure not to reject research protocols that may lead industry sponsors to take their studies elsewhere [8].

Proposals to address these issues include having a dedicated pre-research initiation ethics review incorporated in study protocols. This would allow investigators to specifically identify perceived ethical concerns (i.e., communications, conflicts of interest, cultural differences) for a study in advance in each location proposed as a site [9]. Research disclosures and results should be relayed to participants in their language to ensure transparency. Potential members of the IRB should be drawn from professionals from the various geographies included in the research. However, even research ethics committees based in participating site countries may face limitations relating to insufficient ethical training and expertise or conflicts of interest related to colleagues or institutional support, similar to within the United States [10]. Ongoing educational efforts and reviews are especially critical to ensuring ethical propriety in multisite, multinational clinical trials.

References

1. Souba WW, Wilmore DW, Buchman TG. Surgical research. San Diego, Calif.: Academic Press; 2001. xxxii, 1460 p., [16] p. of col. plates p.
2. Sharrott GW. Ethics of clinical research. Am J Occup Ther. 1985;39(6):407–8.
3. Emanuel EJ, Wendler D, Grady C. What makes clinical research ethical? JAMA. 2000;283 (20):2701–11.
4. Request for Comments on the Draft NIH Policy on the Use of a Single Institutional Review Board for Multi-Site Research. National Institutes of Health (NIH). December 2014. http://grants.nih.gov/grants/guide/notice-files/NOT-OD-15-026.html.
5. Caulfield T, Ries NM, Barr G. Variation in ethics review of multi-site research initiatives. Amsterdam Law Forum. 2011.
6. Loue S, Pike EC. Case studies in ethics and HIV research. New York, NY: Springer; 2007. Available from: doi:10.1007/978-0-387-71362-5.
7. Li R, Barnes M, Aldinger CE, Bierer BE. Global clinical trials: ethics, harmonization ad commitments to transparency. Harvard Public Health Review. 2015;5.
8. Coleman CH, Bouesseau MC. How do we know that research ethics committees are really working? The neglected role of outcomes assessment in research ethics review. BMC Med Ethics. 2008;9:6. doi:10.1186/1472-6939-9-6. PubMed PMID: 18373857; PMCID: PMC2324094.
9. MRCT Workshop Meeting Summary "Ethics Committee Panel (A. Davis)" Nov 20, 2011.
10. Ellenberg SS FT, Demets DL. Data monitoring committees in clinical trials: a practical perspective. USA: Wiley. 2003.

Chapter 23
Trial Advertising

Jennifer Tseng and Peter Angelos

The U.S. Food and Drug Administration (FDA) defines direct advertising to research subjects as the use of newspaper, radio, TV, bulletin boards, posters, and flyers to solicit study participants. Not included are communications to health professionals, news stories or publicity intended toward other audiences (i.e., potential investors). The FDA considers direct advertising "to be the start of the informed consent and subject selection process" [1]. Advertisements are not the only source of patient information, but they are the first and sometimes lasting impression of clinical trials to participants. If the advertisement emphasizes the material rewards over the health risks, the clinical trial's possible adverse events may be downplayed in the subject's mind [2]. Thus, as an extra safety aspect, advertisements should be reviewed and approved by the appropriate institutional review board (IRB). The FDA expects the IRB to ensure truth in advertising and to ensure that there is no coercion of research participants [1].

Advertising deemed to be misleading by the FDA includes claims, "either explicitly or implicitly, that the drug, biologic or device is safe or effective for the purposes under investigation" or that "the test article is known to be equivalent or superior to any other drug, biologic or device." Moreover, advertising is prohibited from employing the term "new" as this implies "newly improved products of proven worth" [1].

Despite these cautionary notes, a recent study of Internet advertisements found that a significant percentage of Internet advertisements were ethically troubling in terms of wording or publication displays. Internet marketing uses web sites devoted to clinical trials, clinical trial databases, and direct email solicitation [3]. Use of

J. Tseng (✉) · P. Angelos
Department of Surgery, The University of Chicago Medicine,
5841 S. Maryland Avenue, Chicago, IL 60637, USA
e-mail: jennifer.tseng@uchospitals.edu

P. Angelos
e-mail: pangelos@surgery.bsd.uchicago.edu

© Springer International Publishing AG 2017
K.M.F. Itani and D.J. Reda (eds.), *Clinical Trials Design in Operative and Non Operative Invasive Procedures*, DOI 10.1007/978-3-319-53877-8_23

variations in typography has been shown to be coercive [4]. The words "free," "no charge," or "no cost" were used as enticements and there was no mention of adverse effects or compensatory response to injuries. Potential solutions may entail a standardized model for advertising as proposed by the World Health Organization, avoiding vagueness and preventing emphasis on remuneration [3, 5].

References

1. Dickert N, Grady C. What's the price of a research subject? Approaches to payment for research participation. N Engl J Med. 1999;341(3):198–203. doi:10.1056/NEJM199907153410312.
2. Phillips TB. Money, advertising and seduction in human subjects research. Am J Bioeth. 2007;7(2):88–90. doi:10.1080/15265160701307621.
3. Bramstedt KA. Recruiting healthy volunteers for research participation via internet advertising. Clin Med Res. 2007;5(2):91–7. doi:10.3121/cmr.2007.718. PubMed PMID: 17607043; PMCID: PMC1905931.
4. Childers TLJJ. All dressed up with something to say: effects of typeface semantic associations on brand perceptions and consumer memory. J Consum Psych. 2002;12:93–106.
5. Clinical Trials Advertising Toolkit. Wake Forest Baptist Health. January 2015. http://www.wakehealth.edu/uploadedFiles/User_Content/AboutUs/Contact_Us/Departments/Creative_Communications/Brand_Center/Downloads/Advertising_Toolkit.pdf.

Chapter 24
Payment to Research Participants

Jennifer Tseng and Peter Angelos

Payments to research subjects help alleviate the cost of time and resources for participation. Payments can come in the form of money, gifts, free medical care, or travel reimbursement. Compensation can have positive effects. Compensation has been shown to increase survey response rates and willingness to participate [1]. The United States has a longstanding tradition of paying human subjects, with famous surgeons such as William Beaumont in the 1800s and Walter Reed in the early 20th century providing monetary compensation to study their subjects [2]. The National Institutes of Health has regularly paid "normal" healthy volunteers for participation since the 1950s.

The U.S. Food and Drug Administration permits advertisements of payment to subject participants, however payments and the amount must not to be emphasized (such as with larger or bold type) [3]. The Council of Organizations for Medical Sciences advises that payments not be so significant that volunteers "take undue risks," as this violates free choice [4]. A distinction needs to be made between coercion and inducement. Coercion is an extreme influence controlling a person's decision violating autonomy and is hence inherently unethical. An inducement is a motivating factor that is not inherently coercive but can become so in certain negative circumstances; thus, an inducement is not necessarily unethical. The distinction also depends on the socioeconomic status of the subject, as one person's undue inducement may hardly solicit the interest of someone with higher means. Macklin attempted to clarify the ethical ambiguity of the term inducement by

J. Tseng (✉) · P. Angelos
Department of Surgery, The University of Chicago Medicine,
5841 S. Maryland Avenue, Chicago, IL 60637, USA
e-mail: jennifer.tseng@uchospitals.edu

© Springer International Publishing AG 2017
K.M.F. Itani and D.J. Reda (eds.), *Clinical Trials Design in Operative and Non Operative Invasive Procedures*, DOI 10.1007/978-3-319-53877-8_24

separating it into two different types: due versus undue inducement. Due induce-ments are usually based on an established, reasonable fee-for-service schedule, often at minimum hourly wage with additional small compensation amounts for providing laboratory samples or to participate in a more unpopular study. Undue inducements cause subjects to lie, deceive, or conceal [5]. An example of undue inducement would be monetary recompense far exceeding a wage the subject would earn with other gainful employment. Emanuel highlighted four key features of undue inducements: that they produce a positive good, are irresistible, produce bad judgment or they cause an action causing substantial risk of serious harm [6].

Several concerns arise when considering payments to research participants. Participants may conceal information for concern of possible disqualification from the study. Some argue against all inducements that expose patients to risks under concern that they lead to inequity in the research process [7]. A skewed sample may occur when money attracts lower income individuals [8]. Furthermore, payments for research involving children should be approached with extra caution. Payments may alleviate the cost and inconvenience of allowing children to participate in research, but they may also sway parental decision-making [1].

Dickert and Grady proposed three models for payment. The market model is based on the economic model of supply and demand, with payment justified by the need to pay subjects for recruitment. The wage payment model is based on standard wage payment for unskilled labor, compensating for time and effort. The reim-bursement model provides compensation for expenses incurred and lost wages, but is problematic in leading to unequal payments of subjects depending on their income. The wage payment model is the most ethically favorable option as it reduces undue inducement and standardizes payment [3].

In keeping with the ethical principle of nonmaleficence–that is, to avoid harming others–if harm comes to research subjects due to their participation in a clinical trial, the International Ethical Guidelines for Biomedical Research Involving Human Subjects recommends "free medical treatment for such injury" and com-pensation for any disability. In case of death, the research participant's dependents are ethically entitled to compensation. Research subjects should not be asked to waive their right to compensation. Whether the pharmaceutical company, organi-zation, institution, government, or investigator is liable for these costs should be determined when designing the study [4]. However, these are ethical rather than legal mandates [9]. In 2012, only 16% of academic medical centers in the United States compensated research participants injuries, and none did so for lost wages or suffering [10]. Personal health insurance still remains the main source of com-pensation in the event of injury. Although other countries, the NIH Clinical Center, and the University of Washington have transitioned to "no fault" schemes of payment for injured subjects, the vast majority of medical centers are still laying the burden of compensation on the individual researcher [11]. It is incumbent on every researcher to be fully aware of the compensation plan at his or her institution and research subjects must be fully informed of what options for compensation will be available in the event of a research-related injury.

References

1. Bentley JP, Thacker PG. The influence of risk and monetary payment on the research participation decision making process. J Med Ethics. 2004;30(3):293–298. PubMed PMID: 15173366; PMCID: PMC1733848.
2. Lederer SE. Subjected to science: human experimentation in America before the Second World War. Baltimore: Johns Hopkins University Press; 1995. xvi, 192 pp.
3. Dickert N, Grady C. What's the price of a research subject? Approaches to payment for research participation. N Engl J Med. 1999;341(3):198–203. doi:10.1056/NEJM199907153 410312.
4. Council for International Organizations of Medical. S. International ethical guidelines for biomedical research involving human subjects. Bull Med Ethics. 2002;182:17–23.
5. Macklin R. On paying money to research subjects: 'due' and 'undue' inducements. IRB. 1981;3(5):1–6.
6. Emanuel EJ. Ending concerns about undue inducement. J Law Med Ethics. 2004;32(1): 100–5.
7. McNeill P. Paying people to participate in research: why not? A response to Wilkinson and Moore. Bioethics. 1997;11(5):390–6.
8. Wilkinson M, Moore A. Inducement in research. Bioethics. 1997;11(5):373–89.
9. Pike ER. Recovering from research: a no-fault proposal to compensate injured research participants. Am J Law Med. 2012;38(1):7–62.
10. Group TL. Task Order Proposal No. 2: care/compensation for injures in clinical research. Draft of the final report prepared for the Department of Health and Human Services Office of the Assistant Secretary for Planning and Evaluation. Falls Church, VA: The Lewin Group. May 18, 2005.
11. Elliott C. Justice for injured research subjects. N Engl J Med. 2012;367(1):6–8. doi:10.1056/NEJMp1205623.

Chapter 25
Conflict of Interest

Jennifer Tseng and Peter Angelos

A conflict of interest is a source of bias. Conflicts of interest have been defined as "a set of conditions in which professional judgment concerning a primary interest tends to be unduly influenced by a secondary interest" [1]. They erode public trust in the medical researcher. The most commonly perceived conflict of interest pertains to financial support for the researcher. NIH funding has declined recently in support of clinical trials, and as a result, clinical trials are increasingly launched and supported by pharmaceutical companies. The physician or researcher thus gains monetarily by being an investigator on a drug trial [2]. Presentations and publications require declaration of industry financial backing for transparency regarding these conflicts of interest. In some extreme cases, study sponsors have tried to change results or stop publication [3, 4]. In academic settings, promotion and ambition toward tenure and professional standing can be just as influential as monetary support.

The dual role of physician–scientist may create conflicts as the physician's duty as a healer sometimes contradicts the scientist's role as a researcher. Conflicts of interest are not inherently unethical but the physician–scientist's actions can cause concerns [2]. The Association of American Medical Colleges (AAMC) released guidelines to help ameliorate these conflicts of interest: full disclosure, aggressive monitoring and misconduct management [5]. Full disclosure applies to both individual and family financial and professional interests. Institutional review boards (IRBs) play a key role in research monitoring and determining if and to what extent conflicts of interest exist.

J. Tseng (✉) · P. Angelos
Department of Surgery, The University of Chicago Medicine,
5841 S. Maryland Avenue, 60637 Chicago, IL, USA
e-mail: jennifer.tseng@uchospitals.edu

P. Angelos
e-mail: pangelos@surgery.bsd.uchicago.edu

© Springer International Publishing AG 2017   215
K.M.F. Itani and D.J. Reda (eds.), *Clinical Trials Design in Operative
and Non Operative Invasive Procedures*, DOI 10.1007/978-3-319-53877-8_25

The disclosure of conflicts of interest by researchers must not only occur when presenting the results of the research, but even more importantly, research participants must be informed prior to their participation if the researchers have conflicts of interest. It is a central responsibility of the IRB at each institution to monitor conflicts of interest and ensure that research participants are made aware of potential conflicts in the informed consent process.

Among the major concerns in the arena of conflicts of interest in research is that the company sponsoring a trial may have an impact on the results of the trial. Although there is a clearly described association between research sponsorship and study outcomes, the association has not been demonstrated with statistical significance [6, 7]. The Consolidated Standards of Reporting Trials (CONSORT) guidelines require disclosure of study funding [8]. The International Committee of Medical Journal Editors (ICMJE) also recommends disclosure of financial ties between authors and sponsors [9]. However, trial funding and conflict of interest remains self-reported and thus may be underreported. Procedural specialties rely heavily on technology and partnerships with industry are common and are not by themselves unethical. However, readers of publication results should be aware of these relationships, since such relationships can influence readers' perceptions [10, 11]. Bridoux et al. found that more than half of the over 650 surgical studies they reviewed between 2005 and 2010 did not reveal funding sources and three-quarters did not disclose conflicts of interest [12]. Journal editorial staff members also have different ways of including statements regarding conflicts of interest, research funding and independent control of data/manuscript contents [13]. Movement toward a more uniform policy of editorship and publication regarding conflicts of interest may influence authors to be more consistent in this important aspect of transparency.

References

1. Thompson DF. Understanding financial conflicts of interest. N Engl J Med. 1993;329(8):573–6. doi:10.1056/NEJM199308193290812.
2. Souba WW, Wilmore DW. Surgical research. San Diego, CA: Academic Press; 2001. xxxii, 1460 pp.
3. McCarthy M. Sponsors lose fight to stop thyroxine study publication. Lancet. 1997;349 (9059):1149. doi:10.1016/S0140-6736(97)23016-3.
4. Constantinou G, Melides S, Modell B. The Olivieri case. N Engl J Med. 2003;348(9):860–3; author reply -3. doi:10.1056/NEJM200302273480919. PubMed PMID: 12606746.
5. Guidelines for dealing with faculty conflicts of commitment and conflicts of interest in research. July 1990. Association of American Medical Colleges Ad Hoc Committee on Misconduct and Conflict of Interest in Research. Acad Med. 1990;65(7):487–496. PubMed PMID: 2242216.
6. Momeni A, Becker A, Bannasch H, Antes G, Blumle A, Stark GB. Association between research sponsorship and study outcome in plastic surgery literature. Ann Plast Surg. 2009;63 (6):661–4. doi:10.1097/SAP.0b013e3181951917.

7. Voineskos SH, Coroneos CJ, Ziolkowski NI, Kaur MN, Banfield L, Meade MO, Chung KC, Thoma A, Bhandari M. A, systematic review of surgical randomized controlled trials: part 2. Funding source, conflict of interest, and sample size in plastic surgery. Plast Reconstr Surg. 2016;137(2):453e–61e. doi:10.1097/01.prs.0000475767.61031.d1.

8. Moher D, Hopewell S, Schulz KF, Montori V, Gotzsche PC, Devereaux PJ, Elbourne D, Egger M, Altman DG. Consolidated standards of reporting trials G. CONSORT 2010 explanation and elaboration: updated guidelines for reporting parallel group randomised trials. J Clin Epidemiol. 2010;63(8):e1–37. doi:10.1016/j.jclinepi.2010.03.004.

9. Drazen JM, de Leeuw PW, Laine C, Mulrow CD, DeAngelis CD, Frizelle FA, Godlee F, Haug C, Hebert PC, James A, Kotzin S, Marusic A, Reyes H, Rosenberg J, Sahni P, Van Der Weyden MB, Zhaori G. Toward more uniform conflict disclosures: the updated ICMJE conflict of interest reporting form. Ann Intern Med. 2010;153(4):268–9. doi:10.7326/0003-4819-153-4-201008170-00261.

10. Chaudhry S, Schroter S, Smith R, Morris J. Does declaration of competing interests affect readers' perceptions? A randomised trial. BMJ. 2002;325(7377):1391–1392. PubMed PMID: 12480854; PMCID: PMC138516.

11. Schroter S, Morris J, Chaudhry S, Smith R, Barratt H. Does the type of competing interest statement affect readers' perceptions of the credibility of research? Randomised trial. BMJ. 2004;328(7442):742–743. doi:10.1136/bmj.38035.705185.F6. PubMed PMID: 14980983; PMCID: PMC381324.

12. Bridoux V, Moutel G, Schwarz L, Michot F, Herve C, Tuech JJ. Disclosure of funding sources and conflicts of interest in phase III surgical trials: survey of ten general surgery journals. World J Surg. 2014;38(10):2487–93. doi:10.1007/s00268-014-2580-5.

13. Forbes TL. Author disclosure of conflict of interest in vascular surgery journals. J Vasc Surg. 2011;54(3 Suppl):55S–8S. doi:10.1016/j.jvs.2011.06.019.

Part V
Considerations Specific to Surgical or Procedural Trials

Chapter 26
Quality Control in Procedural Studies

Nicole E. Lopez and Lawrence T. Kim

Quality Control in Procedural Studies

What Is Quality?

The concept of quality control was originally developed in reference to manufacturing processes during the 1930s. In this context, quality has generally been defined as the ability of a product or service to satisfy a customer's needs [1]. Increasingly, these approaches have been applied to health care and in particular clinical trials [2, 3]. In clinical trials, a similar though slightly nuanced version of quality has been recognized, where quality represents the ability to effectively and efficiently answer a question about risks and benefits of a particular medical product or procedure, while protecting human subjects [4].

Several groups have attempted to standardize the process in order to more consistently achieve quality as an endpoint. The International Council on Harmonisation (ICH), a multinational organization founded in 1990 with the objective to address safety, quality, and efficacy in the development and authorization of medicinal products has been responsible for creating Good Clinical Practice (GCP) guidelines [5]. These guidelines are compulsory in US trials, and have set international guidelines to ensure uniform ethical and quality standards for pharmaceutical development [6]. In addition to assuring the rights, safety, and welfare of clinical trial subjects, GCP also aims to improve and assure the quality of data produced in clinical trials [7].

Similarly, the Clinical Trials Transformation Initiative (CTTI), a public–private partnership established by the US Food and Drug Administration and Duke University in 2007, was founded with the intent to develop and encourage practices

N.E. Lopez · L.T. Kim (✉)
Division of Surgical Oncology, Department of Surgery, University of North Carolina,
170 Manning Dr, CB #7213, Chapel Hill 27599-7213, NC, USA
e-mail: Lawrence_Kim@med.unc.edu

© Springer International Publishing AG 2017
K.M.F. Itani and D.J. Reda (eds.), *Clinical Trials Design in Operative and Non Operative Invasive Procedures*, DOI 10.1007/978-3-319-53877-8_26

221

that increase the quality and efficiency of clinical trials [8]. This group has characterized quality as the ability to effectively answer the intended question about the benefits and risks of a medical product (therapeutic or diagnostic) or procedure, while assuring protection of human subjects [8].

The guidelines and interventions provided by these groups and others with similar goals have effectively established protocols for pharmaceutical investigation with clear procedures to ensure quality in pharmacologic trials. However, the challenge to assure quality in procedural trials can be far greater.

Why Is Quality Important?

Ensuring the quality of clinical trials is imperative for two critical reasons: (1) protection of human subjects and (2) ensuring the reliability of trial data [6]. Providing proper quality assurance in randomized trials is paramount to safeguarding the rights and safety of trial participants. Equally important, though somewhat theoretical, quality assurance procedures aim to minimize biases that skew trial results, potentially protecting the safety of an exponentially greater number of future patients [9].

What Is the Current State of Quality in Surgical Trials?

Randomized controlled trials (RCT) and meta-analyses of RCTs provide the highest quality data to establish causation in interventional studies [10]. They are the gold standard for clinical trials and the crux of evidence-based medicine (EBM), however, in surgery, RCT are rare [11, 12]. In 2012, Wenner et al. [13] reported that only 7.6% of publications evaluating invasive procedures used a comparative clinical trial design and methods to control bias. This was consistent with prior reports from Wente et al. [14] and Chang et al. [15], who concluded that randomized controlled trials accounted for only 3.4 and 7.9% of publications in surgical journals, respectively. To further dilute this number, among RCTs published in surgical journals, the procedure itself is rarely the focus of the study, more commonly perioperative medical management [14]. These figures are helpful in explaining the findings of several authors, who have determined that in comparison to medical practices, surgical practices are less than half as likely to be guided by evidence derived from RCTs [16–18].

While the scarcity of RCT highlights a clear limitation in the quality of surgical trials, poor quality of data provided by surgical RCTs represents a second, and equally concerning problem. In his above-mentioned publication, Wenner et al. found also that even among the small number of surgical RCTs, many lacked critical aspects of trial design [13]. Ahmed Ali et al. [19] confirmed these findings, concluding that, overall, the methodological quality of surgical trials is low, with only approximately 1 in 5 European or North American trials meeting standards to qualify for low risk of bias. Thus, the results of the majority of surgical RCTs are at high risk of bias and therefore, they provide poor quality of data.

The low number of RCTs and the poor quality of data from surgical RCTs are independently worrisome. However, together, they create an even more troublesome scenario, in which the paucity of RCTs in surgery leads to an exaggerated enthusiasm for adoption of practices supported by biased results from small, poorly designed RCTs [20].

What Are the Challenges to Performing High-Quality Surgical RCTs?

Complexity of Systems Effecting Procedural Interventions

The complexity of surgery and other interventional, process-based fields presents challenges in controlling the multitude of variables that can affect outcomes of interest [21]. In procedural fields, results are dependent upon patients, providers, and surroundings, as well as the interactions between them [22]. Patients present with differing constellations of disease, past medical histories, and risk factors. Providers have specific skill sets, training backgrounds, and levels of experience that influence preferences and decision-making. Each institution has multiple teams (anesthesia, pain services, nursing) who may be responsible for caring for a patient, as well as varying infrastructures based on specific institutional goals and values.

Determining which components are most important to outcomes of interest and quantifying to what extent each contributes may be difficult, or even impossible. This makes deciding which components to standardize in trials problematic. Even if individual elements can be identified, standardizing them can be impractical or impossible. As such, controlling for institutional differences in these supporting systems can present an almost insurmountable challenge. Despite the importance of these influences, the difficulty of identifying and quantifying how each aspect contributes to outcomes often results in trial designs that disregard these factors [22]. As such, procedural trials tend to have poor internal validity in comparison to pharmaceutical trials [12].

Difficulty Establishing Appropriate Timing of Trials for Procedural Studies—A Threat to Equipoise

The issue of timing is not commonly recognized among the difficulties in performing procedural trials. Nonetheless, timing is perhaps the first hurdle to overcome. While pharmaceutical trials have a well-defined 4-tier track with specified goals to be accomplished at each step, the hierarchy of procedural trials remains both poorly defined and unregulated. This lack of regulation has allowed for an environment where procedural practices are in constant evolution, such that incremental modifications can result in the development of novel procedures and techniques, occurring in step-wise fashion and over time (i.e., coronary artery bypass, transplantation, and minimally invasive surgery) [23]. The success of this process in pioneering many important advances in procedural fields makes it difficult to predict the optimal timing of studies, in order to preserve equipoise while minimizing negative effects on progress.

Since measurable benefits in the improvement of existing techniques are likely the result of successive modifications in aggregate, rather than due to any single modification, requiring an RCT for each small step would significantly slow progress [20]. Similarly, studying novel techniques too early in their development may hinder advances by dismissing procedures prematurely. This can occur when evaluating new procedures before they are adequately refined, or when assessing data from providers who are still in their learning curve. On the other hand, waiting too long to perform a trial can result in unnecessary harm to patients, as with the popularity gained by such procedures as gastric freezing for peptic ulcer disease and prophylactic portocaval shunt in patients with esophageal varices [24].

Timing is also imperative for the preservation of equipoise; the popularization of procedures is generally accompanied by a loss of equipoise, which inhibits patient accrual into trials, preventing completion of studies once procedures have been disseminated [25]. This predicament is best described by Bruxton's law, which states "It is always too early (for rigorous evaluation) until, unfortunately, it's suddenly too late" [26]. One author proposes an S-curved model to describe this phenomenon, explaining that the maximal rate of uptake of a procedure occurs at approximately 20% adoption, likening this inflection point to Malcom Gladwell's "Tipping Point" [27, 28]. This argument emphasizes the importance of identifying and studying new techniques in a critical window, which occurs at some point after the technique has adequately matured, but before there is widespread acceptance of a procedure. Unfortunately, there is no reliable means by which to predict at what time point this critical window occurs.

Recruitment

Adequate recruitment is required to ensure the integrity and validity of a study. However, recruitment into surgical trials has been regarded as unreliable and in one study less than 3% of eligible patients were entered into surgical trials [29, 30]. Both patient and provider factors contribute to the difficulty of recruiting patients into surgical trials.

As discussed above, loss of equipoise can lead to poor patient accrual. A systematic review performed by Abraham et al. in 2006 showed that having a preference for one form of therapy was the most common patient reported reason for non-entry into surgical RCTs [31]. Other frequently cited patient-related reasons for non-entry were difficulty understanding the premise of the trial, dislike of the randomization process, and concerns about negative outcomes or disease recurrence. Providers, on the other hand, cited difficulty following complex protocols and follow-up requirements as the most common reason for non-entry of eligible patients into RCTs. Still, preference for one procedure over another or a specific dislike for another procedure was the second most common reason for not entering eligible patients into RCTs, again highlighting the importance of loss of equipoise in this critical aspect of trial design [31].

Crossovers

In addition to problems with recruitment, loss of equipoise can also increase the likelihood of crossovers. Crossovers can have negative effects on the sensitivity and specificity of a trial in its ability to detect differences in treatment effect, thus threatening the validity of the study. As such, every effort should be made to reduce crossovers when possible. Trials investigating medical management versus surgical intervention are particularly susceptible to crossovers and can be greater than 50% [32–34]. They are often due to change in patient conditions leading patient and provider to decide patients to move from the medical arm to surgical arm. These occurrences may be unavoidable; however, crossovers can also be the result of enrolling patients or providers with strong opinions for one treatment over another, or when providers are more comfortable with one procedure in comparison to another [35]. To avoid needless crossover, attempts should be made to refrain from enrolling either patients or providers with fervent inclinations. Furthermore, once crossovers have occurred, the influence of this effect should be minimized by performing data analysis based on intention to treat principles. Though there are no flawless mechanisms for evaluating the true treatment effect, using an intention to treat analysis is the standard approach, as it preserves randomization, minimizing bias [33].

Procedural Learning Curve

As previously discussed, both procedure and provider learning curves contribute to the complexity of interventional trials and the difficulty of obtaining quality results. Addressing the learning curve has been regarded as among the most difficult of obstacles to overcome in creating RCT for interventional procedures [11]. There are few options for identifying the correct time in procedural development for a study to occur, but controlling and adjusting for provider learning curves is slightly more feasible. Strategies to reduce the effect of the surgeon learning curve can be addressed in either the study design or in the analytic approach [11].

Approaches for addressing the learning curve in trial design include requiring a pre-specified minimum number of cases, delivering or requiring general training for all participating providers, evaluating unedited video footage of procedures or subjecting procedures to evaluation under direct observation prior to accepting proceduralists to enter the study, requiring outcomes consistent with good clinical practice, and determining quality scores for resected specimens [12]. Each of these practices has limitations; therefore, they are often employed jointly to maximize benefit.

Lack of Surgeon Training in Methodology

The poor quality of data generated by surgical trials has also been attributed to lack of surgeon training in proper methodology. There is little in the way of direct data to support this premise; however, NIH funding to surgical researchers has been notably less than that of non-surgeon scientists [36]. Evidence to confirm that this difference is secondary to a disparity in education is lacking [37]. However, if surgeons are poorly trained in research methodology it might be argued that the lack of surgeon training in methodology is not the principle problem, but rather a symptom of a history and culture that have embraced clinical autonomy and practice by opinion rather than evidence [38]. Therefore, the importance of efforts focusing on the education of surgeons regarding clinical trials methodology may change our understanding, efforts, and culture to improve the quality of trials as well as the data gathered from trials in surgical interventions [39, 40].

Poor Trial Reporting

Proper reporting of trial data is imperative to transparency, critical review, accurate interpretation, and appropriate application of trial results [41]. Poor reporting in trials can lead to errors in determining the true efficacy of interventions [42, 43]. Unfortunately, reporting in procedural trials has been shown to be grossly inadequate [41, 43]. It should be noted, however, that this deficit is not specific to procedural trials. In 1996 the Consolidated Standards of Reporting Trials (CONSORT) Statement was issued by teams from the US and Canada to address shortcomings in the reporting of trial findings in RCTs. The purpose of the statement, which was revised in 2010, was to provide a standard system for trial reporting aimed at reducing bias in results [44, 45]. Accordingly, several studies have confirmed improvement in the quality of reporting with the use of CONSORT guidelines [46–48]. While the CONSORT guidelines were perhaps initiated with pharmacologic trials in mind, it has been the suggestion of several authors that the principles and checklist set forth by CONSORT would be of great benefit in improving the quality of results in non-pharmacologic trials as well [43, 49].

How Can Trial Design Be Modified to Address Some of the More Difficult Challenges Faced in Performing High-Quality Surgical RCTs?

Tracker Trials

Tracker trials can be a helpful solution to the challenge of determining appropriate timing for procedural trials in order to balance delaying studies until procedures are adequately developed with the chance of losing equipoise. This trial design compares multiple new procedures or technologies with the standard, allowing for comparison of different components of treatment as well. Continuous analysis of the data facilitates early identification of procedural strategies that are performing poorly so that harmful treatments might be discarded expeditiously, with eventual identification of the best performing treatment [50]. Notably, the UK Endovascular Aneurysm Repair (EVAR) Trials used some concepts of tracker trial methodology to compare EVAR with either best medical management or surgical management [51]. Other advantages of this strategy include the ability to study developing procedures while maintaining equipoise, the capacity to include all providers and all treatment centers, and flexibility in the incorporation of similar procedures as they appear [50].

Standardization of Procedures

Standardization of processes has become increasingly prevalent in health care. By defining critical steps and outlining them for providers, standardization of processes can reduce errors, identify areas for improvement, and facilitate training. In surgery this movement is evidenced by establishing standards for pre-operative deep vein thrombosis (DVT) prophylaxis and timing of antibiotic prophylaxis. However, standardizing the invasive procedure itself is difficult, if even possible. To assist with this process, one group has proposed a hierarchical taxonomy consisting of "tasks, sub-tasks, and elements" which together, describe what providers do, how they do it, with which tools, and the associated outcomes [52].

A similar system for surgical standardization was recently implemented in the D2 lymphadenectomy and surgical quality control trial (KLASS-02-QC), in which investigators aimed to establish an objective assessment of the quality of D2 lymphadenectomy [53]. Prior to enrolling patients, experts used a 22-item checklist, consisting of benchmarks for completeness of dissection, to evaluate technical quality of unedited videos of procedures by potential surgeons. These experts were approved based on answers provided on a questionnaire regarding their experience and patient volume.

Upon review of the videos, a committee determined evaluation criteria and whether a surgeon was competent to participate in the trial based on demonstration of compliance with criteria on the video submission. Additionally, the committee made annotated video samples of their expectation for a complete lymphadenectomy and required that lymphadenectomy be performed in accordance with these videos. Surgeons were allowed to let preference guide parts of the procedure not under investigation such as reconstruction method, reconstruction instrument use, and insertion of drains.

Such standardization has been proposed in neurosurgery and ophthalmology; however, the costs of such undertakings can be prohibitive, limiting the capacity for widespread application of the principles necessary to attempt procedural standardization in clinical trials [54, 55].

Expertise-Based Trial Design

Changing the design of the study can also assist with minimizing learning curve effects, resulting in improved validity and integrity of RCTs in procedural fields [35]. For example, expertise-based trials reduce learning curve effects by selecting only experts to perform trial procedures. Thus, rather than requiring each participating provider to deliver all procedures under investigation, patients are randomized to providers depending upon procedure expertise. This design has been most often applied when comparing two skill-based interventions or when comparing two interventions performed by providers in differing specialties, such as coronary artery bypass grafting (CABG) by cardiac surgeons versus placement of drug eluting stents (DES) by interventional cardiologists [56]. Despite the fact that expertise-based trials eliminate some of the challenges of performing traditional RCTs in skill-based interventions, employing this methodology has failed to gain popularity [35, 57].

Randomization and the Components of Randomization that Are Challenging in Procedural Studies, but Vital to Maintaining Quality in Procedural RCTs

Randomization

The purpose of randomization is to prevent selection bias. While randomization can be difficult in pharmacologic studies, it is especially challenging in interventional trials. There are several reasons for this. First, ethical considerations regarding both placebo/sham surgeries make randomization to this type of control limb controversial [58, 59]. Indeed, many find sham surgery difficult to justify except in the case of very benign interventions. Sham surgery has been performed successfully and meaningfully in randomized trials, however, and has led to major reconsiderations of indications for procedures. For example, in a trial of interventions for osteoarthritis of the knee, sham surgery was found to be equivalent to arthroscopic debridement or arthroscopic irrigation [60].

Another major barrier to randomization in procedural trials is a perceived lack of equipoise, either on the part of the subject or sometimes the proceduralist. Either party may perceive the novel procedure as better. For the participant, this may be due to advertising or other biased information received prior to being presented with participation. Bias may also be due to conscious or unconscious bias in the investigator. For example, either being the inventor, or an early adopter may heavily invest the investigator in a novel procedure.

Randomized trials also struggle in the case of rare diseases. Performing randomized trials in these situations is impractical and a non-randomized design is often necessary to pursue any meaningful conclusions. In this instance, patients should be carefully matched by prognostic factors, and propensity scores with multivariable analysis of data performed to diminish the bias introduced by an inability to randomize patients. Additionally, while RCTs are expected to result in equal distributions of patients with differing prognostic variables in large trials, when participant number is less than 200, equal distribution is less likely. In these instances minimization should be employed to assist in distributing patients according to prognostic features [61]. For quality control issues, the method for randomization should be described upfront and should not be altered.

Allocation Concealment

When randomization is part of the study design, allocation should be performed as near to the intervention as possible to ensure both that patients are candidates for either procedure and also to minimize crossover. This is particularly pertinent in procedural trials, as they may be more susceptible to crossover, secondary to loss of equipoise of providers and patients.

Thus, optimally, consent for all possible interventions should be performed pre-operatively and allocation performed intra-operatively, once it is confirmed that the patient is a candidate for either procedure or the provider will perform either procedure. Further, to avoid intentional or unintentional bias in randomization, a third party should always perform randomization. This strategy can help ensure concealment of allocation, safeguarding the benefits of randomization in limiting selection bias.

Blinding

Allocation concealment should not be more difficult in procedural trials; however, blinding can certainly pose a challenge. In many cases, blinding in procedural trials is not feasible. As with many aspects of study design, the purpose of blinding is to limit bias. Specifically, blinding limits ascertainment bias (performance and detection bias). In fact, this aspect of trial design has perhaps become so revered as to have gained a meaning almost synonymous with quality data and avoidance of bias. However, blinding is not tantamount to quality of a trial; indeed, trials that are blinded may not be high-quality trials. The converse is also true; unblinded trials may be scientifically strong despite a lack of blinding [62]. This is particularly important to remember in procedural trials, in which this benchmark is inherently difficult, or impossible to achieve. In these instances certain measures may be taken to reduce observer bias. For example, though it may not be possible to blind providers, those assessing outcomes can generally be blinded. Alternatively, independent personnel, who have no vested interest in outcomes, can perform assessments. Similarly, assessment by multiple personnel can also limit potential for bias. Finally, in order to more precisely evaluate the quality added to the trial by blinding, the CONSORT statement suggests comprehensive reporting of blinding including who was blinded and how this was carried out [63].

Selection of Outcome Measures

When possible, using objective outcome measures can also reduce bias since subjective outcomes are more susceptible to measurement or observer bias [12, 64].

Systematic Solutions

With so many distinct challenges in interventional trials, investigators have proposed outlines for unique study processes for surgical trials. In 2002 McCulloch proposed a framework for surgical research consisting of prospective monitoring of data collection, using quality control techniques to assess technical innovations including the associated learning curves, variation, and surgical quality. He suggested an early non-randomized phase to allow for these evaluations and give a more precise indication of when an RCT is appropriate as well as a more informed estimate of adequate sample size. Additionally, he called for more collaboration to promote larger RCTs. Finally, he suggested the need for acceptance of alternative study designs in surgical trials [20].

Nearly 10 years later he and his colleagues published a series of papers proposing the IDEAL framework, which specifically addresses methods, quality metrics, and standards to strive for in procedural studies [22, 65–67]. In this strategy, McCulloch et al. describe a five-phase process designed and specified for procedural trials, meant to be analogous to the four-stage process outlined for pharmaceutical trials: (1) Innovation, (2a) Development, (2b) Exploration, (3) Assessment, and (4) Long-term study. They proposed this outline in hopes of improving the standardization of surgical trials to produce higher quality data in support of surgical interventions. Similarly, adhering to guidelines such as CONSORT and PRISMA for surgical RCTs and meta-analysis, respectively, can improve the quality of data obtained from procedural trials [64, 68].

Conclusion

The quality of surgical trials suffers on multiple fronts. In order to provide patients with the best possible care based on high-quality evidence, the reliability of data must be improved. Here we have discussed design measures to consider before, during and after the conduct of a surgical trial that can be used to limit bias and improve the quality of data in procedural trials.

References

1. Shewhart WA. Economic control of quality of manufactured product. New York: D. Van Nostrand Company, Inc.; 1931.
2. Kopach-Konrad R, Lawley M, Criswell M, et al. Applying systems engineering principles in improving health care delivery. J Gen Intern Med. 2007;22(Suppl 3):431–7.
3. Institute of Medicine (U.S.). Committee on Cancer Clinical Trials., National Academies Press (U.S.), Institute of Medicine (U.S.). Board on Health Care Services., NCI Cooperative Group Program (National Cancer Institute). A national cancer clinical trials system for the 21st century: reinvigorating the NCI Cooperative Group Program. Washington, D.C.: National Academies Press; 2010:xviii, 297 p.
4. Toth-Allen J. Building quality into clinical trials–an FDA perspective. In: Office of Good Clinical Practice OotC, ed; 2012.
5. International Council for Harmonisation (ICH). History. 2016. http://www.ich.org/about/history.html on June 4 2016.
6. Bhatt A. Quality of clinical trials: a moving target. Perspect Clin Res. 2011;2(4):124–8.
7. Group IEW. ICH harmonised tripartite guideline: guideline for good clinical practice E6(R1). International Conference on Harmonisation of Technical Requirements for Registration of Pharmaceuticals For Human Use, 1996.
8. Clinical Trials Transformation Initiative. Mission Statement. http://www.ctti-clinicaltrials.org/who-we-are/mission on May 24, 2016.
9. Baigent C, Harrell FE, Buyse M, et al. Ensuring trial validity by data quality assurance and diversification of monitoring methods. Clin Trials. 2008;5(1):49–55.
10. Centre for Evidence-Based Medicine (CEBM). Oxford centre for evidence-based medicine— levels of evidence (March 2009). http://www.cebm.net/oxford-centre-evidence-based-medicine-levels-evidence-march-2009/ on June 5 2016.
11. Cook JA. The challenges faced in the design, conduct and analysis of surgical randomised controlled trials. Trials. 2009;10:9.
12. Farrokhyar F, Karanicolas PJ, Thoma A, et al. Randomized controlled trials of surgical interventions. Ann Surg. 2010;251(3):409–16.
13. Wenner DM, Brody BA, Jarman AF, et al. Do surgical trials meet the scientific standards for clinical trials? J Am Coll Surg. 2012;215(5):722–30.
14. Wente MN, Seiler CM, Uhl W, Buchler MW. Perspectives of evidence-based surgery. Dig Surg. 2003;20(4):263–9.
15. Chang DC, Matsen SL, Simpkins CE. Why should surgeons care about clinical research methodology? J Am Coll Surg. 2006;203(6):827–30.
16. Howes N, Chagla L, Thorpe M, McCulloch P. Surgical practice is evidence based. Br J Surg. 1997;84(9):1220–3.
17. Ellis J, Mulligan I, Rowe J, Sackett DL. Inpatient general medicine is evidence based. A-team, nuffield department of clinical medicine. Lancet. 1995;346(8972):407–10.

18. Kenny SE, Shankar KR, Rintala R, et al. Evidence-based surgery: interventions in a regional paediatric surgical unit. Arch Dis Child. 1997;76(1):50–3.
19. Ahmed Ali U, van der Sluis PC, Issa Y, et al. Trends in worldwide volume and methodological quality of surgical randomized controlled trials. Ann Surg. 2013;258(2): 199–207.
20. McCulloch P, Taylor I, Sasako M, et al. Randomised trials in surgery: problems and possible solutions. BMJ. 2002;324(7351):1448–51.
21. van der Linden W. Pitfalls in randomized surgical trials. Surgery. 1980;87(3):258–62.
22. Ergina PL, Cook JA, Blazeby JM, et al. Challenges in evaluating surgical innovation. Lancet. 2009;374(9695):1097–104.
23. McKneally MF, Daar AS. Introducing new technologies: protecting subjects of surgical innovation and research. World J Surg. 2003;27(8):930–4; discussion 4–5.
24. Salzman EW. Is surgery worthwhile? Arch Surg. 1985;120(7):771–6.
25. Black N. Why we need observational studies to evaluate the effectiveness of health care. BMJ. 1996;312(7040):1215–8.
26. Buxton M. Problems in the economic appraisal of new health technology: the evaluation of heart transplants in the UK. In: MF D, ed. Economic appraisal of health technology in the European Community. Oxford, UK; 1987. P. 103–118.
27. Wilson CB. Adoption of new surgical technology. BMJ. 2006;332(7533):112–4.
28. Gladwell M. The tipping point: how little things can make a big difference. 1st ed. Boston: Little, Brown; 2000.
29. Allen PJ, Stojadinovic A, Shriver CD, Jaques DP. Contributions from surgeons to clinical trials and research on the management of soft tissue sarcoma. Ann Surg Oncol. 1998;5(5): 437–41.
30. Jack WJ, Chetty U, Rodger A. Recruitment to a prospective breast conservation trial: why are so few patients randomised? BMJ. 1990;301(6743):83–5.
31. Abraham NS, Young JM, Solomon MJ. A systematic review of reasons for nonentry of eligible patients into surgical randomized controlled trials. Surgery. 2006;139(4):469–83.
32. Prasad KS, Gregson BA, Bhattathiri PS, et al. The significance of crossovers after randomization in the STICH trial. Acta Neurochir Suppl. 2006;96:61–4.
33. Peduzzi P, Detre K, Wittes J, Holford T. Intent-to-treat analysis and the problem of crossovers. An example from the veterans administration coronary bypass surgery study. J Thorac Cardiovasc Surg. 1991;101(3):481–7.
34. Weinstein JN, Tosteson TD, Lurie JD, et al. Surgical vs nonoperative treatment for lumbar disk herniation: the spine patient outcomes research trial (SPORT): a randomized trial. JAMA. 2006;296(20):2441–50.
35. Devereaux PJ, Bhandari M, Clarke M, et al. Need for expertise based randomised controlled trials. BMJ. 2005;330(7482):88.
36. Mann M, Tendulkar A, Birger N, et al. National institutes of health funding for surgical research. Ann Surg. 2008;247(2):217–21.
37. Solomon MJ, McLeod RS. Should we be performing more randomized controlled trials evaluating surgical operations? Surgery. 1995;118(3):459–67.
38. Rothenberger DA. Evidence-based practice requires evidence. Br J Surg. 2004;91(11): 1387–8.
39. Sprague S, Pozdniakova P, Kaempffer E, et al. Principles and practice of clinical research course for surgeons: an evaluation of knowledge transfer and perceptions. Can J Surg. 2012;55(1):46–52.
40. Fischer L, Bruckner T, Diener MK, et al. Four years of teaching principles in clinical trials–a continuous evaluation of the postgraduate workshop for surgical investigators at the study center of the German Surgical Society. J Surg Educ. 2009;66(1):15–9.
41. Madden K, Arseneau E, Evaniew N, et al. Reporting of planned statistical methods in published surgical randomised trial protocols: a protocol for a methodological systematic review. BMJ Open. 2016;6(6):e011188.

42. Moher D, Pham B, Jones A, et al. Does quality of reports of randomised trials affect estimates of intervention efficacy reported in meta-analyses? Lancet. 1998;352(9128):609–13.

43. Jacquier I, Boutron I, Moher D, et al. The reporting of randomized clinical trials using a surgical intervention is in need of immediate improvement: a systematic review. Ann Surg. 2006;244(5):677–83.

44. Altman DG. Better reporting of randomised controlled trials: the CONSORT statement. BMJ. 1996;313(7057):570–1.

45. Moher D, Hopewell S, Schulz KF, et al. CONSORT 2010 explanation and elaboration: updated guidelines for reporting parallel group randomised trials. BMJ. 2010;340:c869.

46. Plint AC, Moher D, Morrison A, et al. Does the CONSORT checklist improve the quality of reports of randomised controlled trials? A systematic review. Med J Aust. 2006;185(5):263–7.

47. Moher D, Jones A, Lepage L, Group C. Use of the CONSORT statement and quality of reports of randomized trials: a comparative before-and-after evaluation. JAMA. 2001;285(15):1992–1995.

48. Devereaux PJ, Manns BJ, Ghali WA, et al. The reporting of methodological factors in randomized controlled trials and the association with a journal policy to promote adherence to the consolidated standards of reporting trials (CONSORT) checklist. Control Clin Trials. 2002;23(4):380–8.

49. Adie S, Harris IA, Naylor JM, Mittal R. CONSORT compliance in surgical randomized trials: are we there yet? A systematic review. Ann Surg. 2013;258(6):872–8.

50. Lilford RJ, Braunholtz DA, Greenhalgh R, Edwards SJ. Trials and fast changing technologies: the case for tracker studies. BMJ. 2000;320(7226):43–6.

51. Brown LC, Epstein D, Manca A, et al. The UK endovascular aneurysm repair (EVAR) trials: design, methodology and progress. Eur J Vasc Endovasc Surg. 2004;27(4):372–81.

52. Armstrong T, Yu D, Frischknecht A, et al. Standardization of surgical procedures for identifying best practices and training. Work. 2012;41(Suppl 1):4673–9.

53. Kim HI, Hur H, Kim YN, et al. Standardization of D2 lymphadenectomy and surgical quality control (KLASS-02-QC): a prospective, observational, multicenter study [NCT01283893]. BMC Cancer. 2014;14:209.

54. Feldon SE, Scherer RW, Hooper FJ, et al. Surgical quality assurance in the ischemic optic neuropathy decompression trial (IONDT). Control Clin Trials. 2003;24(3):294–305.

55. Taussky P, Lanzino G, Cloft H, Kallmes D. A checklist in the event of aneurysm perforation during coiling. AJNR Am J Neuroradiol. 2010;31(7):E59.

56. Hannan EL, Wu C, Walford G, et al. Drug-eluting stents vs. coronary-artery bypass grafting in multivessel coronary disease. N Engl J Med. 2008;358(4):331–41.

57. Cook JA, Elders A, Boachie C, et al. A systematic review of the use of an expertise-based randomised controlled trial design. Trials. 2015;16:241.

58. London AJ, Kadane JB. Placebos that harm: sham surgery controls in clinical trials. Stat Methods Med Res. 2002;11(5):413–27.

59. Edward SJ, Stevens AJ, Braunholtz DA, et al. The ethics of placebo-controlled trials: a comparison of inert and active placebo controls. World J Surg. 2005;29(5):610–4.

60. Moseley JB, O'Malley K, Petersen NJ, et al. A controlled trial of arthroscopic surgery for osteoarthritis of the knee. N Engl J Med. 2002;347(2):81–8.

61. Treasure T, MacRae KD. Minimisation: the platinum standard for trials? Randomisation doesn't guarantee similarity of groups; minimisation does. BMJ. 1998;317(7155):362–3.

62. Schulz KF, Grimes DA. Blinding in randomised trials: hiding who got what. Lancet. 2002;359(9307):696–700.

63. Schulz KF, Altman DG, Moher D, Group C. CONSORT 2010 statement: updated guidelines for reporting parallel group randomised trials. PLoS Med. 2010;7(3):e1000251.

64. Boutron I, Moher D, Altman DG, et al. Extending the CONSORT statement to randomized trials of nonpharmacologic treatment: explanation and elaboration. Ann Intern Med. 2008;148(4):295–309.

65. Meakins JL. Surgical research: act 3, answers. Lancet. 2009;374(9695):1039–40.

66. Barkun JS, Aronson JK, Feldman LS, et al. Evaluation and stages of surgical innovations. Lancet. 2009;374(9695):1089–96.
67. McCulloch P, Altman DG, Campbell WB, et al. No surgical innovation without evaluation: the IDEAL recommendations. Lancet. 2009;374(9695):1105–12.
68. Moher D, Liberati A, Tetzlaff J, et al. Preferred reporting items for systematic reviews and meta-analyses: the PRISMA statement. BMJ. 2009;339:b2535.

Chapter 27
Pilot Studies

Ryan E. Ferguson and Mary T. Brophy

Introduction

Pilot studies are fundamental components of the research process that are conducted to examine the feasibility of an experimental approach for a subsequent larger study. The high cost of traditional explanatory clinical research (i.e., randomized controlled trials) and the restriction of financial support for funding agencies accounts for an increasing interest in pilot studies and the demand for pilot data prior to full-scale funding of a trial. Despite the increasing demand for pilot studies from funding agencies and the relative ubiquity of the design in academic settings, training on the design, planning, and execution of pilot studies is often missing in formal training programs for clinical science researchers [1]. To our knowledge, very few epidemiology or biostatistics text books cover the material in the necessary detail. Some texts mention design in passing and few provide more than cursory details, and relatively few textbooks dedicate an entire chapter to the topic. The objective of this chapter is to provide a detailed examination of the key issues of the design and conduct of pilot studies done in a clinical research setting.

R.E. Ferguson (✉) · M.T. Brophy
Massachusetts Veterans Epidemiology Research and Information Center, Boston Cooperative Studies Program Coordinating Center, VA Boston Healthcare System, 150 South Huntington Ave (151-MAV), Boston 02130, MA, USA
e-mail: ryan.ferguson@va.gov

M.T. Brophy
e-mail: mary.brophy@va.gov

© Springer International Publishing AG 2017
K.M.F. Itani and D.J. Reda (eds.), *Clinical Trials Design in Operative and Non Operative Invasive Procedures*, DOI 10.1007/978-3-319-53877-8_27

What Is a Pilot Study?

Pilot studies are preparatory studies that are designed to "test the performance characteristics and capabilities of study designs, measures, procedures, recruitment criteria, and operational strategies that are under consideration for use in a subsequent, often larger, study" [1]. Pilot studies, then, are the vanguard for a full-scale clinical research study. Table 27.1 provides a description of types of clinical trials by 'phase' of drug development. Traditionally, pilot studies are restricted to inform Phase III or IV studies. Pilot studies are **not** first-in-human studies, early phase safety trials, or Phase 1–2 studies.

We will focus our discussion on pilot studies that are being conducted for Phase III clinical investigations as defined in Table 27.1. This restriction in scope is consistent with the recent recommendation from the British Medical Research Council which explicitly recommends the use of feasibility studies prior to the conduct of Phase III trials, especially those that include complex interventions [2]. Restriction of the discussion in this chapter to Phase III pilot studies is not meant to imply that pilot and feasibility studies cannot be done in other settings. In fact, they can be done in a variety of research areas (i.e., drug development, population science, genomic analysis, etc.) and across multiple study designs (i.e., randomized trial, prospective cohort studies, etc.) and are routinely used in qualitative research as well.

Classification of Pilot Studies

Pilot studies can be broadly categorized into four classifications: Process, Resources, Management, and Scientific [3].

Table 27.1 Phases of clinical investigation

Phase	Objective
I	To investigate the pharmacokinetics of a drug and to identify a dose that can be tolerated with minimal toxicity. Usually not randomized; small sample size
II	To assess preliminary evidence on clinical efficacy. Can be randomized or non-randomized; usually small sample size
III	To compare the efficacy and safety of two (or more) interventions, usually the investigational agent and a placebo. Studies are usually randomized; very large sample sizes
IV	To assess the post-marketing experience of the drug (e.g., long-term safety profile, drug–drug interactions, etc.). Studies are often non-randomized; often very large sample sizes

Process—this rationale applies when pilot studies assess the feasibility of key procedures that will take place in the main trial such as consent refusal rates given different types of informed consent documents or procedures as well as the overall accrual rates for the protocol. Draft case report forms (e.g., data collection forms) are often piloted prior to implementation to assess ease of completion, skip pattern and conditionality of questions. The intent is to iteratively improve quality through revisions.

Resource—this rationale applies to pilot studies that assess time and resource issues that are important to the main trial. For example, time for the completion of a subject interview can be assessed to understand how this will impact workload requirements of the study staff and ultimately factor into recruitment potential for the site. Resource piloting is also helpful to assess the availability and use of equipment needed for the trials, especially if the equipment is shared with the clinical staff.

Management—this rationale applies when the objective is to assess the potential human and data management issues that may arise in the main trial and provide opportunity to maximize data integrity and use of human resources. Pilot studies focused on management issues will often assess the challenges that study personnel will encounter when conducting different aspects of the main trial. Examples of key questions addressed include Are participating centers able to see patients within expected visit time interval? Are sites able to collect and capture the data?

Scientific—this rationale assesses study outcomes such as treatment effect size and variance around the estimate allowing for 'fine tuning' of the research hypothesis. In limited circumstances additional parameters such as drug safety and dosing can be assessed. Often, important rates associated with the analysis will be estimated in these pilot studies (i.e., missing data rates and participant attrition rates) and used to inform the analytic plan of the main trial.

Pilot studies have become increasingly more common in recent years and are often required by some sponsors to secure funding [4]. The National Heart, Lung, and Blood Institute (NHLBI) of the National Institutes of Health has an established funding mechanism (R34) specifically for the conduct of pilot studies in preparation of a larger, more robust clinical trial. The guidance from the NHLBI suggests that pilot studies should only be done to address gaps in knowledge that are required for the conduct or the design of the main trial.

In general, pilot studies present opportunities to clarify and sharpen the research hypotheses to be studied; identify potential barriers to study completion; evaluate performance of the trial systems and their acceptability to trial participants and providers; and enhance data integrity and human subjects' protections.

Internal Versus External Pilot Studies

Pilot studies may be classified as *internal* or *external*, each with its advantages and disadvantages. External pilot studies are those that are done completely independently of the main trial to assess its feasibility. They have their own specific aims, data collection procedures, and analytical plan. Data from external pilot studies should not be merged with data from the main trial [5]. Merging the data may create a selection bias and will inflate the type 1 error for the study. Figure 27.1 shows a graphical representation of the abbreviated workflow for an external pilot study.

Internal pilot studies are adaptive trials that are primarily designed to allow for re-estimation of sample size calculations of the main trial [3]. In this type of study, the main trial is planned using the best available data and is initiated on a pre-specified number of trial participants. Sample size is recalculated using the observed outcome rate and effect size seen in the pilot sample. If the originally calculated sample is large enough (or too big) then the original estimate will stand [5]. The principal advantage of internal pilot studies is that the design allows for sample size estimation without increasing the time for the conduct of the full trial [5]. All data collected from the initial patients can be used in the main trial and no effort (or data) is lost. Figure 27.2 shows a graphical representation of an internal pilot study. A major disadvantage of the internal pilot design is that other feasibility factors cannot be assessed as the pilot phase is, in fact, part of the main trial. In addition, the type 1 error will be slightly inflated as the pilot subjects and the main trial participants are considered to be independent when combined in the final analysis [5]. As long as the alpha level is controlled, internal pilot study designs offer flexibility and power [6].

Fig. 27.1 Abbreviated workflow for an external pilot study

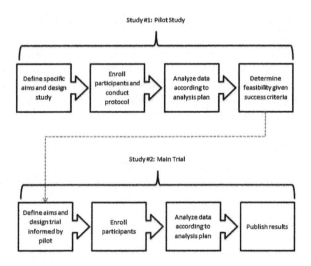

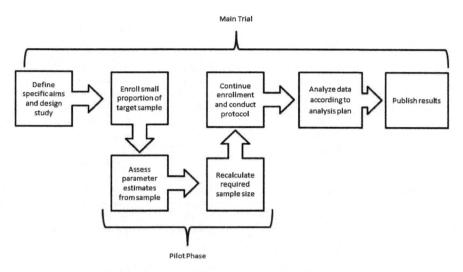

Fig. 27.2 Abbreviated workflow for an internal pilot study

Statistical Considerations

Design and Analytic Plan

The design of pilot studies should be guided by the same principles as the parent clinical trial particularly when feasibility of the parent study is the central issue. Pilot studies must have a well-elucidated statistical analysis plan with carefully constructed strategies for achieving each of its aims. The analysis plan should clearly identify the outcomes, the measures, and the acceptance criteria for each critical element. This axiom is true for all pilot studies regardless of classification and does not imply that formal analysis with inferential statistics is needed. Consider for example, a study investigating proper hydration levels to prevent contrast-induced nephropathy in diabetics receiving an angiography that underwent feasibility piloting within a large healthcare institution. Table 27.2 provides example questions that each category of pilot study may ask as well as sample outcomes that should be included in an analytic plan. As stated above, pilot studies will focus on feasibility; consequently, hypothesis testing on efficacy and safety endpoints are inappropriate analytic procedures for a pilot study analytic plan. As a result of the focus on feasibility, the analysis plan for a pilot will rely heavily on point and interval estimation and should only involve limited, if any, hypothesis testing (more on this below).

Table 27.2 Example analysis plans and acceptance criteria for each pilot classification

Category of pilot study	Example aim	Possible outcome	Sample acceptance criteria or analytic plan
Process	To assess the feasibility of the enrollment	% of eligible patients receiving an angiography that are consented	$\geq 20\%$ of eligible patients are consented into the protocol
Resource	To assess the resource requirements for the baseline participant interview	Time to completion	Successful interviews will be those conducted in less than 20 min (on average) across a sample of 20 patients
Management	To test whether the post-procedure hydration protocol can be implemented within the clinical care workflow	Proportion of consented patients receiving the post-procedure hydration protocol	$\geq 90\%$ of consented patients receive 100% of the hydration protocol within 3 h of the procedure
Scientific	To estimate the variance around the event rate within the healthcare system	Outcome (event) rate	Occurrence and distribution of the event rate with in 96 h of the procedure

Sample Size

Sample size estimation is often incorrectly viewed as 'not essential' for pilot studies because there will be limited hypothesis testing and restricted used of inferential statistics. However, this is a misconception that focuses only on the use of inferential statistics. Instead, sample size should be sufficiently large to obtain precise point estimates and confidence interval estimates for the parent study. Therefore, there is a very real need to have a clear and well-reasoned rationale for the number of participants to be included in the pilot study. The justification must be deeply rooted in the analytic plan and aligned with each of the aims of the pilot study. The choice of the appropriate sample size, then, will be driven by sound judgement and the aims of the pilot with specific consideration to the issues of practical feasibility and not by considerations related to power.

In 2005, Cook et al. [7] reported the results of a pilot study done in preparation for a large-scale study on the prophylaxis of thromboembolism. The pilot focused entirely on feasibility and reported recruitment rates, rates of protocol adherence, and an assessment of workload. The total sample of 120 participants from 16 intensive care units was selected (1) in order to obtain an estimate (with confidence intervals) of the proportion of people that would meet eligibility criteria and; and (2) to allow for an adequate sample (with at least 3 from each ICU) to refine protocol and screening procedures prior to full-scale deployment. All rates observed in the pilot study were then compared to rates that were specified a priori and "feasibility" of the larger trial was determined based on these "acceptance criteria."

There are no explicit rules or guidelines for the appropriate sample size of a pilot study. It should be large enough to provide point estimates and confidence intervals with sufficient precision to reduce statistical uncertainty but in practice they are typically too small to achieve this goal. A recent report from Billingham et al. looked at sample sizes in 79 funded trials recorded within the United Kingdom Clinical Research Network database and found that among pilot and feasibility studies the mean sample size for studies with dichotomous and continuous endpoints was only 36 (range: 10–300) and 30 (range: 8–114) per arm, respectively [8].

Power Calculations and Hypothesis Testing

While pilot studies are underpowered for testing of parent study hypothesis, they should be adequately sized to test operational issues and guide decisions about how the parent study will be conducted. Examples include the following: Is the RNA assay more accurate and more precise than the antigen assay? Is the taste of a particular dietary supplement acceptable to at least 95% of the target population? [1]. In these cases the power of the hypothesis test will depend on the choice of the sample and will be a function of the hypothesized parameter values. It is therefore very useful to calculate power with different sample sizes and to present power curves in the analytic plan. The biostatistical and hypothesis testing literature is rife with examples and formulae to guide calculations of the appropriate sample or power for given parameter estimates.

In summary, pilot studies are an important preparatory step in the progression of research that is hypothesis driven, but the studies themselves may not test a hypothesis. It is appropriate to focus on the level of precision for a given estimate (i.e., the statistical uncertainty and confidence interval) and not necessarily on the power level of a testing procedure.

A Cautionary Tale on the Use of Pilot Study Data to Guide Power Calculations

Kraemer et al. (2006) have shown that pilot studies can generate unreliable, unrealistic, and biased sample sizes for the larger parent trials because they are limited by small samples themselves [3, 9]. As a result, the parameter estimates generated by pilot studies should be used with extreme caution when estimating effect size within a larger population. Parameters generated from pilot studies may not have been estimated with sufficient accuracy to serve as the basis of power calculations or to serve as a basis for decision making on whether the main trial should be funded [9]. The authors report that the two likely outcomes of using pilot study data to drive power computation are as follows:

1. The study proposal will be aborted even when the actual effect is clinically significant.
2. If not aborted, the study sample estimated from the pilot data will be too small and will result in a study that is underpowered to detect the effect sizes of clinical significance.

In short, studies that calculate sample size that are based on effect sizes that are estimated from pilot studies will "likely" end in failed clinical trials and result in wasted resources. Therefore, the results of pilot studies should be used with caution as the data can potentially mislead sample size calculations.

Ethical Considerations

Informed Consent

There is a long standing history of debate on the ethical considerations of conducting underpowered research. In particular, underpowered studies are considered unethical because such studies will not adequately test their underlying hypotheses and they will be "scientifically useless" [10] yet will expose participants to both risks and burdens. However, similar discussion for pilot studies is lacking in this literature [10]. While pilot studies primarily address study feasibility with much less emphasis on statistical power, consideration of the same principles of informed consent is appropriate. Specifically, the consent process for pilot studies must convey the limited scope of the pilot to the subject [10].

Thabane et al. [3] investigated the obligation that researchers have, to patients or to participants in a trial, to disclose the feasibility nature and, hence the "limited" scientific value, of pilot studies. The authors reviewed the most cited research guidelines in the literature (e.g., the Nuremburg code, the Belmont Report, ICH GCP, etc.) and found that pilot studies are not addressed in any of the guidelines [3]. Thabane et al. [3] conclude that "given the special nature of feasibility or pilot studies, the disclosure of their purpose to study participants requires special wording—that informs them of the definition of a pilot study, the feasibility objectives of the study, and also clearly defines the criteria for success of feasibility". In order to fully inform participants, the authors have suggested template language for informed consent documents [3].

Publication

Although pilot studies can be very informative, few are ever published, perhaps because undue emphasis is placed on the statistical significance of findings rather than on feasibility issues that were the primary focus of the pilot study [3].

Underreporting of pilot study data results in publication bias [5] and further compounds the ethical considerations of the conduct of the pilot.

Recommendations for the Conduct of Pilot Studies

1. Keep the next study in mind!
   The pilot should be designed to maximize the information needed for the main trial. The design of the pilot should mimic the main trial as should the study procedures.
2. Maintain methodological rigor.
   The same principles that guide the design of the main study should be followed for a pilot study. The small size and feasibility focus does not remove the obligation to generate accurate and precise data.
3. Clearly define aims, objectives, and the definitions of success.
   The aims, the objectives, and the design should all be aligned. Acceptance criteria and definitions of success should be clearly articulated a priori as should a clear plan to use the data generated by the pilot study.
4. Align analysis plan with objectives and design of study.
   The analysis should be mainly descriptive and contain very limited hypothesis testing. If hypothesis testing is used, results should be treated as preliminary and not definitive. Sample size must be justified in the analysis plan.
5. Must convey limited value to participants.
   Ethical principles demand informed consent and notification of the limited value of the pilot study.
6. Publish the results.
   Results from all pilot studies should be reported. Reporting of results should follow the guidelines adapted from the CONSORT Statement by Thabane et al. in 2010. Reporting will help to reduce the impact of publication bias and will contribute by advancing the scientific community.

References

1. Moore CG, Carter RE, Nietert PJ, Stewart PW. Recommendations for planning pilot studies in clinical and translational research. Clin Transl Sci. 2011;4(5):332–7.
2. Craig P, Dieppe P, Macintyre S, Michie S, Nazareth I, Petticrew M. Developing and evaluating complex interventions: the new medical research council guidance. BMJ. 2008;29 (337):a1655.
3. Thabane L, Ma J, Chu R, Cheng J, Ismaila A, Rios LP, Robson R, Thabane M, Giangregorio L, Goldsmith CH. A tutorial on pilot studies: the what, why and how. BMC Med Res Methodol. 2010;10(1):1.
4. Leon AC, Davis LL, Kraemer HC. The role and interpretation of pilot studies in clinical research. J Psychiatr Res. 2011;45(5):626–9.

5. Lancaster GA, Dodd S, Williamson PR. Design and analysis of pilot studies: recommendations for good practice. J Eval clin Pract. 2004;10(2):307–12.
6. Wittes J, Brittain E. The role of internal pilot studies in increasing the efficiency of clinical trials. Stat Med. 1990;9(1–2):65–72.
7. Cook DJ, Rocker G, Meade M, Guyatt G, Geerts W, Anderson D, Skrobik Y, Hebert P, Albert M, Cooper J, Bates S. Prophylaxis of thromboembolism in critical care (PROTECT) trial: a pilot study. J Crit Care. 2005;20(4):364–72.
8. Billingham SA, Whitehead AL, Julious SA. An audit of sample sizes for pilot and feasibility trials being undertaken in the United Kingdom registered in the United Kingdom clinical research network database. BMC Med Res Methodol. 2013;13(1):1.
9. Kraemer HC, Mintz J, Noda A, Tinklenberg J, Yesavage JA. Caution regarding the use of pilot studies to guide power calculations for study proposals. Arch Gen Psychiatry. 2006;63 (5):484–9.
10. Halpern SD, Karlawish JH, Berlin JA. The continuing unethical conduct of underpowered clinical trials. JAMA. 2002;288(3):358–62.

Chapter 28
Surgeon Training and the Learning Curve

Kamal M.F. Itani

Introduction

With every intervention, procedure, interpretation of a test or even new medical treatment, there is a learning curve. This learning curve differs among providers based on background, training, skills, environment, and available support as well as the similarity of the new intervention to older ones. In addition, moving beyond the learning curve to experienced provider in a new intervention is open to interpretation based on the observer, his/her background within the field, and the observer status on the learning curve for that intervention.

When testing a new intervention in a prospective randomized trial, the investigators will have to decide on the level of expertise of each participating investigator, their standing on the learning curve, the level of expertise that each has to achieve prior to enrolling patients, and how it is measured and ethical considerations related to patients and society. This chapter will discuss each of these points and how to address them within a large prospective randomized clinical trial.

Definition

The learning curve has been defined as the time it takes and/or the number of procedures an average surgeon needs to perform independently in order to reach a reasonable outcome [1]. Others have represented the learning curve as the relationship between experience with a new procedure or technique and an outcome

K.M.F. Itani (✉)
Department of Surgery, VA Boston Health Care System, Boston University
and Harvard Medical School, VABHCS(112A), 1400 VFW Parkway,
West Roxbury, MA 02132, USA
e-mail: kitani@va.gov

© Springer International Publishing AG 2017   245
K.M.F. Itani and D.J. Reda (eds.), *Clinical Trials Design in Operative
and Non Operative Invasive Procedures*, DOI 10.1007/978-3-319-53877-8_28

variable such as operating time, complication rate, hospital stay, or mortality [2]. A learning curve may also be operationally defined as an improvement in performance over time. It therefore implies a baseline performance, an improvement over time which can happen at various rates of speed, and a plateau in performance afterwards. The speed with which a plateau is achieved is dependent on the initial performance level and the rapidity with which the improvement occurs up to the plateau. It is to note that depending on the learning curve phase, lack of investigator equipoise might exist favoring traditional interventions during the baseline or improvement phase and possibly favoring the newer intervention during the plateau phase.

(a) Baseline performance
Baseline performance depends on the individual baseline skills and familiarity with similar interventions or exposure to similar interventions in the past. For example, an orthopedic surgeon performing hip or knee replacements might be comfortable with one or two prostheses that are commonly used. However, when a new prosthesis is introduced into practice, it might require a new set of skills some of which overlap with the old ones and some which are totally new. The level of overlap is also dependent on the type of prosthesis the surgeon was using.

(b) The improvement phase
The improvement phase is also dependent on each individual surgeon's background with the technology, learning abilities, as well as the environment in which they practice. The environment might have other experts able to provide feedback about progress, a larger volume of patients to be treated with the newer intervention, the availability of cadavers, animal labs, or simulators to practice. All of these will factor into the speed at which the plateau is reached.

(c) Plateau phase
During the plateau phase, the individual is considered familiar, comfortable, and experienced in performing the newer intervention and should be able to teach it to others interested in acquiring these skills. The assessment that the individual is at the plateau phase is arbitrary and can be a function of reported volume, time, observation, or a combination of all the above. Any auditor of this new technology should be at the plateau phase.

Selection of Investigators in a Trial

Participation in clinical trials requires that investigators have proven capability and knowledge in the conduct of the research-related operations and ideally at the plateau phase. Parameters for how many operations the surgeon is required to perform must be established with assessment of a defined outcome measure. In some cases, certification might be done by submitting a record of operative and pathology results. Alternatively, the surgeon might be required to submit videos that could be audited and reviewed. For other operations, observation by a proctor can confirm that the surgeon is ready to perform the operation as part of a clinical trial. Techniques and operations that are already part of the surgeon's skills still need to be assessed to measure the surgeon's ability to perform the operation in accordance with the requirements of the study. As mentioned in the chapters on investigators meetings (Chap. 37) and site visits (Chap. 38), the principal investigator must budget for training, including providing funds to train sub-investigators, stipends, and travel for proctors.

In the prospective randomized trial comparing laparoscopic to open inguinal hernia with mesh, the laparoscopic technique was relatively new and had little to moderate penetration in clinical practice. It was arbitrarily decided with the help of experts that each surgeon participating in the trial should have a minimum experience of 25 cases performed laparoscopically, a videotaped laparoscopic repair reviewed by the principal investigator before the start of the study, and random videos of the procedure sent for auditing during the course of the study [3]. A post hoc analysis of the data looking at the influence of volume, age, and time since board certification revealed that a volume of 250 cases was necessary to achieve with the laparoscopic repair the same level of recurrence and complications as the open repair [4]. It became clear that most surgeons participating in the trial were still in the improvement phase. This trial clearly demonstrated the steep learning curve for performing laparoscopic inguinal hernia repairs and that these operations are best performed by surgeons at the plateau phase of the learning curve in order to achieve the desired outcome.

In the prospective randomized trial evaluating laparoscopic assisted vs. open resection of stage 2 or 3 rectal cancer on pathologic outcomes [5], a credentialing committee was established to review unedited videotapes, operative reports, and pathology reports of 46 participating surgeons at 35 institutions. The mechanism of credentialing of participating surgeons is described in an online supplement of the published study [6]. In addition a random audit performed for the first 100 laparoscopic cases was confirmatory of expertise in techniques used throughout the trial. The principal investigators wanted to ensure that all participating surgeons in this trial were at least at the plateau phase for each of the surgeries included in that trial. This resulted in a 93% compliance in the rate of total mesorectal excision, an important goal of the study and a reflection of the high quality of surgery performed in that study.

Auditing Results

It is the responsibility of the principal investigator and the executive committee to audit and monitor any new surgical procedure. Stopping rules must be in place to remedy or remove a surgeon who is not performing as expected with regard to the technical requirements of the intervention or if placing patients at risk. A priori decisions need to be made with regard to whether the data from surgeons who are removed will be used in the final analysis of the results.

Auditing can occur through live visits to investigator sites, videotapes, or close monitoring of outcomes.

Statistical Considerations

Various statistical methods have been reported in the assessment of the learning curve [7]. Commonly used data are split into arbitrary groups and the means compared by chi-squared test or ANOVA. Some studies have data displayed graphically with no statistical analysis. Others use univariate analysis of experience versus outcome. Some studies use multivariate analysis techniques such as logistic regression and multiple regression to adjust for confounding factors. A systematic review concluded that the statistical methods used for assessing learning curves have been crude and the reporting of studies poor [8]. Recognizing that better methods may be developed in other nonclinical fields where learning curves are present (psychology and manufacturing), a systematic search was made of the nonclinical literature to identify novel statistical methods for modeling learning curves. A number of techniques were identified including generalized estimating equations and multilevel, or hierarchical, models. The main recommendation was that given the hierarchical nature of the learning curve data and the need to adjust for covariates, hierarchical statistical models should be used. Ramsay et al. [8] went further to suggest Bayesian hierarchical modeling in order to adjust for effect sizes for learning.

Biau et al. [9] suggested the cumulative summation test for learning curve that allows quantitative and individual assessment for the learning curve. The cumulative summation test has been applied to the learning curve and is designed to indicate when a process deviates from an accepted level of performance.

Other statistical tools available to address the learning curve include the intraclass correlation coefficient. In multicenter trials, data from the same center are more similar than those from different centers. These similarities which often include the level of the center as a whole on the learning curve induce a correlation between data, known as the center effect. This center effect is assessed by the intraclass correlation coefficient [10].

Finally, an expertise-based approach to trial design, where health professionals only deliver an intervention in which they have expertise, has been proposed as an alternative. An expertise-based trial design should be considered but its value seems context-specific, particularly when the control and the intervention under study differ substantially or are delivered by different health professionals [11].

Ethical Consideration

There is no doubt that patients undergoing procedures earlier during the learning curve are at greater risk for adverse events than patients operated on during the plateau phase of the learning curve or by experienced surgeons. Information related to the new procedure and the learning curve of the surgeon should be included in the informed consent and discussed with the patient. This can by itself bias the patient against the procedure and preclude a subject from participating in a trial for fear of undergoing a new procedure by a less-experienced surgeon.

There is also the dilemma of potentially promising procedures that are difficult to learn, replicate, or teach. Such procedures are of limited generalizability and risky to test within the context of a multicenter trial.

Conclusion

When testing a new intervention, principal investigators have a responsibility to evaluate the learning curve and the status of each investigator on the learning curve. Participating subjects should be informed of the expertise level of the investigator caring for them. Lack of equipoise among investigators or bias against a new procedure by patients may be introduced based on the learning curve of the investigator. Frequent monitoring and auditing should be in place to avoid exposing patients to risk and compromise the results of the trial. Various statistical tools are also available to address variability resulting from the learning curve.

References

1. Subramonian K, Muir G. The learning curve in surgery: what is it, how do we measure it and can we influence it? BJU Int. 2004;93(9):1173–4.
2. Michel LA. Epistelogy of evidence-based medicine. Surg Endosc. 2007;21(2):145–51.
3. Neumayer L, Giobbie-Hurder A, Jonasson O, Fitzgibbons R Jr, Dunlop D, Gibbs J, Reda D, Henderson W. Veterans affairs cooperative studies program 456 investigators: open mesh versus laparoscopic mesh repair of inguinal hernia. N Engl J Med. 2004; 29;350(18):1819–27.
4. Neumayer LA, Gawande AA, Wang J, Giobbie-Hurder A, Itani KM, Fitzgibbons RJ Jr, Reda D, Jonasson O. CSP #456 investigators: proficiency of surgeons in inguinal hernia repair: effect of experience and age. Ann Surg. 2005;242(3):344–8.
5. Fleshman J, Branda M, Sargent DJ, Boller AM, George V, Abbas M, Peters WR Jr, Maun D, Chang G, Herline A, Fichera A, Mutch M, Wexner S, Whiteford M, Marks J, Birnbaum E, Margolin D, Larson D, Marcello P, Posner M, Read T, Monson J, Wren SM, Pisters PW, Nelson H. Effect of laparoscopic-assisted resection vs open resection of stage II or III rectal cancer on pathologic outcomes: the ACOSOG Z6051 randomized clinical trial. JAMA. 2015;314(13):1346–55.

6. Fleshman J, Branda M, Sargent DJ, et al. Effect of laparoscopic-assisted resection vs open resection of stage II or III rectal cancer on pathologic outcomes: the ACOSOG Z6051 randomized clinical trial. JAMA. 2015 Oct 6;314(13): e-appendix B.
7. Ramsay CR, Grant AM, Wallace SA, Garthwaite PH, Monk AF, Russell IT. Statistical assessment of the learning curves of health technologies. Health Technol Assess. 2001;5: 1–79.
8. Cook JA, Ramsay CK, Fayers P. Statistical evaluation of learning curve effects in clinical trials. Clin Trials. 2004;1:421–7.
9. Biau DJ, Porcher R, Boutron I. The account for provider and center effects in multicenter interventional and surgical randomized controlled trials is in need of improvement: a review. J Clin Epidemiol. 2008;61(5):435–9.
10. Vierron E, Giraudeau B. Sample size calculation for multicenter randomized trial: taking the center effect into account. Contemp Clin Trials. 2007;28(4):451–8.
11. Cook JA, Elders A, Boachie C, Bassinga T, Fraser C, Altman DG, Boutron I, Ramsay CR, MacLennan GS. A systematic review of the use of an expertise-based randomised controlled trial design. Trials. 2015;16(241):1–10.

Chapter 29
Using a Placebo or Sham Procedure as a Control: Ethics and Practicalities

Joshua S. Richman

New surgical treatments are often introduced without proof of efficacy from randomized controlled trials, and some procedures that are perceived to be effective have never been rigorously tested [1, 2]. In the early 2000s the results of two particularly controversial randomized controlled trials of surgical interventions appeared in the New England Journal of Medicine, Published in 2001 the Freed trial tested embryonic stem cell implantation as an experimental cutting-edge therapy for Parkinson's disease compared to a control group without implantation. Unlike most controlled surgical trials, the control group underwent a 'sham surgery' nearly identical to the intervention procedure including four twist drill holes through the frontal bone. However, for patients in the control group, the dura mater was not penetrated. This procedure blinded study participants to whether they received the intervention or not making it possible to account for any placebo effect of the surgical intervention per se.

The following year Mosely et al. published their findings in a study which compared patients with osteoarthritis of the knee randomized to undergo arthroscopic debridement, then a commonly accepted therapy, versus patients randomized to two other groups (1) arthroscopic lavage only, or (2) a 'placebo surgery,' where the surgery was simulated in detail but the actual procedure was limited to three 1-cm incisions in the skin. While the Freed study tested a novel therapy, this study used a design with a 'placebo surgery' to test whether an accepted therapy was, in fact, effective.

Recent years have seen further randomized trials of surgical interventions using placebo or sham surgeries as the control. Two reviews published in 2015 examined randomized controlled trials of surgical procedures where the control group received a placebo, or sham, surgery [1, 2]. Both reviews found that more than half

J.S. Richman (✉)
Department of Surgery, University of Alabama at Birmingham and the Birmingham VAMC, Kracke 217C, 1922 7th Ave South, Birmingham, AL 35203, USA
e-mail: jrichman@uabmc.edu

© Springer International Publishing AG 2017
K.M.F. Itani and D.J. Reda (eds.), *Clinical Trials Design in Operative and Non Operative Invasive Procedures*, DOI 10.1007/978-3-319-53877-8_29

of the studies considered showed significant improvement among the control groups, and the treatment group was superior to the placebo in less than half of the trials. Furthermore, in most of those the difference between intervention and placebo was small. This evidence of significant effects from placebo procedures highlights the need to account for the placebo effect in surgical trials. Nevertheless, placebo-controlled surgical trials remain controversial and can be difficult to conduct.

Blinding and Placebos

Blinding of the randomly assigned treatment in clinical trials is a key design feature to protect the integrity of the trial. Depending on the level of blinding (single or double-blind), it controls for bias due to participants' (single blind) and also researchers' (double-blind) expectations [3]. It has long been recognized in medicine that some accepted therapies are observed to be more effective than no treatment at all but, after rigorous testing, are found to be no more effective than a placebo. In these cases, the effect of the accepted treatment is likely due largely to the patients' expectation of efficacy. The existence of this placebo effect highlights the importance of managing both conscious and unconscious expectations. To minimize the chance that observed differences can be attributed to the placebo effect, when a study compares two or more treatments, care should be taken for them to appear as similar as possible. In some scenarios such as in studies comparing two medications, incorporating a placebo comparator may be simple. For studies comparing two surgical techniques or a surgical technique to a nonsurgical treatment, it may be difficult or impossible to maintain blinding.

Distinctive Aspects of Sham Surgeries or Procedures

The most obvious difference between placebo-controlled trials of medications and procedures is that finding a suitable placebo becomes much more difficult with an invasive surgical procedure involving the use of anesthesia and obvious long-term effects such as scarring. Trials of therapies involving injections or infusions could use saline as a placebo without difficulty because the intrinsic harm is no greater than drawing blood for laboratory tests which is a routing part of medical testing. This qualifies these placebos as posing 'minimal risk.'

There is evidence that the placebo effect is stronger for more invasive procedures than for medications, in turn suggesting that a suitable placebo for a procedure must be more invasive than an injection, and therefore beyond what can be considered to be minimal risk [4]. Summarized evidence from various trials suggested that in placebo-controlled trials, improvement from an injected placebo was greater than from oral placebo, and that sham acupuncture had a greater placebo effect than an oral placebo [4]. The authors presented additional evidence of various novel procedures with early anecdotal success which were later found to be unsupported by controlled trials, making a case that the placebo effect may be stronger when the intervention is more involved than swallowing a pill. They also proposed a design for a prospective randomized trial to compare a placebo procedure (sham acupuncture) to an oral placebo. Subsequently, Kaptchuk conducted the proposed trial in the context of treating arm pain and reported that the sham acupuncture was found to be more effective than an oral placebo [5]. The finding that the placebo effect may be more pronounced for interventions than for oral placebos carries the implication that the inclusion of placebo or sham procedures may be even more important for evaluating surgical interventions than they are for medical interventions. It also highlights the importance and difficulty of designing a realistic and suitable sham procedure to ensure blinding and account for benefits due solely to the placebo effect itself.

Ethics

Reports of preliminary results of the Parkinson's trial sparked an ethical controversy precisely because the sham procedures could not be considered to be harmless, raising questions about whether and in what circumstances sham surgeries could be considered to be ethical and appropriate [6, 7]. The critical analysis by Ruth Macklin identified three main ethical issues to consider: (1) Finding a balance between the highest standards of research design and the highest standards of ethics; (2) uncertainties and disagreements in the analysis of risks and benefits of research; and (3) issues of informed consent.

The first issue, finding a balance between research and ethical standards, considers when placebo controls may be appropriate in surgical trials. There is a general consensus that as with medical trials placebo controls may be acceptable when there is no standard effective therapy. Others add that there may be a stronger argument for a placebo control when the major outcomes are subjective and self-reported such as pain, which is known to be susceptible to the placebo effect [8, 9]. Even in cases where a placebo control seems ethical and the strongest design, the fact that a placebo surgery undeniably causes harm without the expectation of therapeutic benefit seems to conflict with the mandate that ethical research should minimize risk of harm. Macklin [6] concludes that the duty to minimize harm is paramount and that placebo surgery is not ethical. Others argue that in the presence of genuine equipoise, the placebo surgery causes no more harm than the experimental surgery, and possibly less if the experimental surgery is found to be ineffective [8, 10]. They conclude that risk should be minimized within the context of answering the scientific question. The arthroscopy trial is a good example of minimizing harm within the context of the study. Participants randomized to the placebo group were not placed under general anesthesia or intubated and received only three 1-cm skin incisions, and were thus subjected to a less-invasive procedure than the intervention groups [11].

The second issue pertains to analyzing and comparing the risks and benefits of the proposed research, particularly with respect to the risk to the subjects in the placebo group. Here, the opposing viewpoints differ in weighing the risk to the individual versus either that individual's potential benefit or the potential benefit in terms of the knowledge to be gained. In Macklin's analysis of the Parkinson's trial from the individual standpoint, the risk–benefit ratio is at best uncertain and at worst unfavorable [6]. However, others consider the benefit more in terms of the knowledge to be gained, and the potential number of future ineffective surgeries avoided, thus ultimately reducing risks for many [9, 12]. Some authors even suggest considering the expected benefit of the placebo surgery rather than considering only the surgical risks [13]. While there is consensus that the risk of the placebo procedure should be reduced as much as possible without sacrificing the validity of the experimental design, there is little agreement among ethicists on how to decide when the potential benefits outweigh the risks. This is further complicated by the variability in severity of proposed placebo procedures that can range from superficial skin incisions to drilling holes in participants' skulls.

The third issue in Macklin's critique considers whether informed consent in studies using sham procedures is adequate to protect the patient's interests. One point is that informed consent is necessary, but not sufficient for research to be considered ethical. Institutional review boards (IRB) are charged with judging whether the risks are justified by potential benefits and could decide in some cases that they are not, even with consent. A more troubling concern is whether participants are truly capable of rationally providing informed consent to a sham procedure. There is some evidence that patients who seem to have been properly consented do not understand their role in the study. Macklin notes "In one study, people who had been research subjects told interviewers that they had trusted their doctors, believed that their physicians would do nothing to harm them, and thought that the physician–researchers had always acted in their best medical interests." Macklin further reports that patients in the Parkinson's study were told that if randomized to the sham procedure, they would be offered the intervention if it proved to be effective. Ultimately, the intervention resulted in more serious adverse events than expected and was not offered. When told they would not be able to receive the real intervention, some participants expressed anger rather than relief that they had been spared a possibly dangerous and ineffective procedure.

Trials with placebo procedures may subject participants to a problematic degree of deception beyond disclosing the randomized and blinded design at the time of consent. In the Parkinson's study, the surgeon asked patients undergoing the sham tissue transplantation "Are you ready for the implant now?" This active deception, even in the context of the study, could mislead patients into thinking that they had actually received the intervention despite the randomized design. This highlights variability among sham procedures. Such a statement would not be relevant in the arthroscopy trial where all procedures were done with the participant under sedation or anesthesia. The Parkinson's study could also have used more neutral terminology asking instead 'Are you ready to proceed' to minimize any specific deception. It is thus unclear whether participants truly understand their role in the study, the possibility that the procedure received may not be in their best interest, and the full extent of blinding. Thus, even seemingly satisfactory informed consent procedures may fail to ensure that participants understand the risks and benefits of the study.

Practical Considerations and Guidelines

In 2002 the Council on Ethical and Judicial Affairs of the American Medical Association published a report titled "Surgical 'placebo' controls" in the Annals of Surgery which gave a cogent overview of the ethical and practical considerations and provided a five-point recommendation [9].

First: A placebo surgery should be considered only when no other experimental design could provide the necessary evidence. It recognizes that placebo or sham procedures are ethically controversial, to be used only when truly necessary.

Second: Particular attention should be paid to the informed consent process. The risks of procedures should be carefully explained, and the randomized design emphasized. This should carefully explain the differences between study arms along with the importance of blinding and the fact that the participant should not know which treatment was received. Additional measures may be employed to ensure that consent is truly informed, such as an additional neutral witness or a trained monitor present during the consent process. The arthroscopy trial went so far as to require that consenting participants write the following statement in their own chart: "On entering this study, I realize that I may receive only placebo surgery. I further realize that this means that I will not have surgery on my knee joint. This placebo surgery will not benefit my knee arthritis" [11]. In that trial only 44% of patients consented to participate suggesting that the consent process was effective. The fact that among each of the three study arms approximately 13% of participants thought they had received the placebo procedure demonstrates both that the blinding was effective and that even with stringent informed consent procedures participants may still tend to overestimate the likelihood that they will receive the experimental treatment.

Third: The use of a surgical placebo is not justified when the experimental procedure being tested is a modification of an already accepted procedure. In this case the suitable control group is the accepted procedure. An example would be comparing robotic surgery versus laparoscopy for a standard procedure or inguinal hernia repair with and without mesh.

Fourth: A surgical placebo group may be considered when testing an experimental procedure to treat a condition that has no accepted surgical treatment or to test an accepted surgery when its efficacy has come into question. However, this is only appropriate when the relevant outcomes are likely to be susceptible to the placebo effect and the risks of the placebo procedure are relatively minor. As a general rule, outcomes that can respond to the placebo effect tend to be patient self-reported outcomes such as pain, or other related outcomes such as functional tests, which can be influenced by patient's perceptions and expectations. This can also extend to physiological measures like blood pressure [14]. Determining whether the risks of the placebo procedure are sufficiently low requires careful thought and is ultimately subjective. The case of the arthroscopy trial where the placebo procedure involved three small skin incisions and minimized anesthesia risks presents a clear case of low risk. On the other hand, in the Parkinson's trial, the placebo procedure was more invasive, potentially pushing the boundary of acceptable risk. Whether a placebo surgery can be designed to maintain blinding and to have an acceptably low risk will depend on the procedure being tested. In the case of a complicated procedure with a prolonged recovery time, it may not be feasible.

Fifth: When there is an acceptable and effective nonsurgical treatment and withholding or forgoing that treatment could cause injury, then the nonsurgical treatment should be offered to all arms of the surgical trial. This is consistent with both the conduct of the Parkinson's trial where standard medical therapy was continued throughout the trial.

Conclusion

There is ample evidence that surgical patients can experience a placebo effect, and that this placebo effect may be even more pronounced than for a medical placebo. Some previously accepted, and seemingly effective, surgical procedures have been shown in placebo-controlled trials to be no more effective than a sham procedure. Therefore, a rigorous evaluation of the efficacy of some surgical procedures will require a carefully designed randomized trial where the control arm includes a placebo or sham procedure and appropriate blinding to account for the placebo effect. Nevertheless, although the 'best' experimental design may require a placebo surgery, the fact that any surgery causes some harm and increases the risk to control participants raises ethical concerns that must be addressed to justify the use of a placebo procedure. For a placebo-controlled surgical trial, there must be no surgical treatment that is known to be superior to placebo and there must be true equipoise between the experimental and placebo procedures. The use of placebo controls in surgical trials requires increased attention to designing a placebo procedure to maintain blinding while minimizing risk, along with scrupulous attention to the informed consent process.

References

1. Holtedahl R, Brox JI, Tjomsland O. Placebo effects in trials evaluating 12 selected minimally invasive interventions: a systematic review and meta-analysis. BMJ Open. 2015;5(1): e007331.
2. Wartolowska K, Judge A, Hopewell S, Collins GS, Dean BJ, Rombach I, Brindley D, Savulescu J, Beard DJ, Carr AJ. Use of placebo controls in the evaluation of surgery: systematic review. BMJ. 2014;348:g3253.

3. Schulz KF, Grimes DA. Blinding in randomised trials: hiding who got what. Lancet. 2002;359(9307):696–700.
4. Kaptchuk TJ, Goldman P, Stone DA, Stason WB. Do medical devices have enhanced placebo effects? J Clin Epidemiol. 2000;53(8):786–92.
5. Kaptchuk TJ, Stason WB, Davis RB, Legedza AR, Schnyer RN, Kerr CE, Stone DA, Nam BH, Kirsch I, Goldman RH. Sham device v inert pill: randomised controlled trial of two placebo treatments. BMJ. 2006;332(7538):391–7.
6. Macklin R. The ethical problems with sham surgery in clinical research. N Engl J Med. 1999;341(13):992–6.
7. Stolberg SG. Ideas & trends; sham surgery returns as a research tool. The New York Times. 1999.
8. Rogers W, Hutchison K, Skea ZC, Campbell MK. Strengthening the ethical assessment of placebo-controlled surgical trials: three proposals. BMC Med Ethics. 2014;15:78.
9. Tenery R, Rakatansky H, Riddick FA Jr, Goldrich MS, Morse LJ, O'Bannon JM 3rd, Ray P, Smalley S, Weiss M, Kao A, Morin K, Maixner A, Seiden S. Surgical "placebo" controls. Ann Surg. 2002;235(2):303–7.
10. George AJT, Collett C, Carr A, Holm S, Bale C, Burton S, Campbell MK, Coles A, Gottlieb G, Muir K, Parroy S, Price J, Rice ASC, Sinden J, Stephenson C, Wartolowska K, Whittall H. When should placebo surgery as a control in clinical trials be carried out? Bull Royal Coll Surg Engl. 2016;98(2):75–9.
11. Moseley JB, O'Malley K, Petersen NJ, Menke TJ, Brody BA, Kuykendall DH, Hollingsworth JC, Ashton CM, Wray NP. A controlled trial of arthroscopic surgery for osteoarthritis of the knee. N Engl J Med. 2002;347(2):81–8.
12. Miller FG. Sham surgery: an ethical analysis. Sci Eng Ethics. 2004;10(1):157–66.
13. Brim RL, Miller FG. The potential benefit of the placebo effect in sham-controlled trials: implications for risk-benefit assessments and informed consent. J Med Ethics. 2013;39(11):703–7.
14. Bhatt DL, Kandzari DE, O'Neill WW, D'Agostino R, Flack JM, Katzen BT, Leon MB, Liu M, Mauri L, Negoita M, Cohen SA, Oparil S, Rocha-Singh K, Townsend RR, Bakris GL, Investigators SH-. A controlled trial of renal denervation for resistant hypertension. N Engl J Med. 2014;370(15):1393–401.

Chapter 30
Patient Recruitment and Retention in Procedural Trials

Drew Moghanaki and Tomer Z. Karas

Introduction

Invasive procedures for human disease are often pioneered during eras when there are no better options. Over time, they commonly evolve to become the standard of care for years, decades, or even generations. Historical examples include Halsted's radical mastectomy for breast cancer, or Billroth's gastric antrectomy for peptic ulcer disease. Even though these treatments may have been associated with high rates of morbidity and mortality, they were widely accepted as the optimal treatment at that time due to a lack of more effective alternatives.

Fortunately, the field of medicine is rarely static and newer treatments are commonly explored. Once their promise is demonstrated, they might even become widely available without randomized trials. When this happens, debates often ensue over the role of the newer procedure with regards to its degree of benefit, or even equivalence, when compared to the established standard. Eventually, efforts to compare the outcomes of newer procedures with historical controls are undertaken. However, the results are commonly rejected given the limitations of retrospective study designs. As a consequence, disagreements about the ideal standard of care can become polarizing, particularly when newer procedures are resource intensive. The controversies might be amplified only further when the livelihood of practitioners who deliver the older standard may be in jeopardy.

D. Moghanaki (✉)
Radiation Oncology Service, Hunter Holmes McGuire VA Medical Center,
1201 Broad Rock Blvd, Richmond, VA 23249, USA
e-mail: drew.moghanaki@va.gov

T.Z. Karas
Surgical Service, Bruce W. Carter VA Healthcare System, Miami,
1201 NW 16 Street (112), Miami, FL 33125, USA
e-mail: tomer.karas@va.gov

© Springer International Publishing AG 2017
K.M.F. Itani and D.J. Reda (eds.), *Clinical Trials Design in Operative and Non Operative Invasive Procedures*, DOI 10.1007/978-3-319-53877-8_30

259

Nonetheless, inspired by the opportunity to generate high quality scientific evidence to guide clinical recommendations, phase III trials are often designed to resolve questions about the advantages of newer procedures. They are admirable in their endeavor, but studies that aim to enroll patients in randomized procedural studies are often difficult to complete. The primary reasons relate to clinician and patient biases that contribute to concerns, albeit at times irrational, about random assignments to disparate treatments. That is, preferences and prejudices among both clinicians and patients commonly interfere with the concept of equipoise. This can occur even when the greater medical community accepts the uncertainty of differences in outcomes between the treatments being studied. Fortunately, increasing a clinical trial team's awareness of these challenges, and reviewing strategies that can optimize recruitment, can be helpful to facilitate the success of any randomized clinical trial that compares a promising new treatment to an older established standard of care.

Clinician Preferences and Biases

Clinicians may not always endorse the idea of recruiting patients to a randomized trial that challenges a well-accepted standard of care. An unwillingness to support ongoing studies is often observed even among individuals who had provided verbal or written agreements to participate. Common reasons typically relate to personal biases about the newer investigational, or the older control treatment.

To be fair, it is only natural for clinicians to develop a fondness for a given treatment, particularly if it is widely accepted and one they have mastered to deliver. However, these preferences can become engrained and difficult to influence by the time newer treatments emerge. They might even persist in the face of evidence that suggests alternative approaches might be better for patient outcomes. It is valuable to recognize that such dismissive behaviors are not always made consciously. Instead, a bias for established paradigms is a well-recognized human tendency [1]. It has been studied by behavioral scientists and found to be particularly noticeable under conditions of uncertainty when the evidence that supports a new idea is unfamiliar. As the Nobel laureate Daniel Kahneman has described, individuals commonly prefer mental shortcuts to beliefs that are more readily recalled whenever a new idea requires intellectual processing. This behavior, referred to more formally as an "availability heuristic," is often exacerbated in medicine when a clinician's influences are limited to discussions at medical conferences within their own specialty, reading journals that echo common beliefs, and communication with like-minded peers.

Clinicians may also have cognitive biases that sustain opposition to new ideas, even after there is increased awareness about the potential advantages of a novel treatment. One example that can be observed among those who are used to delivering a standard of care procedure is referred to as "choice-supportive bias" [2]. It is described as a behavior where an individual's decisions are believed to be more ideal because they are the one recommending it. With limited insight, this can contribute to an "overconfidence effect" that clouds judgment even when objective information exceeds the accuracy of their subjective beliefs.

In addition to personal uncertainties about the potential advantages of a new treatment, the influences of financial remuneration also deserve attention. These relate to scenarios where clinical trials are undertaken in fee-for-service healthcare systems. In these settings, trials that randomize patients to treatments that are offered by different clinical teams typically present a risk for lost revenue that might affect daily clinical operations. Consequently, clinicians who are offered opportunities to participate in a randomized clinical trial often face tough financial decisions and may prefer to decline participation. There are no simple remedies for this dilemma, unless clinicians are salaried or share revenue with others participating in the trial.

Patient Preferences and Biases

While it is critical to recognize the biases of participating clinicians, it is equally important to understand the potential prejudices that may influence patients' willingness to enroll. Several major influences are highlighted below, with solutions for each provided later in this chapter.

The Idea of a Clinical Trial Can Be Overwhelming

This is even before the concept of randomization is introduced. When patients first learn about their treatment options, they are usually still concerned with understanding the nature of their illness. Once addressed, they may prefer to focus on learning whether or not there is a need for treatment in the first place. Next, they frequently seek to learn what additional options might be available, how other people are usually treated, and then focus on the hope that they are eligible to receive the "standard of care" treatment. The amount of information that is gathered is often overwhelming and difficult to process, particularly among those without a background in healthcare. Patients with low health literacy levels are even more daunted. They may seek clarification during their healthcare visits, but often forget to ask their questions in front of their clinicians. Worse, there may be insufficient time in a busy clinical environment to have all of their questions answered.

Thus, it comes as no surprise that patients who are approached about participation in a clinical trial often struggle with the idea, particularly if they have never heard about this option previously. The concept can be obtuse, especially if it is introduced only after standard treatment options have been reviewed. This is because the idea of anything "alternative" might simply be too difficult to comprehend. Some may even develop the misconception that they will be the "guinea pig" subject of an experiment that concerns itself with benefits to the medical community without regard to the patients themselves. Whenever any of these concerns arise, cognitive dissonance may paralyze a patient's decision making capacity to consider enrollment in a trial that is presented as "optional." Patients may seek to simplify the situation by redirecting discussions to just learn about what people normally receive (i.e., the standard of care). In this situation, efforts by clinicians to provide more information about the investigational strategy are rarely helpful, unless time is taken to appreciate the patients' level of health literacy and develop a thorough understanding of the patients' beliefs and values.

Patients May Have a Prejudice for More, or Less, Invasive Treatments

As with clinicians, patients also have preconceived notions that influence their decisions. For example, they may have for years thought that more, or less invasive treatments, were a better overall approach in medical care. Some may prefer invasive procedures that are aggressive and definitive, whereas others may be terrified about undergoing major surgery even if the less invasive alternative is presented as less effective [3]. Next, if they have a life-threatening condition and the current standard of care does not offer much hope, they may actually prefer the experimental treatment and reject the idea of anything standard. As a result, patients may develop a preference for one of the study treatment arms, particularly if the risks are dissimilar. Some may even guide their decisions on the opportunity to be the one who chooses their treatment, as this preserves the perception of control over their care.

Patients Are Commonly at Risk for Misinformation About Clinical Trials

A less commonly recognized reason that patients decline participation in clinical trials relates to their exposure to inaccurate information upstream of recruitment. By the time patients are approached to participate in a clinical trial, they have typically had multiple discussions with various individuals about how best to manage their disease. Well-intended clinicians along the referral pathway often spend considerable amounts of time teaching patients about the current standard of care, particularly if unfamiliar with the option of an available trial.

In addition to misinformation from referring physicians, patients are also at risk for receiving misguided advice from nonclinical staff or other patients, commonly in waiting rooms. For those without acquaintances in healthcare, they may even turn to help from neighbors, friends, and family who often resort to anecdotal personal stories without sufficient details. Patients may have had exposure to a documentary about their condition, though the investigational treatment they are being offered is usually too new to have been covered. Brief television stories might provide an introduction in the realm of clinical trials, but rarely yield meaningful insights. Patients may seek information from print, Internet websites, or blogs, but are often unsophisticated in their ability to discern peer reviewed and accurate information from opinion and hearsay.

Strategies to Improve Recruitment and Retention

Fortunately, most patients seek and rely upon the advice of their clinicians for guidance. They are often willing to learn about the potential advantages of each treatment offered in a trial, and usually acknowledge that they lack sufficient background to independently choose one treatment or the other. When a study is presented in a balanced manner, patients commonly recognize that the clinicians' equipoise is based simply on not knowing which treatment is better and that the current clinical trial is underway to determine just that. Furthermore, they are commonly reassured to learn that studies have ethical oversight so that they will not be treated as "guinea pigs." Patients actually often agree to enroll in trials simply for the opportunity to help future patients with similar illnesses. With awareness of personal biases and the risks of misinformation, the following recommendations are offered to help overcome the aforementioned challenges commonly encountered during the recruitment of patients onto randomized procedural trials:

1. **Assure clinician buy-in**. It is always important to be aware of participating clinicians' biases whenever a clinical trial compares different treatments. When the treatments entail different specialties, then the potential influences of specialty biases should be addressed. When it becomes difficult to get buy-in from recruiting physicians, it may be beneficial to add an unbiased physician from another related field to the study team. For example, in comparing lung cancer resection to stereotactic radiation, a pulmonologist or medical oncologist who performs neither procedure, but has a deep understanding of the pathology, would be an ideal "non-combatant." Their neutral position might lend an opportunity to facilitate more meaningful discussions about equipoise since they might not have any "skin in the game." When such neutral parties double as referring physicians, they may also have useful insights into the nuances and biases of clinicians along referral pathways, and can thus help with designing a recruitment strategy. Furthermore, these clinicians will be better poised to introduce the trial to their patients at earlier opportunities along the recruitment pathways.
   Another issue that can help with recruitment is addressing the potential impact of lost revenue when patients might be randomized to receive treatment by different physicians. One might consider opportunities for revenue sharing, something that might require discussions with department chairmen and/or

financial officers. It is recognized that a study team might ultimately be unable to resolve recruiting clinicians' concerns about remuneration. If identified, it might be important to stop and recognize that recruitment is unlikely to be successful in such a clinical environment. In this situation, the study team might consider conducting the trial within salaried healthcare systems such as the Department of Veterans Affairs, Kaiser Permanente, or Mayo Clinics which typically do not build in financial incentives to treat.

2. **Establish group equipoise along referral pathways**. As discussed above, patients are commonly curious about their illness and may seek information from multiple sources. Subsequently, patients will be more likely to enroll when equipoise is preserved throughout the entire recruitment pathway. Thus, it is important for the study team to reach out to those who counsel potential study participants upstream of recruitment since they can impact patients' willingness to participate in a clinical trial. As this often includes nonphysicians, as well as nonclinical staff, study teams should consider reaching out to any individual in the healthcare system from whom a patient may seek advice. Mapping out the potential referral pathways is a useful starting point to identify and query individuals who may often have an influence. Investigators will often identify individuals who are not up to date on the clinical question being studied. This offers an opportunity to develop targeted education strategies that are typically more effective when discussed in person. It also helps curate additional educational strategies that can include lectures in individual departments or grand rounds. These efforts are often productive, but may need to be repeated regularly, particularly in settings where staff turnover may be high or the clinical issue being studied is relatively uncommon.

3. **Approach patients in a manner that emphasizes building trust**. This might be one of the most important elements that help with recruitment. Kindness, empathy, and the simple skill of listening to patient concerns are some of the most valuable skills that can build the trust needed for a patient to accept the idea of enrollment in a clinical trial. However, to build trust, it is important for patients to have easy access to the study team. Thus, it is valuable to provide patients with a point of contact, such as a research coordinator, who can be readily reached whenever a patient has questions about the study. This can be particularly helpful when patients are overwhelmed with too much information and have questions that they may otherwise turn to their friends, family, or the Internet for answers. By opening direct channels for communication, coordinators can help patients rest assured that the clinical trial is designed to identify the best treatment for them, and that both treatments are thought to be beneficial for them.

4. **Utilize educational strategies that are patient-centric**. Recent and ongoing research has led to the development of decision aids that help patients understand complicated clinical information. At times, these tools may even be used to recruit patients to a clinical trial. It is unclear how helpful each can be for a given patient, given individuals have a wide array of learning styles. For example, some prefer simplified summaries whereas others seek more rigorous evidence. Many patients dislike written materials and prefer direct dialog with their clinicians. Meanwhile,

certain novel decision aids such as the Question Prompt Lists for Clinical Trials (QPL-CT) might be particularly helpful [4]. The QPL-CT is a validated instrument that provides patients with 33 questions in 11 categories to select from before meeting with clinicians to learn about the option of enrollment in a clinical trial. A shorter 22 item version is currently under development. Each of the questions in the QPL-CT covers sensitive and difficult topics such as prognosis, diagnosis, issues surrounding end of life care, improved outcomes, and human subjects' protection. It helps empower patients to seek information that is most important for them. It consequently reduces time spent on topics that may be boring, discomforting, or of less value to a particular patient.

5. **Consider strategies that safeguard patients from bias.** It is often considered that treating physicians will be more successful with recruitment to a clinical trial if they temper their enthusiasm about any one particular treatment. It is thus more useful to present a more balanced view of the risks and benefits of each. If they take a lead to foster such equipoise among their staff, they can even energize a research team to be more effective with accrual. However, there is always a risk that subjective biases may creep back into the subconscious thinking process of recruiting physicians, particularly if they are the ones delivering the protocol-defined treatment. Even when subliminal, any perceived loss of equipoise can negatively impact clinical staff and patients' willingness to participate [5, 6]. Thus, it might be valuable to consider recruitment strategies that minimize this risk of treating clinicians' biases.

A recent series of phase III clinical trials that each aimed to answer a similar research question, but all closed prematurely due to poor accrual, provides valuable insight into the risk of clinician biases as well as the aforementioned challenges. Each trial was designed to randomize operable early stage lung cancer patients between surgical resection and stereotactic radiotherapy; however, accrual was very poor. It was noted retrospectively that patients were typically recruited in thoracic surgery clinics, commonly after they had completed their evaluations and had been found to be eligible for surgery, the current standard of care. Clinical trial monitors had identified that patients were typically eager to learn if they would be eligible for surgery, and were uncomfortable with a last minute option to be randomized to something different. It was also found that at times the clinical trial was discussed as a less attractive option since it might randomize patients to a "non-standard" treatment. Following the lessons learned, a new generation of randomized trials were eventually opened with modified recruitment strategies. The current ongoing studies that aim to randomize early stage lung cancer patients between surgical resection and stereotactic radiotherapy include the STABLE-MATES (NCT02468024), SABRTooTH (NCT02629458), and VALOR (NCT02984761) trials. Each uses a more patient-centric recruitment model, as described below.

The recruitment schema for STABLE-MATES utilizes a pre-randomization technique where patients are randomized to either treatment prior to their consent in a process known as the Zelen design. The main goal is to minimize the cognitive demand required for patients to learn about each treatment, and to protect them from having to weigh the options of two or more different treatments. In this study design, patients are randomized before they learn about the study. Once approached, they are given the choice to accept the assigned treatment, or receive treatment off-protocol. If they agree, they next meet with either their thoracic surgeon and/or radiation oncologist to learn about the treatment they were randomized to receive. They may be informed about the alternative treatment, but may not necessarily see the other specialist.

In a similar fashion, the SABRTooTH study safeguards patients from specialty biases all together by restricting contact with thoracic surgeons and/or radiation oncologists until pulmonologists can complete the consent and randomization process. As in the STABLE-MATES study, patients will only need to see the clinician who will deliver the treatment they are randomly assigned to receive. Alternatively, the VALOR study team focuses on building trust between patients and the entire study team. As a part of this, the study coordinators actually disclose that the patients may experience bias. Following an initial consent process, research navigators help to foster equipoise between the two treatments, and counsel patients before each mandatory clinical appointment with their thoracic surgeon and radiation oncologist. They even offer an opportunity to accompany them at these visits. Throughout the screening process, they serve as a direct point of contact to help with scheduling and coordinating appointments. This affords an opportunity to provide ongoing emotional support during the difficult times faced by any patient with a new diagnosis of lung cancer.

The benefit of close engagement with study coordinators was demonstrated in the ProtecT trial from the UK that successfully randomized 1643 prostate cancer patients between surgery, radiotherapy, and active monitoring [7]. Through early engagement of patients with research nurses, even before PSA screening, the study ultimately randomized 62% of its eligible patients [8]. This exceeded the 15% accrual rate in the similar PIVOT randomized trial of prostatectomy versus watchful waiting that recruited patients once they were diagnosed [9].

6. **Consider continuous learning strategies**. Despite extensive efforts to address the predicted challenges of any clinical trial, it is common for unidentified issues to arise only after it is activated. For this reason, it is advised that research teams meet frequently to share their insights with recruitment. Study team leaders should routinely solicit feedback from as many individuals as possible. This can include clinicians upstream of recruitment, as well as patients themselves willing to provide their perspectives. The short list of strategies, as summarized in Table 30.1, can provide a framework for each meeting. In trials conducted at multiple centers, strategies from successful (high-recruiting) centers can be shared with centers that have been less successful in an ongoing process to augment accrual rates. For such an approach to be successful, it will be important for the entire study team to remain agile. In this way, a committed flexibility to adapt one's recruitment strategies will allow the team to more readily address any unforeseen challenges to make changes in a timely manner.

Table 30.1 Strategies to optimize recruitment

1. Assure clinician buy-in
2. Establish group equipoise along referral pathways
3. Approach patients in a manner that emphasizes building trust
4. Utilize educational strategies that are patient-centric
5. Sustain strategies that safeguards patients from bias
6. Include continuous learning strategies

Conclusions

The enrollment of patients into randomized procedural trials commonly faces challenges that are related to biases and prejudices of both physicians and patients. Further complicating matters is the risk of misinformation that clouds judgment along the recruitment pathway. The success of any trial may therefore hinge upon strategies to address these potential interferences, such as those provided in this chapter.

References

1. Kahneman D. Thinking, fast and slow. 1st pbk. ed. New York: Farrar, Straus and Giroux. 2013.
2. Mather M, Johnson MK. Choice-supportive source monitoring: do our decisions seem better to us as we age? Psychol Aging. 2000;15:596–606.
3. McNeil BJ, Weichselbaum R, Pauker SG. Fallacy of the five-year survival in lung cancer. N Engl J Med. 1978;299:1397–401.
4. Brown RF, Bylund CL, Li Y, Edgerson S, Butow PN. Testing the utility of a cancer clinical trial specific Question Prompt List (QPL-CT) during oncology consultations. Patient Educ Couns. 2011;88:311–7.
5. Huddart RA, Hall E, Lewis R, Birtle A. Life and death of spare (selective bladder preservation against radical excision): reflections on why the spare trial closed. BJU Int. 2010;106:753–5.
6. Van Schil PE, Van Meerbeeck J. Surgery or radiotherapy for early-stage lung cancer—a potential comparison bias. Lancet Oncol. 2013;14:e390.
7. Hamdy FC, Donovan JL, Lane JA, et al. 10-Year outcomes after monitoring, surgery, or radiotherapy for localized prostate cancer. N Engl J Med. 2016;375:1415–24.
8. Lane JA, Donovan JL, Davis M, et al. Active monitoring, radical prostatectomy, or radiotherapy for localised prostate cancer: study design and diagnostic and baseline results of the ProtecT randomised phase 3 trial. Lancet Oncol. 2014;15:1109–18.
9. Wilt TJ, Brawer MK, Barry MJ, et al. The Prostate cancer Intervention Versus Observation Trial:VA/NCI/AHRQ Cooperative Studies Program #407 (PIVOT): design and baseline results of a randomized controlled trial comparing radical prostatectomy to watchful waiting for men with clinically localized prostate cancer. Contemp Clin Trials. 2009;30:81–7.

Chapter 31
Equipoise in Interventional Trials

Judy C. Boughey

Equipoise in Interventional Trials

Introduction to Equipoise

The principle of equipoise is the ethical basis for clinical trial research involving randomized patient assignment to different treatments. Clinical equipoise means that there is an uncertainty in the expert medical community about whether one treatment is superior to the other treatment. The term clinical equipoise was first used by Benjamin Freedman in 1987. Equipoise is critical from an ethical standpoint as it would be an ethical dilemma for an investigator to design or randomize a patient to a clinical trial where they have evidence or conviction that the intervention in one of the trial arms is superior to the other. Thus, the basis for randomized clinical trial design requires that there is no decisive evidence that the intervention being studied is superior or inferior to the alternative intervention or lack of intervention.

Definitions of Equipoise

Equipoise is the situation where the intervention and the comparison group are not known to be superior or inferior to each other. This applies both for the control and experimental group and is a key requirement for a randomized controlled trial (RCT). A true state of equipoise exists when there is no good basis for a choice

J.C. Boughey (✉)
Department of Surgery, Mayo Clinic, 200 First Street SW,
Rochester, MN 55905, USA
e-mail: Boughey.judy@mayo.edu

© Springer International Publishing AG 2017   269
K.M.F. Itani and D.J. Reda (eds.), *Clinical Trials Design in Operative
and Non Operative Invasive Procedures*, DOI 10.1007/978-3-319-53877-8_31

between the two or more treatment options being evaluated. Thus, there exists a true state of uncertainty, also known as an honest null hypothesis.

It has been debated as to who should have equipoise in the design of clinical trials. To some, the individual doctors being genuinely unsure which treatment is best for the patient, thus, following the uncertainty principle is felt to be acceptable for randomization in a clinical trial. To others, the level of "clinical equipoise" requires collective professional uncertainty regarding the intervention and is felt to be the strongest ethical criteria. In essence, society believes that uncertainty regarding the interventions is necessary for a randomized trial; the point of discussion being whether it is based on the uncertainty of the individual physician or group uncertainty across the medical community/experts.

Personal equipoise refers to the beliefs of the medical provider and exists when the physician involved in the research study has no preference or is truly uncertain about the overall benefit or harm offered by the two treatments available for their patient. If a physician believes, thinks he knows or has good reason to believe that a certain intervention is better than an alternative therapy, he cannot ethically participate in the comparative trial and will not be successful in discussing this randomized trial with patients. Ethically, the physician is obligated to provide the best recommendation to each of his patients. The definition of clinical equipoise, which is genuine uncertainty within the expert medical community regarding the intervention, allows conduct of randomized controlled trials as the equipoise is defined to be across the expert medical community and not necessarily on the part of the individual physician treating the patient. In this situation, the physician can approach the patient for participation in a clinical trial; although, if the investigator has a strong enough bias, a balanced discussion with the patient is less likely and the patient is most likely to feel comfortable enrolling in the clinical trial.

Clinical equipoise is defined as uncertainty across a group of experts who honestly are not in agreement regarding which intervention is superior. The choice of an adequate comparative control is an important aspect of clinical trial design to address the clinical equipoise question. Clinical equipoise is evaluated and vested during the review of a protocol which often requires a rigorous review by multiple committees such as through the National Cancer Institute cooperative group mechanism and other national trial networks and multicenter mechanisms. This review process ensures that across national experts there is true uncertainty about the superiority of one intervention versus another and does not allow clinical trials that contain highly biased proposals to move forward; thus, protecting patients from a randomized controlled trial where one arm contains an inferior treatment. At the level of the individual physician supporting the clinical trial, the discussion between the treating physician and the patient is important and in situations where the physician believes that one treatment is superior to the other, often the clinical trial may not be proposed to the patient or in the process of the discussion, the patient may sense the treating physician's bias or preference for one of the treatment arms and therefore decide not to enroll in the clinical trial but elect to be treated with the intervention that the physician feels is the superior option.

Equipoise Must Be Continually Assessed Throughout the Trial

The importance of clinical equipoise in interventional trials is also reflected in the importance of a data safety monitoring board (DSMB) and annual continuing reviews by the IRBs, such that if during the conduct of the trial sufficient evidence is obtained to demonstrate that the intervention being tested or the lack of intervention is superior or inferior, this would result in the trial being suspended and the superior intervention recommended for all patients. Annual review of ongoing clinical trials is also important to ensure that the clinical equipoise related to the question being studied is maintained and that additional data is not available from other studies conducted across the country or internationally that would impact the status of equipoise regarding the intervention being tested.

Clinical equipoise with uncertainty across the expert community allows conduct of a clinical trial up until the point that enough evidence is obtained that documents a superiority of one arm over the other. This reflects the importance of the data safety monitoring board as an independent body to review the ongoing results of the clinical trial and recommend to the trial sponsor that the trial be discontinued at any time point should data reflect that one arm is statistically superior to the other arm of the clinical trial [1].

Importance of Equipoise for Patients and Clinical Trial Accrual

The success of randomized clinical trials is highly dependent on patient enrollment. From a patient's perspective, when considering enrollment in the clinical trials, patients look for and expect a guarantee they will not knowingly receive an inferior treatment or knowingly be harmed, and that with participation in the clinical trial, they have the opportunity to receive the most favorable treatments available. The status of equipoise regarding the interventions in a clinical trial makes it easier for physicians to discuss clinical trials with patients and makes it easier for patients to consider participation in these clinical trials.

With equipoise being a crucial component of all randomized controlled trials, patient enrollment in clinical trials is easier and additionally institutional review boards are able to approve the study. With patient enrollment and IRB approval, a clinical trial can be successfully conducted, allowing discovery and/or validation of new interventions. If the chances of treatment success are too high or too low, patients would be reluctant to enroll in the clinical trials and would prefer to be managed outside of the clinical trial with the superior intervention. In this setting, advancement of clinical practice would be hindered and new interventions or technologies would not be discovered or validated.

Equipoise and Clinical Trial Success

With appropriate equipoise in the trial design, by definition in a randomized clinical trial, the chances of success with a new intervention across all trials should be 50:50 (one to one). However, by definition, the fact that the optimal treatment success rate is 50:50, indicates that a significant portion of clinical trials will have negative findings and limits the proportion of breakthrough interventions that ultimately change this clinical practice. By definition, there are limits to the advances that can be made and ultimately across all clinical trials success rate is expected to be around 50 percent. It is because the progress in surgery and interventional procedures often rests on data from prospective randomized trials to validate the feasibility, safety, and efficacy of the intervention that the ability to design a clinical trial with equipoise in the intervention is critical to enable patients willingly to participate in these interventional trials [2].

Challenges for Surgical and Interventional Trials

Treatments in general surgery are half as likely to be based on randomized controlled trial evidence as treatments in internal medicine. This is due to many factors. Many of the current operations were introduced well before randomized trials became established in medicine, unlike many modern drugs which have been developed in a far more recent era. Additionally, evaluation and acceptance of new surgical procedures do not fall under FDA regulation, unless the procedure involves use of a device or other regulated aspects of treatment. Thus, new surgical techniques can come into widespread use with less formal evidence of safety and efficacy than is provided by a randomized clinical trial. Once a surgical procedure/intervention is accepted into clinical practice as standard care, testing this intervention against placebo (withholding intervention) becomes difficult. In essence, due to the long history of surgical intervention and limited regulatory authority for many surgical conditions, the basis of a surgical standard for many diseases has been established in the absence of randomized clinical trials. However, although it was established in the absence of clinical trials, it is now no longer ethical to study the benefit of the surgical procedure against placebo in a randomized trial.

One example of such situation would be the role of appendectomy for patients with appendicitis. This is probably one of the most long-standing operations performed by general surgeons and thus when a patient presents with appendicitis, the standard of care is an operative appendectomy. Currently, this surgical dogma is beginning to be challenged with consideration of antibiotics and avoiding surgical intervention. Although to many this seems like a step back, it is an important question to assess. Equipoise in this situation has been challenging, although with increasing reports from small series on patient outcome from management with oral antibiotics without operative intervention, the clinical equipoise is being established as the basis for a randomized controlled trial.

There are also additional challenges for clinical trials in invasive operative and nonoperative procedures with a significant one being the lack of funding since pharmaceutical companies tend to invest in clinical trials evaluating the performance of drugs; however, the availability of funding for interventional-based trials is more limited. Many of these interventions that should be studied involve changes in the technique of the intervention and manufacturers of devices are often less interested in financially supporting this kind of study.

Interventional procedures and operations are complex procedures and are all associated with a training curve. Thus, the quality of the performance of a surgical procedure/intervention changes with the degree of experience of the operator. Quality performance requires frequent repetition over time. Thus, it is not feasible to randomize between a familiar operation that a surgeon has been performing for many years and an unfamiliar operation which is a completely new procedure for the surgeon. This would introduce bias against the new procedure as the quality outcomes would improve with repetition of performing the procedure multiple times over and over. Therefore, the best way to approach randomization between two interventions is to ensure that the procedures, in both arms are performed by surgeons/interventionalists that are comfortable and competent with both procedures, having performed them both multiple times and being comfortable with good outcomes from this procedure. In some trials comparing surgical procedures, the same surgeon at a study site is not required to perform both procedures. Rather the surgeon who had adequate experience with either procedure could perform that procedure in the trial.

Surgeons are more likely than internal medicine physicians to have levels of pre-existing bias favoring particular intervention or treatment approaches. Surgeons are less likely to be consciously uncertain which of two treatments is better. This is a nature of the personality of most surgeons and that surgeons are comfortable making important decisions quickly, sometimes with incomplete information as is required in the operative setting.

Surgeons in general appear more comfortable recruiting patients for cancer chemotherapy trials but are often more reluctant to enroll patient in trials evaluating surgical techniques. The multiple challenges related to interventional/surgical trials are reflected by the relatively low number of surgical/interventional trials. Taking surgical oncology, for example, surgical oncology research represents only 9% of all cancer research and of the published surgical oncology research only 6% is clinical trials [3]. There has been a steady decrease in funding for clinical trials and also a decrease in the number of NIH grant applications from surgical faculty members as well as a decrease in the number of funded grants awarded to surgeons. In a study from 2001 to 2011 of North American Surgical Oncology Research, only 10.5% (1049) of a total of 9961 cancer trials evaluated cancer and surgery. Of these, 898 were interventional studies with surgery as a variable in only 125 studies (1.3% of all cancer trials) [4].

Intervention null trial designs are important to evaluate when considering designing the clinical trial with the highest likelihood of success in terms of accrual and providing the appropriate information and comparison for clinical impact. Studies that randomize an individual patient to an intervention versus no intervention will often be far more challenging both from the standpoint of clinical equipoise as well as patient enrollment than a clinical trial that randomizes a patient to one intervention compared to another intervention. There are many critical questions when considering a clinical trial design focused on a surgical intervention. First of all, if this intervention involves a component subject to FDA regulation, does that component have marketing approval as it will be used in the trial or does it require any special approval by FDA before the research can be conducted? Is this ethical to randomize a patient between this intervention and another treatment and is there appropriate clinical equipoise across experts in the medical field. Given the length of time that it takes for clinical trial development and conduct, considering the time frame of this intervention will be important. Is it anticipated that the new intervention being evaluated could be obsolete over the time course of conduct of the clinical trial. If this is likely, the clinical trial is unlikely to be successful in changing clinical practice. Other aspects that should be considered include the timing of the intervention, the length of the intervention, and any special tests required to evaluate prior to the intervention or after performing the intervention.

Comparison Group

When designing a clinical trial to evaluate the effectiveness of an invasive therapeutic procedure, the options for the comparative arm could involve a nonoperative therapy, an alternative invasive procedure, or potentially a sham procedure. Sham procedure often provides the best comparator; however, it can be far more challenging to conduct, especially as this can involve operative room fees and potentially putting the patient under anesthetic and maybe even making an incision on the skin. When the comparator is a sham procedure, it allows random allocation between the two groups thus controlling for selection bias. It allows blinding of patients and therefore controlling for expectancy bias. It also allows blinding of the outcome assessor in that the physician or healthcare members seeing the patient in follow up can be successfully blinded to which arm the patient was enrolled in and it also minimizes crossover between arms of the study, preserving the best attributes of random allocation. In comparison, a nonoperative comparison group struggles with many of these components. It does allow the random allocation in a randomized controlled trial, however, patients cannot be blinded between an operative intervention and nonoperative therapy, and similarly the people assessing the outcome generally cannot be blinded and there is significant potential for crossover between the two arms. The randomized trial that randomizes between two interventions probably provides the compromise between nonoperative therapy and a comparative sham procedure. The alternative invasive procedure does allow the random allocation based on randomized control trial design. In some cases, it can allow blinding of the patients to which arm they were in depending on the alternative invasive intervention and it may also allow blinding of the healthcare members assessing outcomes. It does preserve the attributes of random allocation and minimizes the number of patients wishing to crossover between interventions.

If we look at some examples of large randomized controlled trials in the past that have changed clinical practice, one example is the NSAPB B-06 trial. At that time, there was true clinical equipoise in treatment options at the time of the trial conduct. The control group was total mastectomy, which was the standard procedure at the time. The interventions in the other arms were ethical and different from the control arm, thus, being justifiable and meaningful. This trial changed the clinical options to allow for both breast conservation surgery and mastectomy to be surgical options for women with early-stage breast cancer. The surgeon's experience was not well documented in the study and it may well be that some of the surgeons who had not performed many lumpectomies at that time were early in their learning curve. The large number of surgeons participating in the trial, which was a multicenter cooperative group trial, ensures that the results are generalizable to larger patient populations.

As we enter an era of more advanced technique and also advanced technology, surgical credentialing prior to participation in the clinical trial is critically important to maintain the integrity of the results generated. The VA randomized trial looking at open inguinal hernia repair with mesh versus laparoscopic inguinal hernia repair with mesh had a requirement that each surgeon performed at least 25 procedures of the intervention they were performing, open hernia or laparoscopic hernia, prior to participating in the clinical trial. Additionally, pretrial submission of a video of laparoscopic hernia case was required for central review prior to participation in the trial. This surgical credentialing and evaluation is a way to control for the learning curve with the introduction of a new interventional procedure. This trial highlights an important dilemma with new operative procedures. The transition from open surgical repair to laparoscopic surgical repair can occur without adequate evaluation with clinical trials as in the case of laparoscopic cholecystectomy whose growth was primarily driven by patient requests rather than validation of prospective surgical outcomes.

For surgical procedures, the protocol should include clear documentation of all of the critical steps of the surgical procedure to ensure that the intervention is performed in a similar fashion across all patients participating in the study. In looking at the United Kingdom trial on reflux, they randomized patients to surgery versus medical therapy. However, the surgical intervention recommended routine crural repair and nonabsorbable synthetic suture; however, the type of fundoplication performed was at the discretion of the surgeon. This can introduce a significant variability across the surgical procedure and therefore impact the results of the clinical trial. Thus, for interventional studies, specifics regarding the critical steps of the procedure are important to be outlined in the protocol, similar as for drug intervention studies the dose–dose interval and dose adjustments are clearly dictated in the protocol. The American College of Surgeons Operative Standard Manual is the first textbook designed to outline the minimum intraoperative requirements for oncologic procedures to standardize the surgical approach and can be used for clinical trials standardization [5]. One way to improve the standardization across the interventional trial arms is to require surgeon credentialing prior to clinical trial participation and require submission of videos of the procedure for central review. For surgical resection procedures, photographic documentation of the resected specimen along with standardized pathological assessment of the specimens are important components to include. Similarly standardized imaging of the patient prior to surgical intervention and well-described eligibility criteria are critical.

References

1. Freedman B. Equipoise and the ethics of clinical research. N Engl J Med. 1987;317(3):141–5.
2. Djulbegovic B. The paradox of equipoise: the principle that drives and limits therapeutic discoveries in clinical research. Cancer Control. 2009;16(4):342–7.
3. Purushotham AD, Lewison G, Sullivan R. The state of research and development in global cancer surgery. Ann Surg. 2012;255(3):427–32.
4. Menezes AS, Barnes A, Scheer AS, Martel G, Moloo H, Boushey RP, Sabri E, Auer RC. Clinical research in surgical oncology: an analysis of ClinicalTrials.gov. Ann Surg Oncol. 2013;20(12):3725–31.
5. Nelson H, Hunt KK, Blair S, Chang GJ, Halverson A, Katz MHG, Matthew H.G. Katz, Posner M. Operative standards for cancer surgery. 2015: Wolters Kluwer. p. 332.

Part VI
Regulatory Considerations

Chapter 32
Setting up a Clinical Trial Research Office

Kamal M.F. Itani

Introduction

The success of a clinical trial is dependent on the organizational infrastructure set by the principal investigator. The principal investigator and the executive committee are responsible for the management of a large personnel spread across multiple institutions, multiple committees, a large budget and responsibilities for the safety and privacy of enrolled subjects and the integrity of the data. The following chapter describes how to set that infrastructure in place, a schematic representation of which is presented in Fig. 32.1.

Chair's Office

The chair's office, also known as the clinical coordinating center, should consist of the study chair who is usually the principal investigator (PI) for the whole study, the national nurse coordinator who leads the site coordinators, and an administrative assistant if budgeted. The PI and national nurse coordinator usually are not the site investigator and coordinator for their own site to maintain separation between the clinical coordination and data collection. This responsibility is usually to others within their center. It is advantageous for the PI's center to be enrolled within the study in order for both the PI and the National nurse coordinator to have firsthand experience with all issues related to the study.

K.M.F. Itani (✉)
Department of Surgery, VA Boston Health Care System/Boston
University and Harvard Medical School, VABHCS(112A),
1400 VFW Parkway, West Roxbury, MA 02132, USA
e-mail: kitani@va.gov

© Springer International Publishing AG 2017
K.M.F. Itani and D.J. Reda (eds.), *Clinical Trials Design in Operative and Non Operative Invasive Procedures*, DOI 10.1007/978-3-319-53877-8_32

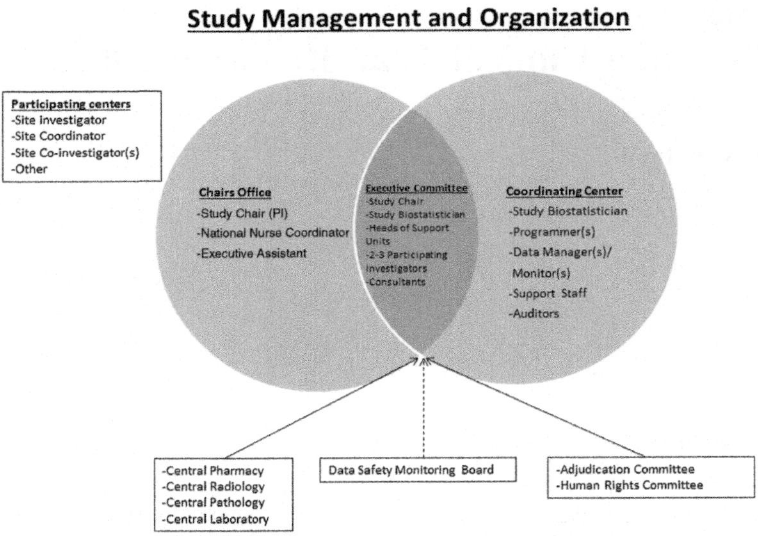

Study Management and Organization

Participating centers
-Site Investigator
-Site Coordinator
-Site Co-investigator(s)
-Other

Chairs Office
-Study Chair (PI)
-National Nurse Coordinator
-Executive Assistant

Executive Committee
-Study Chair
-Study Biostatistician
-Heads of Support Units
-2-3 Participating Investigators
-Consultants

Coordinating Center
-Study Biostatistician
-Programmer(s)
-Data Manager(s)/ Monitor(s)
-Support Staff
-Auditors

-Central Pharmacy
-Central Radiology
-Central Pathology
-Central Laboratory

Data Safety Monitoring Board

-Adjudication Committee
-Human Rights Committee

Fig. 32.1 Clinical trial study infrastructure

Once the study is approved and funded, the first order of business is to recruit a National nurse coordinator who will work closely with the PI and the coordinating center on all aspects of the study.

The identification of participating centers and the timeline for recruitment, institutional review board approval (central and local) as well as progress of the study are all delineated within the original proposal. The chair's office will have to make every effort to comply with the timelines.

One of the first activities of the chair's office is to put together a study operations manual, also known as a manual of procedures, for the study as a whole. The operating guidelines manual will describe step by step all activities of the study and the delegation of study tasks and training of each individual within the study. This manual is intended to provide complementary information to that which is found in the study protocol and to provide additional details on specific study procedures. In the event of personnel turnover or in case of a sudden emergency, any study personnel should be able to obtain information about any step or role within the study from the operating guidelines manual.

The chair's office should also set the date for the first investigator's meeting which should coincide with the time that all or most of the participating sites' personnel are in place. The meeting should include at least every site investigator, co-investigator if the budget allows, site coordinators, members of the coordinating center, members of the executive committee including representatives of all support units such as radiology, laboratory, pathology, and consultants as well as members of the adjudicating committees. During the meeting, the PI and coordinating center staff will cover all aspects of the study, step by step, review of the study protocol, recruitment strategies, retention of participants, data tools, and the operations manual. For specific procedures or surgeries, the details and material are agreed on by the investigators with hands on training through videos, mannequin, or cadavers (as deemed necessary) occurring during that initial meeting. The site coordinators will have their own training session on all aspects of the data entry tools. A review session on good clinical practices for human research should be included during that meeting.

It is during that first meeting that all staff meet each other, understand each other's roles, and the tone, expectations and details of the study are set. All possible questions should be answered. It is not infrequent during this first meeting that questions might not be answered or that a step within the protocol might not be realistic based on consensus by the investigators. These issues can be taken back to the executive committee, who can provide an answer or decide to proceed with a protocol amendment that will require IRB approval. Yearly face-to-face meetings can be held if budgeted and deemed necessary for the proper progress of the study.

The chair's office will then organize monthly conference calls with all site investigators and coordinators to discuss challenges, learn from each other, and respond to questions. These conference calls might be held more or less frequently depending on the difficulties encountered and the progress of the study.

The national nurse coordinator should have a separate conference call with the site coordinators at least monthly to discuss issues related to recruitment, screening strategies, data entry and transmission, participant follow up, and retention.

It is also very beneficial for the chair's office to publish a newsletter at least quarterly that provides information about each site's recruitment, overall study progress, responses to frequently asked questions, and to feature one site each time.

Study Coordinating Center

The study coordinating center, sometimes known as the biostatistical and data coordinating center, is led by the lead biostatistician who interacts frequently and closely with the chair's office. The study coordinating center allocates various staff to the study including a programmer, data manager, other statisticians, and support staff depending on the size of the study [1].

The randomization process and tools for enrolling patients are built by the coordinating center which will then monitor screening at each participating center, recruitment, data quality, protocol compliance, and participant retention. The coordinating center will provide reports as well as any concern to the Chair's office prior to an executive committee meeting. The coordinating center will also prepare various reports including safety and efficacy to be reviewed by the independent data monitoring committee at their regularly scheduled meetings. Data requested by other committees to adjudicate end points or other issues can be provided as long as it does not compromise the integrity of the results and any blinding of the participating staff.

Executive Committee

The executive committee, sometimes known as a steering committee, is led by the study chair with participation of the lead biostatistician, 2–3 principal investigators, the national nurse coordinator, key consultants, and the heads of any supporting unit (radiology, pharmacy, etc…).

The executive committee acts as the management group and decision-making body for the operational aspects of the study. They usually meet on a monthly basis and as needed to review compliance with timelines, recruitment strategies, additional efforts and retention of study participants. Based on feedback during the site investigator conference call, the committee makes decisions about protocol amendments and takes actions on medical centers whose performance is unsatisfactory. The executive committee makes decisions about site visits to review compliance with protocol or observe a procedure or surgery. Depending on the concerns at a specific center, the executive committee might decide to dispatch the study chair, a consultant or site PI, or a multidisciplinary team to review and report on any issue of concern.

The executive committee refers cases to the adjudication committee in case the outcome is not clear or to the human rights committee in case of a safety breech or ethical concern. Those committees report back to the executive committee for action.

Data Safety Monitoring Board

The data safety monitoring board (DSMB) is an independent oversight committee organized by the study sponsor. It is responsible for monitoring the progress of the study. The lead biostatistician provides the DSMB unblinded reports on the efficacy and safety outcomes according to a prespecified plan. The DSMB also considers new scientific information from sources outside the study that may impact whether the study should continue. The DSMB is a recommending body that communicates its recommendations to the study sponsor. If the sponsor accepts the recommendations of the DSMB, the sponsor then communicates that information to the study executive committee. However, the study investigators do not receive any discussions concerning unblinded data. The DSMB is covered in more detail in Chap. 39.

Supporting Units

Different studies might require different services to support various functions of the study. Medications might be dispensed through a central pharmacy if the study drug is experimental or not on the market; for devices and implants, these might be distributed through central supply on a case by case basis or through limited batches to ensure proper handling, storage, and compliance with expiration dates. Specialized laboratory testing such as special histologic staining for genetic markers and biomarkers might be sent to central laboratories for standardization purposes. This will require training for proper handling of human specimen and safe shipping in accordance with the International Air Transportation Association (IATA) regulations. Radiologic testing can be done locally but might require reading in a central location by dedicated staff for standardization purposes. Representatives from any of those areas should be on the executive committee available to discuss any issue, challenges or progress.

Other Committees

An adjudication committee or ends point committee consisting of various experts in the field under investigation should be in place. It is not uncommon for disagreements to arise when an outcome is determined by clinical interpretation and the necessity for an unbiased opinion to adjudicate that outcome.

Although the IRB provides oversight over all aspects of the study, it is important to have a human rights committee especially with procedural and surgical trials to ensure ethical and safe conduct of all aspects of the protocol without bias, avoiding un-blinding especially when the control consists of a sham operation or procedure. In some instances, a DSMB may include one or more members who are ethicists and patient advocates in lieu of having a separate human rights committee.

A publications committee might be established for large trials with the potential for several sub-studies. However, it is not unusual for the executive committee to also act as the publications committee if a separate one was not established. All requests for publication by any member of the study should be channeled through that committee for approval and release of the data. Before submission, the publications committee reviews any manuscript for accuracy, authorship and proper credit.

Large complex trials may also have additional committees responsible for various aspects of study conduct, such as recruitment and retention, and quality control.

Site Investigator's Research Office

The site investigator's office mirrors the set up in the chair's office. The site PI recruits the site coordinator as well as co-investigators to help with all aspects of the study. The site PI should designate one or multiple co-investigators as his/her delegate when absent from the study site. The co-investigators should be familiar with the protocol and the study operations manual. One or several of them will attend the investigators' meetings and will be trained in all aspects of the study procedure or surgery. The PI is responsible for maintaining up to date files, consents and IRB approvals, will report protocol deviations at the site and all adverse and serious adverse events to the chair's office within the allowable timeframe and is responsible for securing data safety and protecting personal health information for each patient. The site PI must also provide information that the IRB requires to fulfill its oversight role, such as serious adverse events and documentation on the informed consent process. The site PI will also identify ancillary staff in radiology, laboratory, pathology as well as other specialties needed for the study. Communication with and availability to study subjects is essential at each study site.

Although strategies for recruitment and retention of study subjects are delineated by the chair's office, it is ultimately the responsibility of the site investigator to implement a plan that best fits the culture and environment of a particular site.

It is also critical that study personnel at each site participate in the scheduled conference calls and meetings and remain apprised of all changes and issues pertaining to the study.

Summary

In summary, the organization of the Chair's office, the various committees, the study coordinating center and the ongoing consistent communication from that office and response to various questions, challenges, and issues are critical to the success of that study. The cost of a large prospective randomized trial usually in the millions of dollars, the large number of participating sites, personnel, and most importantly patients place a tremendous responsibility on the study chair's office to make sure that every aspect of the study is attended to in a fair, equitable, and responsible fashion.

Reference

1. Williford WO, Krol WF, Bingham SF, Collins JF, Weiss DG. The multicenter coordinating center statistician: "More than a consultant". Am Stat. 1995;49(2):221–5.

Chapter 33
Regulatory Considerations: The Clinical Research Coordinator

Marie Campasano and Kamal M.F. Itani

The Clinical Research Coordinator, also known as Nurse Research Coordinator, Research Coordinator or Study Coordinator has a critical role in the conduct and success of a clinical trial. It has been said that the coordinator is the "heart and soul" [1] of a clinical trial. Although all responsibilities fall on the Principal Investigator (PI) [2], the Clinical Research Coordinator manages and oversees the day-to-day operation to ensure that all aspects of the clinical trial run smoothly from initiation to completion of the research study.

Professional Background

In 2007, the National Institutes of Health Clinical Center (NIHCC) issued the results of a role delineation project, *Building the Foundation for Clinical Research Nursing Domain of Practice for the Specialty of Clinical Research Nursing*. The document described the scope of research practice in nursing and framed it within two roles [3]: Clinical Research Nurses (CRN) and Research Nurse Coordinators (RNC). In certain settings those roles are not mutually exclusive. The CRN

M. Campasano (✉)
Department of Surgical Service, VA Boston Healthcare,
1400 VFW Parkway, MS 112, West Roxbury, MA 02132, USA
e-mail: Marie.Campasano@VA.gov

K.M.F. Itani
Department of Surgery, VA Boston Health Care System/Boston University and Harvard
Medical School, VABHCS(112A), 1400 VFW Parkway, West Roxbury, MA 02132, USA
e-mail: kitani@va.gov

© Springer International Publishing AG 2017   285
K.M.F. Itani and D.J. Reda (eds.), *Clinical Trials Design in Operative
and Non Operative Invasive Procedures*, DOI 10.1007/978-3-319-53877-8_33

functions within a research unit, such as the NIHCC, research units in Clinical Translational Science Award sites, General Clinical Research Centers (GCRCs), or specialty care programs with a clinical research focus [3]. Their role is to provide and support all the clinically related activities of a study protocol. The RNC, however, is primarily responsible for study coordination and data management with a central focus on managing subject recruitment, integrity, and compliance with regulatory requirements and reporting [3]. The NIH Role Delineation Project defines five dimensions—distinct categories of activities—within the specialty practice of research nursing.

Clinical Practice

Direct nursing care is provided to participants in clinical research, with support to their families, and significant others. Care requirements are established by the scope of study, the clinical condition of the patient, and the requirements and clinical effects of research procedures and include functions such as history and physical exam, administration of study drugs, monitoring of effect and specimen collection, handling, and processing [3].

Study Management

The Research Coordinator ensures compliance with all steps of the protocol, accurate data collection and form completion. He/she maintains communication with the sponsor, IRB and different regulatory bodies [3].

Care Coordination and Continuity

Coordination of research activities without interfering with required clinical care and needs is an essential function of the clinical research coordinator, who should also achieve a relationship with referring and primary care providers [3]. Examples of activities under this dimension include the education of all caring for the patient on the study protocol, coordinating the scheduling of the study participants' visits, acting as the case manager for study participants, and answering participants' and providers' questions and concerns.

Human Subjects Protection

The Research Coordinator facilitates the informed participation of participants from diverse backgrounds in clinical research [3]. As an example, he/she makes the initial and ongoing informed consent process easier for the study participants by explaining the study protocol and answering questions and concerns. The Research Coordinator also works with the Principal Investigator and the rest of the team to address any potential ethical conflicts.

Contributing to the Science

The Research Coordinator is in a unique position to make observations during the conduct of a study that can lead to protocol amendments to minimize risks to participants, improve flow of the study or lead to new research ideas. In addition, the Research Coordinator will keep participants apprised of new findings resulting from a study and how it affects them.

Education and Training

Traditionally, the Research Coordinator's role was filled by a registered nurse. More recently others such as advanced practice nurses (NP), physician assistants (PA), and foreign-trained physicians who may choose not to obtain medical licensure in the United States have fulfilled the role of research coordinators and made significant contributions to the conduct of Clinical Trials. Historically Study Coordinators, Research Coordinators, and Nurse Research Coordinators have learned the duties of the position "on the job" being initially oriented and mentored by the Principal Investigator, by another site coordinator, or offsite study personnel [4]. Although this is still accepted today, the complexity and administrative requirements might require more formal training.

Training in clinical research is offered via programs leading to a Certificate, an Associate's Degree or a Bachelor Degree Program. These programs prepare the research candidate for entry-level positions in the field and provide them with certification. Other jobs such as Senior Research Coordinator, and Project Manager, may require a Master's Degree. Associate's Degree Programs in clinical research include general education courses along with specialized clinical research classes and may also include an internship [5, 6].

For a Registered Nurse or others with some medical experience, such as an NP, a PA, or a medical doctor from another country not certified in the United States, a certificate program may suffice. A solid foundation based on years of experience in nursing or the medical field makes the clinical research coordinator (CRC) an excellent candidate. Others who have no medical foundation need to complete an Associate's Degree, Certificate Program that will cover basic courses in medical and research terminology and an introductory level course in clinical research. Example topics in a CRC educational program include clinical research management, drug safety, legal and regulatory compliance, clinical statistics, pharmacology for clinical trials and research ethics. Education in clinical research and clinical experience are required to work as a CRC. Although not mandatory, professional certification is available through the Society of Clinical Research Associates (SOCRA) and the Association for Clinical Research Professionals (ACRP) [7, 8].

Certification

The Clinical Research Professional certification (CRP) offer by SOCRA is available to members of the association who provide evidence of full-time employment in the field of research. The amount of experience the applicant is required to have is contingent upon the level of education and training completed. SOCRA has 3 "Categories" that would make a candidate eligible to take their certification exam:

Category 1. Minimum of two (2) years of fulltime employment as a clinical research professional in the past five years.
Category 2. Holds a degree in "Clinical Research" from an Associate, Undergraduate or Graduate Program and has completed a minimum of one year of full-time experience during the past two years as a Clinical Research professional.
Category 3. Holds an Undergraduate or Graduate Certificate in "Clinical Research" and holds an associate or bachelor degree in a science, health, pharmacy, or related field plus completed a minimum of one year of full-time experience during the past two years as a Clinical Research Professional.

The CRP is available for clinical research coordinators, principal investigators, researchers, and others working in clinical research [7].

A Clinical Research Coordinator certificate is offered by ACRP. To qualify for the ACRP certification, an applicant must provide evidence of an associate or bachelor degree or be a registered nurse (RN) and have a minimum of 3500 h hours of work experience. A high school diploma or experience as an LVN, LPN, medical assistant, or laboratory technician together with 4500 h Hours of related work experience will also meet the requirement. The ACRP offers other certifications, such as Clinical Research Associate (CRA) and Clinical Physician Investigator (CPI). Each certification requires that the applicant meets eligibility qualifications and pass an examination [8].

In addition to training and certifications all research staff engaged in human subject research must complete a Collaborative IRB Training Initiative (CITI) [9] or National Institutes of Health (NIH) course that meets the educational requirements for Human Subjects Protection and Good Clinical Practice [10]. These programs are available online. Different research organizations also require other annual trainings on Privacy and Health Insurance Portability and Accountability Act of 1996 (HIPAA) regulations [11, 12].

Role in Clinical Research

The role of the CRC is complex; The CRC oversees and coordinates the daily activities of clinical research studies, works closely with the clinical multidisciplinary teams and investigators to ensure that all protocol required procedures and study visits occur according to protocol specified guidelines. The CRC works in many different settings including university or private hospitals, and government institutions such as the NIH, Veterans Administration, Centers for Disease Control and Prevention (CDC) and Department of Defense (DOD). They may also be employed in the pharmaceutical industry or private research sites. The CRC needs to have a wide range of skills and knowledge [13]. Prioritizing and decision-making skills are essential for this role. Excellent communication and interpersonal skills are a must since the CRC interfaces with clinicians, patients, sponsor, and the IRB. A range of computer skills are necessary as well. They generally manage participant enrollment and ensure compliance with the protocol and other applicable regulations, ascertaining that Clinical Trials are conducted according to governmental regulations and guidelines, International Conference on Harmonization (ICH) regulations [14], GCP guidelines, site's Standard Operations Procedures (SOPs), and other policies and procedures (Table 33.1).

Table 33.1 Functions of the clinical research coordinator

Prepares site initiation, monitoring, and close-out visits with the study sponsor
Attends investigator meetings
Facilitates the execution of the NDA[a]
Prepares and manages IRB and Ethics Committee documentation[b]
Participates in preparing the study budget and CTA[c]
Participates in the development and execution of the CRADA[d]
Reads and implements protocols, informed consent forms, investigator's brochures, and other study guidelines
Maintains participant data in CRF/eCRF
Trains new personnel/medical staff in protocol implementation and adherence
Aids in the development and implementation of a recruitment strategy
Screens and enrolls subjects
Maintains a recruitment log[e]
Serves as a liaison between study subjects and the Principal Investigator

(continued)

Table 33.1 (continued)

Obtains, in collaboration with the Principal Investigator, the ICF and maintains these forms in regulatory binders
Develops and implements a retention plan for subjects in the study
Monitors for early subject withdrawal
Ensures Principal Investigator performs protocol specific tasks
Randomizes subjects and assigns study numbers
Informs subject and dispenses study medication(s) or device(s)
Manages study finances and subject stipends
Records/Reports all (serious) adverse events to the Principal Investigator, study sponsor and IRB
Documents and explains any premature unblinding of the study drug or investigational product
Manages the receipt, distribution, retrieval and return of all clinical supplies
Ensures that Principal Investigator reviews and signs required study documents
Communicates with and updates the study sponsor regarding study activities
Responds to data queries
Prepares a records retention and storage plan[f]

Abbreviations: *NDA* Non-disclosure Agreement, *IRB* Institutional Review Board, *CTA* Clinical Trial Agreement, *CRADA* Clinical Cooperative Research and Development Agreement, *CRF* Case Report Form, *eCRF* Electronic Case Report Form, *ICF* Informed Consent Form

[a]A legal contract between at least two parties that outlines confidential material, knowledge, or information that the parties wish to share with one another for certain purposes, but wish to restrict access to or by third parties

[b]Original submission, annual renewal, protocol amendments or deviations, adverse events, data safety monitoring board reports, visit reports, participant recruitment tools, and other reports provided by the study sponsor

[c]Include terms for indemnification, confidentiality, publication, intellectual property, insurance, data safety and monitoring boards, subject injury, governing law, and termination clauses [15]

[d]An agreement between a government agency and a private company or university to work together on research and development [16]. In study sites that are part of the Federal Government such as the Veterans Administration

[e]Lists subjects who were contacted for enrollment and reason subject either declined to participate, met exclusion criteria or failed to meet inclusion criteria

[f]Must follow research site's policies and procedures and be in accordance with requirements for the protection of human subjects in research (45CFR 46.115) [17] and the FDA-device policy [18]

Role in Human Subjects Protection

Clinical Trials are critical for enhancing standards of patient care and patient satisfaction with healthcare. The Clinical Research Coordinator is in a unique position to be a patient advocate and study advocate when conducting Clinical Trials. One of the most vital roles of the Study Nurse Coordinator is to ensure the safety and welfare of study subjects. On virtue of his/her education, background and clinical skills, the CRC is able to prioritize the patient's needs and best interests as well as protect their welfare during the trial. Subject advocacy promotes an informed decision to participate in research [19]. By carrying out the objectives of the study protocol, the CRC is also able to advocate for the study to ensure that all steps of the protocol are followed and that scientific goals are met. Because of their central position, holistic perspectives and their commitment to balancing the three advocacies, CRCs are uniquely positioned to advance the goals of human subjects protection and advancement of knowledge.

References

1. Fedor CA, et al. (2006 Remedica). Responsible research a guide for coordinators 1st edition. London/Chicago: Remedica Publishing, 2006 ISBN 1-901346-68-4.
2. US Department of Health and Human Services Food and Drug Administration Center for Drug Evaluation and Research (CDER) Center for Evaluation and Research (CBER) Guidance for Industry E6 Good Clinical Practice: Consolidated Guidance April 1996 ICH. http://www.fda.gov/downloads/Drugs/.../Guidances/ucm073122.pdf. Accessed May 2016.
3. CRN 2010 Domain of Practice Committee 2009. Building the foundation for clinical research nursing: domain of practice for the specialty of clinical research nursing. National Institutes of Health Clinical Center, Nursing and Patient Care Services. Available at: http://www.cc.nih.gov/nursing/crn/DOP_document.pdf. Accessed May 2016.
4. Mueller MR. From delegation to specialization: nurses and clinical trial co-ordination. Nurs Inq. 2001;8(3):182–90.
5. National Institutes of Health. Required education in the protection of human research participants, notice OD-00-039 (June 5, 2000) (revised 25 Aug 2000). Available at http://grants.nih.gov/grants/guide/notice-files/NOT-0D-00-039.html.
6. How do i become a certified clinical research coordinator?. Learn.org. http://learn.org/articles/How_Do_I_Become_a_Certified_Clinical_Research_Coordinator.html. 2003–2016. Accessed 6 June 2016.
7. The Society of Clinical Research Associates. The Society of Clinical Research Associates. 2005. http://www.socra.org/.
8. The Association of Clinical Research Professionals. The association of clinical research professionals. 2005. http://www.acrpnet.org/.
9. Collaborative Institutional Training Initiative. A division of BRANY NY. https://www.citiprogram.org/. Accessed May 2016.
10. National Institutes of Health. National Institutes of Health: required education in the protection of human research participants. 2000. http://grants.nih.gov/grants/guide/notice-files/NOT-OD-00-039.html.
11. National Institutes of Health and Office of Extramural Research. National Institutes of Health, and Office of Extramural Research: OER: peer review and policy issues. 2005. http://grants.nih.gov/grants/peer/peer.htm.
12. U.S. Department of Health and Human Services, et al. U.S. Department of Health and Human Services, Food and Drug Administration, Center for Drug Evaluation and Research, and Center for Biologics Evaluation and Research: guidance for industry, E6 good clinical practice: consolidated guidance. 1996. International conference on harmonisation of technical requirements for registration of pharmaceuticals for human use.
13. Pick A, Liu A, Drew VL, McCaul J. The role of the research nurse. Nursing Times; 107 on line edition, 26 Apr, vol 107 on line edition/www.nursingtimes.net.
14. World Medical Association Declaration of 2004. World medical association declaration of Helsinki: ethical principles for medical research involving human subjects. Verney-Voltaire, France: World Medical Association Declaration of Helsinki; 2004. p. 2004.
15. Non-disclosure agreement. Wikipedia.org. https://en.wikipedia.org/wiki/Non-disclosure_agreement. Accessed May 2016.

16. VHA Directive 1206 Transmittal sheet. Use of a cooperative research and development agreement (CRADA). May 13, 2015.
17. US Department of Health and Human Services. Code of federal regulations tittle 45Part 46.115 protection of human subjects effective, 14 Jul 2009. Accessed 1 June 2016. http://www.hhs.gov/ohrp/regulations-and-policy/regulations/45-cfr-46/.
18. US Food and Drug Administration http://www.fda.gov/MedicalDevices/. Last Updated 06/02/2016. Accessed 06/06/2016.
19. Davis AM, Hull SC, Grady C, Wilfond BS, Henderson GE. The invisible hand in clinical research: the study coordinator's critical role in human subjects protection. J Law Med Ethics. 2002;30(3):411–9.

Chapter 34
Data Collection Forms

William G. Henderson and Marie Campasano

Introduction

Data collection forms are vehicles by which observations and measurements on clinical trial patients are entered into the trial's database so that the data can be analyzed to meet the objectives of the trial. No matter what devices are used to enter data (whether by paper forms, distributed data entry using personal computers, World Wide Web, etc.), the principles of data collection form design are similar. The objectives and design of the clinical trial will dictate the types and content of data collection forms that are required. Although many investigators might feel that the design and use of data collection forms are tedious tasks to be avoided, the design of the forms has a very significant impact on the efficiency and accuracy of data collection, and on the ultimate success of the clinical trial, and, therefore, requires an intense collaborative effort between the surgeon and the biostatistician. The more thought and effort that are given to designing good data collection forms in the planning stages of the clinical trial, the less likely that problems will be encountered regarding needed changes in the forms and resultant data quality issues later in the clinical trial.

W.G. Henderson (✉)
Adult and Child Consortium for Outcomes Research and Delivery Science (ACCORDS)
and Department of Biostatistics and Informatics, Colorado School of Public Health,
University of Colorado Denver, 13199 E. Montview Blvd., Suite 300, Aurora,
CO 80045, USA
e-mail: William.Henderson@ucdenver.edu

M. Campasano
Department of Surgical Service, VA Boston Healthcare, 1400 VFW Parkway,
MS 112, West Roxbury, MA 02132, USA
e-mail: Marie.Campasano@VA.gov

© Springer International Publishing AG 2017
K.M.F. Itani and D.J. Reda (eds.), *Clinical Trials Design in Operative
and Non Operative Invasive Procedures*, DOI 10.1007/978-3-319-53877-8_34

Initial Planning and Organization of Data Collection Forms for a Clinical Trial

Data collection forms should be used in a clinical trial whenever it is planned to use a computer to analyze the data. The data collection forms should be laid out in a clear, logical, and convenient manner so that they can be easily completed by the data collector and easily entered into computer readable form by the data entry operator. It is a good idea to have the data collectors and data entry staff review drafts of the data collection forms before they are finalized.

If the research project is relatively simple (for example, requiring data collection at one time point), it may only require one or two data collection forms for each patient. However, in larger scale studies (for example, where patients have baseline and follow-up data collection, perhaps with multiple areas of data collection at each visit), forms organization becomes more important. In the latter case, it is a good idea to organize the forms in a chronological sequence related to how the typical patient would progress through the study. Individual forms should be devoted to specific content areas; for example, screening and demographic data, medical history, physical examination, laboratory tests, treatment given, etc. Individual forms should not be too long and complex; probably one to four pages per form is the ideal length. In many clinical trials, forms can be subdivided into those completed at baseline, at regularly scheduled follow-up visits, and those to be completed only when a specific event occurs (for example, a nonscheduled interim visit, hospitalization, death, drop-out, etc.). It is helpful to create a chart showing at each study visit which forms are expected to be completed. Each type of form should be given a form name and number.

As an example, we will use VA Cooperative Study #456 (CSP #456, "Tension-Free Inguinal Hernia Repair: Comparison of Open and Laparoscopic Surgical Techniques") [1, 2]. This was a multicenter randomized clinical trial (RCT), conducted between January, 1999, and November, 2003, in 14 VA medical centers (VAMCs). The purpose of the RCT was to compare open tension-free inguinal hernia repair (Lichtenstein method) with preperitoneal tension-free laparoscopic inguinal hernia repair on recurrence rates at 2 years (primary outcome). Secondary outcomes included postoperative complications, pain, time to return to normal activities, health-related quality of life, patient satisfaction, caregiver burden, and cost.

Men presenting to general surgery clinics at the participating VAMCs who were ≥ 18 years of age, had a diagnosis of inguinal hernia, and gave written informed consent were eligible for randomization. Patients in American Society of Anesthesiology classes IV or V, who had a contraindication to general anesthesia, bowel obstruction, bowel strangulation, peritonitis, bowel perforation, local or systemic infection, contraindications to pelvic laparoscopy, a history of repair with mesh, a life expectancy of less than 2 years, or were participating in another clinical trial were excluded. The patients were stratified by type of hernia (primary or recurrent), whether the hernia was unilateral or bilateral, and study site, and then randomized within these strata to one of the two treatment groups.

Patient baseline screening information included sociodemographic data, characteristics of the hernia, a comorbidities checklist, some general health questions, inclusion and exclusion criteria, and stratification and randomization information. These data were collected on all screened patients. After randomization and before intervention, the patients also completed the Standard Form, SF-36, health-related quality of life instrument, and forms evaluating their activity level, pain, and discomfort levels. The patient's caregiver also completed a form addressing their perception of the impact of the hernia on the patient's ability to perform activities of daily living and how much the caregiver had to help the patient.

Operative data included surgeon experience, operating time, details of anesthesia, antibiotics used, characteristics of the hernia, size of mesh, blood loss, Current Procedural Terminology (CPT) codes of other operations performed, and a few specific details about the Lichtenstein or laparoscopic procedure.

Postoperatively, patients were examined at two weeks, three months, and yearly thereafter to determine the presence or absence of a hernia recurrence by a surgeon not involved in the patient's operation; potential recurrences were confirmed by examination by an independent surgeon, by ultrasound examination, or during a second operation.

Secondary outcomes were complications, patient-centered outcomes (pain, health-related quality of life, activity assessment, satisfaction with care, and caregiver burden), and cost. Operative complications were recorded for the intraoperative period, and at two weeks and thirty days after the operation. Patients completed a visual analog scale for pain every day after surgery until their first postoperative visit. The other patient-centered outcomes were collected at the first postoperative visit, at three months, 6 months, and then annually.

Utilization and cost data were collected using patient diaries for the first three months after surgery and from administrative databases up to one year after surgery. These data included inpatient and outpatient utilization.

Tables 34.1 and 34.2 present a summary of the forms used in CSP #456. Table 34.1 includes the clinic visit forms, and Table 34.2 includes the "administrative" and utilization/cost forms. We include form number, form title, when the form was collected, and by whom. The forms were organized by how the typical patient progressed through the study, and also by area of data collection (for example, complications, activities assessment, pain and discomfort, satisfaction with care, etc.). Separate forms were needed for intraoperative, postoperative, and life-threatening complications, because different types of complications were collected at the different time periods (Forms #3–5). The preoperative and postoperative activities assessment (Forms #6–7) could have employed just one form because the assessments used the same activities and scales; but the form instructions were slightly different, so the investigators decided to use separate forms for the preoperative and postoperative assessments. The same was true for the preoperative and postoperative pain and discomfort forms (Forms #9–10). The SF-36 data collection used the same form for the baseline and postoperative periods, so this instrument had one form number (Form #11). The satisfaction with care forms (Forms #12–13) included slightly different questions at different points in time, so two separate forms were used.

Some forms were "administrative" in nature; for example, Form #20 was used to record missed visits or missing forms; Form #21 was used to record the numbers for the forms completed for each patient that were being transmitted to the central data

Table 34.1 Clinic visit forms used in CSP #456, "tension-free inguinal hernia repair: comparison of open and laparoscopic surgical techniques"

Form number	Form title	When collected	Who completed form
1	Patient screening	Baseline	PRA
2	Operative data	At the operation	PRA
3	Intraoperative complications	At the operation	PRA
4	Postoperative complications	2-week postoperative visit	PRA
5	Life-threatening complications	30-days postoperatively	PRA
6	Preoperative Activities Assessment	Baseline	Patient
7	Postoperative Activities Assessment	2 weeks, 3 months, 6 months, annually postoperatively	Patient
8	Activities resumption	6 weeks postoperatively	PRA (telephone call with patient)
9	Preoperative pain and discomfort	Baseline	Patient
10	Postoperative pain and discomfort	2 weeks, 3 months, 6 months, annually postoperatively	Patient
11	SF-36 health-related quality of life	Baseline, 3 months, 6 months, annually postoperatively	Patient
12	Satisfaction with care	2-week postoperative visit	Patient
13	Satisfaction with care	3 months, 1 year postoperatively	Patient
14	Caregiver assessment	Baseline, 2 weeks, 3 months postoperatively	Caregiver
15	Termination	At time of event	PRA
16	Assessment of recurrence	3 months, annually postoperatively	PRA or independent surgeon
17	Long-term complications	3 months, annually postoperatively	PRA
18	Surgeon satisfaction survey	After operation	Operating surgeon

PRA Professional research assistant

Table 34.2 Administrative and utilization/cost forms used in CSP #456, "tension-free inguinal hernia repair: comparison of open and laparoscopic surgical techniques"

Form number	Form title	When collected	Who completed form
20	Missed visit/missing forms	At time of event	PRA
21	Forms submission cover sheet	At time of event	PRA
30	Index admission/inpatient utilization bed section	At operation, 3 months postoperatively	PRA
31	Index admission/inpatient utilization procedures and tests	At operation, 3 months postoperatively	PRA
33	VA outpatient clinic visit	3 months postoperatively	PRA
34	VA outpatient procedures, labs, radiology	3 months postoperatively	PRA
40	Summary of non-VA utilization	At time of event	PRA
41	Non-VA inpatient admission	At time of event	PRA
42	Non-VA outpatient/ER utilization	At time of event	PRA
90	Protocol deviation	At time of event	PRA

PRA Professional research assistant

coordinating center; and Form #90 was used to record protocol deviations. Some forms were completed only when an event occurred; for example, Form #15 (Termination) was completed when a patient died, was lost-to-follow-up, or withdrew consent; and Forms #40–42 were completed if the patient had an episode of health care utilization that was not in the VA system.

Most of the forms were completed by the PRA (Professional Research Assistant) who was employed by the study. Because this study also collected quite a bit of data on patient-centered outcomes, the patients and caregivers completed a significant number of forms (Forms #6–7, and 9–14). It is important that when forms are completed directly by patients or caregivers that their construction and instructions are very clear.

It is also useful to include a form (perhaps Form 0) to give basic locator information for each patient. This might include patient name, address, telephone number, email address, medical record number, social security number, patient study ID number, and the names, addresses, and telephone numbers of a few people who would always know the whereabouts of the patient. These data could be kept in a data file separate from the main study data to maintain privacy of protected health information. These two data files could be linked using the patient study ID number, which might be composed of a site number (if the RCT is multicenter) and a patient number starting with 001 at each site and increasing consecutively as patients are screened for the study.

Identifier Information on Each Form

Each page of each form should contain certain identifier information so that if the pages of a form inadvertently become separated they can be correctly reassembled. This information should include: name of study; form number; form name; page number and total number of pages in the form (for example, "Page 1 of 4"), patient study ID number, and visit number. If the Institutional Review Board allows, it is also helpful to include the patient's initials as a double check to make sure that the form is associated with the correct patient. At the end of each form, there should be space for the signature of the person completing the form and the date that the form was completed. This is useful if a central data coordinating center is reviewing the accuracy of the contents of the form and the person completing the form needs to be contacted about questions or suspected errors.

Selection of Individual Data Items

In planning the data collection for a clinical trial, the investigators must make sure that all important data collection areas and variables are included, but should avoid excessive data collection. As the volume of data collected per patient in a study increases, it becomes increasingly difficult to ensure the accuracy of the data collected. The ideal selection of variables for inclusion in a RCT should at least include these areas: (1) the primary and secondary objectives of the RCT as stated in the protocol; (2) safety issues; (3) the interventions in the RCT (dose, frequency, duration, compliance, surgical techniques); (4) all endpoints or outcomes; (5) variables anticipated to have a high correlation with the outcome variables; that is, predictor variables for the outcomes known from the literature; (6) demographics, disease stage, and other variables to characterize the sample and to use in the reporting of Table. One of the RCT to look at balance of the treatment groups produced by the randomization; (7) selected comorbidities; (8) concomitant treatments; (9) death, date, and cause of death; and (10) some administrative variables (e.g., missed visits, terminations, protocol deviations, reasons for these, etc.).

After the general areas of data collection and the form numbers and titles have been selected, the next step is to select specific data items for each form. One way to do this is to first select the subareas of data collection for each form, and then select specific data items within each subarea. For example, in the screening form #1 in CSP #456, the subareas were sociodemographics, characteristics of the hernia, comorbidities, general health variables, exclusion and inclusion criteria, and stratification and randomization information. Once these subareas were decided upon, specific data items were developed. For example, for the subarea of sociodemographics, the specific data items included race/ethnicity, employment status, marital status, education, health insurance, and availability of a caregiver. The characteristics of the hernia included primary/recurrent, enlargement in past 6 weeks, hernia duration, reducibility, and physical findings. Rather than "reinventing the wheel", it can be helpful to find other studies which have used similar forms and to build upon this experience.

Knatterud et al. [3] have presented a good list of considerations to be made in selecting specific items for data collection:

1. Is there a need to determine whether the experimental treatment may have an effect—either beneficial or adverse—with respect to this item? These are the primary and secondary outcomes or dependent variables of the study.
2. Is the baseline observation for this item likely to be highly correlated with the primary response variable for the study, thus making it a useful variable for assessing comparability of treatment groups at baseline?
3. Is there another item similar to this one and probably highly correlated with it that has already been selected for inclusion on the form? For the most important variables, such as primary and secondary endpoints, it is often useful to build in some redundancy of this kind to provide additional computer edits checks and improve the quality of the data; for less important variables, such redundancy might well be avoided.
4. Does the anticipated quality (i.e., validity and reliability) of the data item warrant its inclusion?
5. Is there likely to be any harm in asking the question or making the measurement?
6. Is the cost of measuring this item and processing it at the data coordinating center commensurate with its anticipated worth to the study?

Frequency of Data Collection

The length of follow-up in a study is related to how long it will take the therapy to work, whether or not long-term as well as short-term effects are of interest, and whether it is anticipated that the effects of therapy will be different at different time periods. The frequency of data collection depends on whether it is anticipated that the therapeutic effects will change rapidly or be relatively stable over a long period. Frequency of data collection in VA cooperative studies has varied from a few weeks or once per month to every six months or every year. When follow-up visits are less frequent than every 6 months, loss to follow-up can be a problem. Interim telephone calls could be used to keep track of patients. In some studies, the response to therapy tends to be relatively volatile when therapy is begun and then becomes more stable when therapy is in a maintenance period. In those situations, one might want to have more frequent data collection in the early stages of a patient's participation and less frequent in the later stages.

Once the frequency of follow-up visits is determined, the investigators need to decide what data areas or items should be collected at each visit. The frequency of data collection could vary from one data type to another. However, one advantage of keeping the frequency the same for all follow-up data items is that it makes it easier for the research assistant to remember what needs to be done at each visit.

Construction of Individual Data Items

There are three basic types of data items—write-in responses with fixed field size (numerical data), multiple choice questions or checklists, and open-ended questions. Numerical data generally require write-in responses. Solid lines should not be used because the data collector does not know how many digits to enter. Also, decimal places and units of the variables should be indicated on the form. Boxes or dashes could be used for each digit. Enough boxes or dashes should be allowed to accommodate the largest conceivable value of the variable. If in doubt, it is better to allow an additional box or dash.

Multiple choice questions are the preferred method for obtaining categorical, nonnumeric data. The forms designer should attempt to list all possible choices and then leave a last checkoff box for "other" just in case a few choices are forgotten. A line could also be used to specify the nature of the "other". The "other" answers need to be organized and coded to be used in statistical analyses.

Open-ended questions requiring written responses should be kept to a minimum because these are challenging to code for statistical analysis. To analyze them, a person must first review them manually, place them into similar categories, and code the categories. If the sample size of the study and frequency of data collection are large, this can be a formidable effort.

Format of Study Forms

One easy way to format study forms is to put all of the questions in a column on the left-hand side of the page and all of the responses in columns on the right-hand side of the page. This works particularly well when the text describing the data items is similar in length (for example, a list of potential comorbidities), and the potential responses to each item are the same (for example, yes, no).

For multiple choice questions if the number of responses is ≤ 3, Knatterud et al. [3] recommend putting the responses on the same line as the question. If the responses number more than three, they recommend that each response be listed on a separate line underneath the question.

Similar questions on different forms or visits should be worded the same way, unless perhaps one is checking for reliability. It is also helpful in dichotomous response questions to have "no" and "yes" always in the same order with the same numerical value to be data entered.

Every data item on a form should be numbered, so that the central data coordinating center can refer to these numbers when querying a specific variable value.

Also, forms often contain record numbers and data field numbers to facilitate data being entered into computer readable form.

Data definitions should be given for every data item. If these are short, they could be included on the data collection form. Alternatively, a separate data dictionary should be included as part of the operations manual for the study.

Pretesting and Revisions to Data Collection Forms

Since all factors cannot be anticipated in the design of data collection forms, pretesting of the forms is very important. Forms should be pretested on a few patients who will not be included in the main study.

All major revisions (for example, shifting large blocks of data from one form to another) should be done prior to starting the main study. Otherwise, this will disrupt the data file and data management programming in a major way. Minor revisions (for example, addition or deletion of a data item) can more easily be done during the course of the study. An added item should be put at the end of the form so as not to disturb the remainder of the items. If an item is deleted, words to that effect could be stamped across the item rather than printing new forms.

Standardization of Forms Across Studies

In any research organization that conducts many studies, it could be advantageous to try to standardize forms and data elements across studies to facilitate the development of forms for new studies and to enable the possibility of comparing data items across studies. Some organizations, such as pharmaceutical companies and cooperative oncology groups, have created libraries of standardized case report pages, each to be used to record data from a particular type of examination, test, or measurement [4]. There are also movements at the National Institutes of Health to standardize data collection across studies [5–7].

References

1. Neumayer L, Jonasson O, Fitzgibbons R Jr, et al. Tension-free inguinal hernia repair: the design of a trial to compare open and laparoscopic surgical techniques. J Am Coll Surg. 2003;196:743–52.
2. Neumayer L, Giobbie-Hurder A, Jonasson O, et al. Open mesh versus laparoscopic mesh repair of inguinal hernia. N Engl J Med. 2004;350:1819–27.
3. Knatterud GL, Forman SA, Canner PL. Design of data forms. Cont Clin Trials. 1983;4:429–40.
4. Hosking JD, Newhouse MM, Bagniewska MS, Hawkins BS. Data collection and transcription. Cont Clin Trials. 1995;16:66S–103S.

5. NINDS Common Data Elements. www.commondataelements.ninds.nih.gov. Accessed 11/03/2016.
6. Health Measures. www.nihpromis.org. Accessed 11/03/2016.
7. CDISC. www.cdisc.org. Accessed 11/03/2016.

Chapter 35
Data Security

Jennifer M. Gabany and Kamal M.F. Itani

Background

Data security is safe-guarded legally by several state and federal regulations as well as local institutional policies. These policies are influenced by the principles reflected in many joint international consensus statements such as the Nuremburg Code, Declaration of Helsinki, Belmont Report, and the International Committee on Harmonization which all emphasize respect for persons and the rights of an individual. The U.S. Food and Drug Administration (FDA) cites 21CFR820.180 for general requirements of storage, confidentiality, and retention of medical records while the Health Insurance Portability and Accountability Act of 1996 (HIPAA) is the core legislation addressing the handling of personally identifiable information collected in the course of providing medical care. This law, enforced in 2003, required the U.S. Department of Health and Human Services to develop regulations protecting the privacy and security of certain health information resulting in the HIPAA Privacy Rule and the HIPAA Security Rule [1]. Three key elements of the privacy rule include:

- De-identified health information is not private or protected health information (PHI), and thus is not protected by the Privacy Rule. PHI generally refers to demographic information, medical history, test and laboratory results, insurance

J.M. Gabany (✉)
Division of Cardiac Surgery Research (112), VA Boston Healthcare System,
1400 VFW Parkway, West Roxbury, MA 02132, USA
e-mail: Jennifer.Gabany@gmail.com

K.M.F. Itani
Department of Surgery, VA Boston Health Care System/Boston University and Harvard
Medical School, VABHCS(112A), 1400 VFW Parkway, West Roxbury, MA 02132, USA
e-mail: kitani@va.gov

© Springer International Publishing AG 2017
K.M.F. Itani and D.J. Reda (eds.), *Clinical Trials Design in Operative and Non Operative Invasive Procedures*, DOI 10.1007/978-3-319-53877-8_35

information and other data that a healthcare professional collects to identify an individual and determine appropriate care.

- PHI may be used and disclosed for research with an individual's written permission in the form of an Authorization.
- PHI may be used and disclosed for research without an Authorization in limited circumstances: under a Waiver of the Authorization, as a limited data set with a data use agreement, work that is preparatory to research, and for research on decedents' information.

Additional legal safeguards provide special protections for studies of highly sensitive topics protected under 38 U.S.C. 7332(b)(2)(B) such as drug abuse, alcohol abuse, HIV infection, and sickle cell anemia when collected data may have the potential to negatively impact a subject and even family members indefinitely.

Protected health information (PHI) is variable in definition but typically refers to information that contains identifiers specific to individuals, such as demographic information specific enough for which there is a reasonable basis to believe it can be used to identify an individual. PHI is individually identifiable information and includes:

- the individual's past, present, or future physical or mental health or condition, the provision of health care to the individual, or
- the past, present, or future payment for the provision of health care to the individual.

HIPAA regulations have standardized a list of 18 elements of identification that constitute a full data set. The following table lists these standard HIPAA elements (see Table 35.1).

To be a completely de-identified data set, or anonymized as more commonly referred to in Europe, all 18 elements of identification must be removed. This de-identification process may be conducted by two different methods to meet HIPAA requirements:

1. Expert Determination Method: A person with appropriate knowledge of and experience with generally accepted statistical and scientific principles and methods for rendering information not individually identifiable: (i) Applying such principles and methods, determines that the risk is very small that the information could be used, alone or in combination with other reasonably available information, by an anticipated recipient to identify an individual who is a subject of the information; and (ii) Documents the methods and results of the analysis that justify such determination, while there is no set expiration of data for this method, experts recognize that technology developments require the quality of de-identification to be assessed after a period of time has passed; or

2. Safe Harbor Method: (i) The 18 identifiers of the individual or of relatives, employers, or household members of the individual, are removed; and (ii) The covered entity does not have actual knowledge that the information could be

Table 35.1 18 elements of HIPAA identification

1. Names
2. All geographical subdivisions smaller than a State, including street address, city, county, precinct, zip code, and their equivalent geocodes, except for the initial three digits of a zip code, if according to the current publicly available data from the Bureau of the Census: (1) The geographic unit formed by combining all zip codes with the same three initial digits contains more than 20,000 people; and (2) The initial three digits of a zip code for all such geographic units containing 20,000 or fewer people is changed to 000
3. All elements of dates (except year) for dates directly related to an individual, including birth date, admission date, discharge date, date of death; and all ages over 89 and all elements of dates (including year) indicative of such age, except that such ages and elements may be aggregated into a single category of age 90 or older
4. Phone numbers
5. Fax numbers
6. Electronic mail addresses
7. Social Security numbers
8. Medical record numbers
9. Health plan beneficiary numbers
10. Account numbers
11. Certificate/license numbers
12. Vehicle identifiers and serial numbers, including license plate numbers
13. Device identifiers and serial numbers
14. Web universal resource locators (URLs)
15. Internet protocol (IP) address numbers
16. Biometric identifiers, including finger and voice prints
17. Full face photographic images and any comparable images
18. Any other unique identifying number, characteristic, or code (note this does not mean the unique code assigned by the investigator to code the data)

used alone or in combination with other information to identify an individual who is a subject of the information. No linkage code should be maintained that would allow the data to be reidentified and the provider of the data should have no clear direct knowledge of methods to reidentify the data.

Covered health entities may use and disclose some information that may be used for research, public health or healthcare operations without an authorization or waiver of authorization if the information is presented as a Limited Data Set. A Limited Data Set excludes 16 of the 18 HIPAA identifiers but allows elements of dates and any other unique identifying number, characteristic, or code (note this does not mean the unique code assigned by the investigator to code the data).

The meaning of the term de-identification has taken on increased scrutiny with technological advances in multiple fields such as genetics, statistics, and computer software with increasingly sophisticated methods that could be used to reidentify data despite privacy preserving data mining. Because of the reidentification risk, some organizations sharing de-identified data may still wish to execute a data use agreement (DUA) with collaborators who wish to use the data to prevent them from attempting to reidentify the subjects [2]. Meanwhile larger meta-analyses are being conducted using de-identified sets of big data. Naessens et al. [3] determined that the addition of the last four numbers of individual social security numbers (SSNL4) to administrative data, accompanied by appropriate data use and data release policies, can enable trusted repositories to link data with nearly perfect accuracy without compromising patient confidentiality and recommended that states maintaining centralized de-identified databases should add SSNL4 to data specifications. This issue of how to share anonymous data will remain at the forefront with the release of the 2013 Institute of Medicine's report [4] on sharing of clinical trial data and the International Committee of Medical Journal Editors published draft proposal on de-identified individual clinical trial participant data sharing [5].

Just as every research project should undergo a risk assessment for the protection of Human Subjects, every project should also have a data risk assessment. In addition to being cost-effective, risk assessments create other advantages for data accuracy and sharing and are considered a necessary tool in the management of data security. Studies of risk models for data de-identification indicate that assigning of a level of risk for reidentification, and customizing a data plan according to this assigned level of risk, contributes to a greater overall quality of research by allowing more data to be shared in original form [6].

Data Security Tools

Secure data should maintain information accurately over time, be accessible upon request, and accessible only to those intended to have access [7]. Protection of data begins with a well trained staff and well written protocol. A standard investigational plan, or study protocol, requires a comprehensive data management plan that details a strategy for collection, storage, sharing, and dissemination of data. This plan should accurately and appropriately reflect privacy and information security rules. Paper and electronic systems create different needs and challenges, both are fundamentally regulated by the same principles governing medical records with the goal of protecting privacy while remaining easily accessible to those who are permitted access. Collection of protected health information (PHI) for research purposes is not included in the exemption of HIPAA requirements for treatment, payment, and usual daily operations of a healthcare facility and therefore specific permission must be obtained for research activities. Three critical tools frequently used by investigators to ensure compliance with privacy rules are a DUA) HIPAA Authorization for Release of Medical Records (HIPAA authorization) and/or Waiver of HIPAA Authorization (HIPAA waiver) for research purposes. The last two require Institutional Review Board (IRB) review and approval prior to initiating any research activities. These documents are typically included with an initial submission to an IRB for review along with a HIPAA Revocation form provided to subjects at the time of consenting for a research study. As part of the review process, the institution's Privacy Board will also review the documents for compliance and provide appropriate language if the documents are incomplete.

Data use agreements are effective in managing PHI when collaborating with external groups. A compliant DUA clearly describes the original source of data, who owns the data, who can view the data, and how the data will be handled when analysis is complete. Typically the Principal Investigator (PI) is considered the owner of the data and collaborators are expected to return the data to the PI when analysis is completed. The DUA should describe how the data is transported from and returned to the collaborator, how the data is stored, whether physically or electronically, and should identify measures taken to keep the data secure such as a double locked office or computer firewall. The DUA should indicate the collaborators will protect the data at the same level of security as the PI's institution requires.

An IRB approved HIPAA authorization is obtained in any research study that collects PHI and provides a detailed description of all intended uses and disclosures by the research team to provide an individual the opportunity to make a fully informed decision before allowing data to be used in the manner described. The following elements are required to be included in all HIPAA authorizations:

- Description of PHI to be used or disclosed (identifying the information in a specific and meaningful manner).
- The name(s) or other specific identification of person(s) or class of persons authorized to make the requested use or disclosure.
- The name(s) or other specific identification of the person(s) or class of persons who may use the PHI or to whom the covered entity may make the requested disclosure.
- Description of each purpose of the requested use or disclosure. Researchers should note that this element must be research study specific, not for future unspecified research.
- Authorization expiration date or event that relates to the individual or to the purpose of the use or disclosure (the terms "end of the research study" or "none" may be used for research, including for the creation and maintenance of a research database or repository).
- A statement that the individual may revoke the authorization in writing with instructions on how to exercise such right and who to contact.
- A statement about the potential for the PHI to be re-disclosed by the recipient and no longer protected by the Privacy Rule.
- Signature of the individual and date. If the authorization is signed by an individual's personal representative, a description of the representative's authority to act for the individual.

Included with every HIPAA authorization is a HIPAA revocation form that clearly describes how a subject may revoke a previously signed authorization for use of PHI. The revocation form is reviewed by an IRB prior to use and must contain instructions in writing on how to withdraw authorization for use of PHI by signing the revocation form and providing this written notice to the PI of the research study. The investigator's name and mailing address must be provided on the form along with the title of the study and the institution. The revocation form is not signed at the time of consenting, however this document must be provided to the subject if a HIPAA authorization is signed. A common error during the consenting process, when multiple pages are being initialed and signed, is to mistakenly sign this form as well, so keeping the revocation document separate from the informed consent form (ICF) and HIPAA authorization is one strategy to avoid this mistake until after signatures have been completed.

The HIPAA waiver is a request by the investigator, to the institution, for the collection of PHI prior to or without obtaining consent from an individual so this document is not signed by research subject, but is approved by the IRB along with the informed consent form (ICF) and HIPAA auth. The HIPAA waiver clearly describes all intended uses and disclosures of PHI by the research team so the institution has the required documentation to remain compliant with state and federal regulations for accounting. A HIPAA waiver may be requested for some of the planned research activities or for the entire study protocol. Often an investigator will request a HIPAA waiver for recruitment purposes only, so an investigator may review the medical record of a potential subject to confirm eligibility for a specific study protocol, significantly minimizing the burden for a patient who has likely already provided this information to the institution multiple times. In some instances, a HIPAA waiver may be requested for the entire protocol such as when no identifiable information is collected and no linkage code exists to reidentify subjects. Limited data sets under a DUA may also qualify in certain circumstances. Three criteria must be met for a waiver of authorization to be approved under the Privacy Rule:

1. The use or disclosure of PHI involves no more than a minimal risk to the privacy of individuals, based on, at least, the presence of the following elements:

   a. adequate plan to protect the identifiers from improper use and disclosure;
   b. adequate plan to destroy the identifiers at the earliest opportunity consistent with conduct of the research, unless there is a health or research justification for retaining the identifiers or such retention is otherwise required by law; and
   c. adequate written assurances that the PHI will not be reused or disclosed to any other person or entity, except as required by law, for authorized oversight of the research project, or for other research.

2. The research could not practicably be conducted without the waiver.
3. The research could not practicably be conducted without access to and use of the PHI.

An investigator submitting a request for IRB initial review is required to provide specific justification for each of the three criteria above, such as the need to accurately identify patients and the need to accurately identify patients that meet eligibility criteria based on information in the medical record. An investigator also needs to include a copy of this approved HIPAA waiver when submitting a request for IRB continuing review.

Amendments to these documents may be submitted to the IRB of record for review and approval during the course of a research project as needed for future subjects and may require previously consented subjects to be re-consented depending on the content under revision.

A powerful security tool that allows electronic sharing of data is public key infrastructure, referred to as PKI, which includes options for encryption and digital identification signatures to maintain a secure and authentic electronic work environment. The Federal Information Processing Standard (FIPS) is the government computer security standard used to accredit cryptographic modules. Emails containing any form of PHI or other types of sensitive data require encryption prior to sending. Employers typically provide personal identification verification (PIV) cards that enable an employee with the appropriate clearance to read an encrypted email when connected to the system. A fact worthy of noting is that many unauthorized access issues begin with an employee who opens an email and accesses an embedded link or replies to the email which opens the system to hacking. Any email asking for sensitive or identifiable information from an unknown source should be deleted as no employer or agency will solicit sensitive information in a manner that exposes the data to risk.

Remote access is increasingly becoming a useful tool for employers struggling with work space issues and a new generation of workers that expect technological advances to improve their daily lives by providing great convenience, but may also expose serious gaps in the security process. Strict permission to remote access capability should be maintained and justification provided for each person before granting this privilege. The PIV card here again is a valuable tool for managing this access along with a two-step verification process. Employees should also be aware that PIV cards with embedded electronic chips contain a great deal of sensitive information and should be carried at all times with a holder that prevents wireless tapping of the employee's information when the card is not in use at the computer terminal.

Data Storage

While methods of data collection are critical to security, storage of data may pose even more concerns, particularly with the utilization of electronic data capture and storage. Currently the FDA requires a paper-based collection of essential documents but clearly recognizes the future direction of electronic-based data management with the Affordable Care Act allotting significant funds specifically for the implementation of electronic medical records systems. Many do not recognize the risk of saving data on a computer hard drive (My Documents, Desktop, C drive) that will someday be moved or exchanged for a new computer. Password protected shared drives with access controlled folders behind an adequate firewall should be set up through the institution's Information Technology department with proper mapping and permissions established at the onset. Any electronic data system should be backed up regularly on a schedule that reflects the content of the data. Critical medical information should be stored on a system that is backed up frequently, such as every 24 h, while a system storing less critical information may be appropriately backed up weekly or monthly.

External storage devices (data sticks, DVDs, memory drives) should only be connected to the system if approved by the institution maintaining the server and should also be scanned for viruses each time the external device is connected to the system. Once disconnected from the system, the device should be stored in the same manner as a sensitive paper document with a double locked filing system including a locked file cabinet in a locked office accessible only to designated members of the study team. If the external data storage device is shared with an external entity under a DUA, the devices should be transported by chain of custody or a secure mailing system with tracking capability such as the United States Postal Service registered mail, UPS, or Fed-ex. Indeed some of the best strategies for data protection focus on simple routine behavior such as logging off when walking away from a computer in use, privacy screens for unexpected walk-ins, and not sharing passwords ever. Any concern for compromised security codes should be reported to a supervisor accompanied with an immediate change in the password.

Conclusion

Security and privacy are essential components in the foundation of all successful growth and development and the protection of research data is no different. The value of this philosophy was not lost on law makers when assigning the Office for Civil Rights with the task of oversight and enforcement of the numerous privacy and security laws that impact core research activities such as patient recruitment and data collection. A commitment to these values by investigators and regulatory agencies is essential to maintaining public trust and the successful recruitment of human subjects for clinical trials, otherwise the cycle of discovery and knowledge in healthcare is lost.

References

1. U.S. Department of Health & Human Services Office for Civil Rights. HIPAA for professionals. Available at: http://www.hhs.gov/hipaa/for-professionals/index.html.
2. Garfinkel SL. De-identification of Personal Information. National Institutes of Standards and Technology U.S. Dept. of Commerce. 2015 Oct. Retrieved from: http://dx.doi.org/10.6028/NIST.IR.8053.

3. Naessens JM, Visscher SL, Peterson SM, et al. Incorporating the last four digits of social security numbers substantially improves linking patient data from de-identified hospital claims databases. Health Serv Res. 2015;50(Suppl 1):1339–50. doi:10.1111/1475-6773.12323.
4. Institute of Medicine. Sharing clinical research data. Workshop summary. Washington, DC: National Academies Press, 2013.
5. Dal-Re R. The ICMJE trial data sharing requirement and participant's consent. Eur J Clin Invest. 2016. doi:10.1111/eci.12694.
6. Prasser F, Kohlmayer F, Kuhn K. The importance of context: risk-based de-identification of biomedical data. Methods Inf Med. 2016;55(4). doi:10.3414/ME16-01-0012.
7. Lee L, Gostin L. Ethical collection, storage, and use of public health data: a proposal for a national privacy protection. JAMA. 2009;302(1):82–4. doi:10.1001/jama.2009.958.

Chapter 36
Remote Monitoring of Data Quality

Jennifer M. Gabany

Definition and Purpose

Before defining risk-based monitoring (RBM), researchers may find it helpful to revisit the International Conference on Harmonisation (ICH) E6, section 5.18 which identified three main criteria for monitoring of research activities as described below [1]. These same principles are reinforced in the Code of Federal Regulations as well (21 CFR 312.50, 812.40, and 812.25) which mandate proper monitoring and written monitoring procedures within a research protocol. These consist of

- Protecting the rights, safety, and welfare of human subjects;
- Ensuring trial data are accurate, complete, and verifiable;
- Ensuring trial conduct is in compliance with the protocol, good clinical practice (GCP), and regulations.

In 2011, the United States Food and Drug Administration (FDA) released draft guidance for a risk-based approach to monitoring for public comment, and a finalized guidance document was released in August 2013. Risk-based monitoring is defined in this document as a remote evaluation carried out by sponsor personnel or representatives (e.g., clinical monitors, data management personnel, or biostatisticians) at a location other than the sites at which the clinical investigation is being conducted. In addition, this approach focuses on detecting "errors that matter." In comparison, on-site monitoring is defined by the FDA as an in-person evaluation carried out by sponsor personnel or representatives at the sites at which the clinical investigation is being conducted [2].

J.M. Gabany (✉)
Division of Cardiac Surgery Research (112), VA Boston Healthcare System,
1400 VFW Parkway, West Roxbury, MA 02132, USA
e-mail: Jennifer.Gabany@gmail.com

© Springer International Publishing AG 2017   313
K.M.F. Itani and D.J. Reda (eds.), *Clinical Trials Design in Operative and Non Operative Invasive Procedures*, DOI 10.1007/978-3-319-53877-8_36

While the main purpose of any monitoring strategy is to protect human subjects and data integrity, current monitoring procedures are varied but typically consist of periodic, on-site, face-to-face visits that involve conducting 100% source data verification. These visits are resource intensive, require skilled and experienced personnel to be truly effective and still may not address risks of systemic errors according to the FDA (2013) [2]. Unique opportunities exist with RBM to increase efficiency and better understanding of data trends. When studied by an experienced statistician, data trends generated by RBM are capable of identifying flaws that are not evident to the human eye or even the most experienced monitor.

Background

The current guidance for RBM was largely born out of a study conducted by the Clinical Trials Transformation Initiative (CTTI) involving a survey of over 200 organizations about current monitoring practices titled: Effective and Efficient Monitoring as a Component of Quality Assurance in the Conduct of Clinical Trials (2011) [3]. In addition, this study reviewed FDA warning letters, 300 other surveys, and expert panel meetings as well as a thorough review of existing literature. From this investigation, CTTI acknowledged a wide variety of monitoring strategies that appeared to reflect the institutions' characteristics. While most research enterprises established the plan and frequency of monitoring based on study design, academic institutions were most likely to make standard practice an exemption from its monitoring plan. Contract research organizations (CROs) were more likely to have standard operating procedures in place to guide their monitoring and industry appeared to just consider study design when establishing a monitoring plan. However, CTTI reported that in general, industry and CROs conducted on-site monitoring visits more frequently.

Study design is obviously an important factor for consideration when determining a monitoring plan; however, other factors may influence the decision-making process of a sponsor. On-site monitoring is considered more useful at the start of a new study and also when a protocol includes new technology or procedures not commonly performed by study staff [4]. Proponents of on-site monitoring emphasize relationship building between sponsors and sites, and more opportunities for education on protocol requirements and enrollment issues. Although sponsors report a 25% cost savings with RBM, others argue that this may just represent cost shifting [5]. In fact, sites are often required to dedicate time to submit certain documentation electronically such as specific screening, enrollment, and follow up data, as opposed to a monitor accessing these documents on-site which allows the study team to continue with normal daily research activities including screening and enrollment. In addition, some argue that on-site monitoring remains a critical tool in identifying several specific types of study issues such as

- identification of data entry errors or transcription errors,
- identification of missing clinical data in source records or case report forms,
- assurance that study source documentation exists,
- familiarity of the site's study staff with the protocol and required procedures, and
- compliance with the protocol and investigational product.

FDA Guidance

Despite the extensive investment in monitoring by research sponsors, several high-profile recalls of FDA approved products over many years led to a comprehensive review of the regulatory approval process. The FDA guidance issued in 2013, clearly places increasing emphasis on RBM when appropriate, which is largely influenced by many factors including the following

- sponsor's use of electronic systems,
- sponsor's access to subjects' electronic records, if applicable,
- timeliness of data entry from paper CRF, if applicable, and
- communication tools available to the sponsor and study site.

The document goes on to state that centralized monitoring processes can provide many of the capabilities of on-site monitoring as well as additional capabilities with the utilization of standard checks of range, consistency, completeness of data, identification of unusual distribution of data, identification of higher risk sites to target for on-site monitoring, and routine review of data in real time. The other important take home message coming from this guidance is that the FDA acknowledges that a variety of monitoring strategies are acceptable and that these strategies should be site- and study-specific and not one style for all [2]. As such, research sponsors began actively implementing centralized analysis of selected high-risk indicators and instituted best practices for remote monitoring of data. Despite the existence of RBM for many years, the clinical trials industry estimates that approximately 50% of sponsors have implemented RBM only in the last two years and approximately 25% have focused solely on phase II studies for the utilization of RBM [5].

Applications

The first step to effective monitoring by any method is the development of a well-designed protocol. Centralized monitoring strategies are designed with the expectation of uniformity in terms, definitions, and procedures used by researchers when collecting data during the conduct of a clinical trial. A clearly written protocol should provide this standardization not only for collecting the data, but also interpreting the data when monitoring and analysis are conducted.

The desire for physician flexibility with the ability to adapt and revise based on intra-operative, or intra-procedural findings during the conduct of operative and non-operative procedures is sometimes essential. However, this can be highly problematic for data integrity and reproducible outcomes in a clinical trial, particularly for multi-center protocols where different investigators at different institutions are expected to practice uniformly. Group training for these types of trials is typically limited to one- or two-day sessions at the launch of the trial. Local site training may continue with the sponsor providing proctors at the time of the investigational intervention as well as additional monitoring through site visits or remote video-monitoring of procedures. The best learning occurs when feedback from the various monitoring tools is given back to the local study teams.

Following the quality of protocol writing, design of the case report form itself is the next largest factor in the development and implementation of a successful RBM. Incomplete source documentation is reportedly the second most commonly cited deficiency in FDA inspections of clinical investigator sites [6]. Electronic case report forms (eCRFs) obviously lend themselves to more effective remote monitoring and may be created automatically from electronic medical record documentation or programmed such that the eCRF is created as the original source document. These electronic formats are capable of capturing a large amount of data queries from automated reference ranges programmed into the system, even before the data is remotely reviewed.

This level of automated data review does not necessarily capture all the necessary elements of the ALCOA acronym for source data verification: Attributable, Legible, Contemporaneous, Original, and Accurate [6], but a high-level centrally conducted statistical analysis may readily accomplish this task. Consider the scenario presented by George and Buyse [7] with the use of a bubble plot to identify fraudulently completed subject self-assessment questionnaires in a large clinical trial. In such a plot each center is represented by a bubble with the horizontal axis proportional to the volume of subjects and the vertical axis representing a data inconsistency score for the centers. Bubbles (centers) above the designated line of consistency had a greater chance of extreme data inconsistency that could not be explained by chance alone. On-site audits revealed no inconsistencies at one identified center as staff presented completed questionnaires and stated they were completed by subjects when in fact, staff had completed those questionnaires without ever showing them to subjects. While nothing looked discrepant about the questionnaires themselves during a monitoring visit, when compared to a large number of other centers it was obvious to a statistician observing the overall pattern of data in the bubble plot that each questionnaire was not answered by different individual subjects. This is just one example of the powerful effect RBM contributes to the overall monitoring plan for a study with proper utilization.

The Veterans Affairs Cooperative Studies Program (CSP) is another good example of how a program-wide adoption of RBM is based on FDA guidance and their own objectives of human subjects protection, data integrity, and efficiency [8].

CSP is a large network of coordinating centers in the VA responsible for conducting large multi-center studies in collaboration with VA investigators. While CSP has been assigning a risk category to studies since 2005, this was dramatically expanded in 2014 to integrate centralized activities for improving the successful conduct of studies. Multiple areas within the CSP program were brought together with the data coordinating centers, including the Site Monitoring and Auditing Resource Team (SMART) and the Clinical Research Pharmacy Coordinating Center (PCC) responsible for safety reporting, regulatory compliance, and product accountability. Each data coordinating center also has a quality assurance nurse specialist on staff, who has access to the electronic medical record of study patients and can conduct source data verification remotely. A variety of internal, centralized activities were initiated including site performance metrics, data falsification detection methods, remote monitoring, good data management practices, and creation of an electronic central study file to collect study documents.

Performance metrics are categorized as administrative (enrollment and randomization numbers, team attendance on conference calls), data integrity (rate of data queries, length of time for open data queries, rate of missing visits), and safety (eligibility errors, protocol deviations, and serious adverse event rates). Parameters of desired metrics are used to identify and classify local study sites that reach medium or high alert status requiring intervention by the data team based on pre-determined thresholds. The risk-based assessment results provide a direct path for corrective action planning and facilitates education with the local study site when presented in appropriate format (i.e., raw data may be distracting and info graphs may expedite the discussion).

In summary, RBM is an effective tool leveraged with recent technological advancements to significantly expand the capability for remote monitoring. While experts in the field of research welcome this powerful tool, many suggest that RBM is only one tool in the many strategies necessary for effective monitoring and efficient conduct of clinical trials. With the unlimited potential yielded by rapid technological growth, RBM is certainly a permanent fixture and necessitates planning in the early stages of protocol development of a large clinical trial.

References

1. International Conference of Harmonisation. E6: guideline for good clinical practice. 1996. Available at: http://www.ich.org/fileadmin/Public_Web_Site/ICH_Products/Guidelines/Efficacy/E6/E6_R1_Guideline.pdf.
2. US Food & Drug Administration. Guidance for industry: oversight of clinical investigations—a risk-based approach to monitoring. 2013. Available at: http://www.fda.gov/downloads/Drugs/.../Guidances/UCM269919.pdf.
3. Clinical Trials Transformation Initiative. Effective and efficient monitoring as a component of quality assurance in the conduct of clinical trials. 2011. Available at: http://www.ctti-clinicaltrials.org/files/Monitoring/Monitoring-Recommendations.pdf.
4. Lightfoot, J. The history of risk-based monitoring. Monitor. 2013;December:15–17.

5. Causey JM. Voices from the field—risk-based monitoring. Clin Res. 2015;29(5):59–62. doi:10.14524/CR-15-4085.
6. Bargaje C. Good documentation practice in clinical research. Perspect Clin Res. 2011;2(2): 59–63. doi:10.4103/2229-3485.80368.
7. George S, Buyse M. Data fraud in clinical trials. Clin Investig (Lond). 2015;5(2):161–73. doi:10.4155/cli.14.116.
8. Veterans Affairs Cooperative Studies Program-wide Adoption of Risk-based Monitoring. 2014. VA CSP RBM Guidance Policy. June 23, 2014.

Chapter 37
Investigators' Meetings

Kamal M.F. Itani

Introduction

Investigators' meetings are scheduled and budgeted events within a clinical trial and will set the tone and direction for the overall trial. Although face-to-face meetings are preferable, more recent technologies allow for virtual meetings through teleconferencing, videoconferencing, or Web conferencing. Face-to-face conferencing allows for investigators and research coordinators to meet, network, and learn from each other and how each site has strategized for recruitment, enrollment, and retention of study subjects, hurdles encountered, and troubleshooting.

As a general rule, face-to-face meetings should be scheduled in a central location that is easily accessible to all investigators. For meetings funded by the federal government, hotel rates and meal allowances for the length of the meetings should meet the government allowable rates for that location.

All Internet-based conferencing should meet the minimum standard for secure conferencing, in case patient-specific information is discussed. Alternatively, no patient-specific information should be discussed.

The principal investigator's office is charged with making all the arrangements for a face-to-face or virtual meeting. Alternatively, for a face-to-face meeting, a meeting organizer can be hired if budgeted.

Several meetings should be planned during the planning and conduct of a clinical trial. These would consist of one or two planning meetings during protocol development, an investigator initiation meeting, a yearly meeting, and a closing meeting.

K.M.F. Itani (✉)
Department of Surgery, VA Boston Health Care System/Boston University and Harvard
Medical School, VABHCS (112A), 1400 VFW Parkway, West Roxbury, MA 02132, USA
e-mail: kitani@va.gov

© Springer International Publishing AG 2017   319
K.M.F. Itani and D.J. Reda (eds.), *Clinical Trials Design in Operative
and Non Operative Invasive Procedures*, DOI 10.1007/978-3-319-53877-8_37

Clinical Trial Planning Meeting

After agreeing on the question, the primary and secondary outcomes, the intervention and the control groups, the principal investigator in collaboration with a biostatistician, and a few interested investigators and experts in the field of study develop a detailed protocol outline. Members of this group will usually constitute themselves as the executive committee of the overall study if funded. After agreement on the outline, it is not unusual for that group to have one or two face-to-face meetings to develop in great detail all aspects of the protocol. The principal investigator is responsible for finalizing the protocol for submission to the funding agency.

Within the VA system, the protocol outline is submitted to the Veterans Administration (VA) Cooperative Studies Program (CSP) as a letter of intent. If the idea and research proposal are approved, members of the study executive committee are funded for a face-to-face meeting to fully develop the protocol. Outside the VA system, it is not unusual for the investigators to meet at their own expense, through institutional funds or by Web conferencing.

This planning meeting is critical for the successful development of a detailed and feasible protocol that meets the requirements of a funding agency.

Study Initiation Meeting

Once a study is approved for funding, the study initiation meeting should take place after all study research personnel are in place. It is preferable for this initial meeting to be a face-to-face meeting for all assigned study personnel from all sites, including the study coordinating center and members of the executive committee.

During the meeting, the study protocol is reviewed in great detail with all investigators and research coordinators allowing ample time for questions and answers. It is not unusual for concerns to be aired and for the executive committee to decide on study protocol amendments based on these concerns and comments made during the meeting. A session should be dedicated to review compliance with research guidelines, ethical issues, and institutional review board (IRB) regulations. Another session should be dedicated to recruitment, enrollment, and retention of study subjects and various aspects of the consent to participate in the study.

The investigators should have a hands-on session on the technical aspects of the intervention whether surgical or nonsurgical invasive procedure. The purpose of this session which might involve videos, cadavers, or other hands-on techniques is to familiarize and standardize all steps of the intervention. As each surgeon or proceduralist might have biases or preferences, it is very important for the principal investigator to emphasize the importance of standardization and for each to maintain equipoise during the conduct of the trial. This session could also include laboratory procedures, if applicable. Minor modifications can be introduced to the procedure based on suggestions, feedback, or consensus of participating investigators.

Training might also be needed if the trial involves a diagnostic device, such as MRI, to determine eligibility in the trial. A trial of a procedure that may benefit or harm cognitive function might require training on a standardized battery of assessments tailored to that type of outcome. Alternatively, the trial might need to provide funding for people already trained in those assessments to perform that function in the trial.

The research coordinators will have a separate session to review in details data acquisition, form completion, interactions with the coordinating center, audits, handling of adverse and serious adverse events and maintaining screening and enrollment log books and regulatory folders.

It is advisable to define a certification standard in advance of the training meeting and develop an assessment procedure to certify that each person conducting the trial is certified according to the standards in the protocol.

Changes in personnel at the study will often require a special training meeting for the new personnel before they can begin recruiting and following study participants.

There may also be a need for personnel from the chair's office and coordinating center to visit a study site that is having problems conducting the trial. These visits may help identify the nature and cause of the problem and aid in finding solutions.

Annual Meeting

It is also advisable to have a yearly face-to-face meeting to review the progress of the study with all sites and study personnel. With dwindling resources and improving technology, it is currently more common to hold these yearly meetings by Web conferencing. The yearly meeting brings all investigators and research personnel together and provides them with additional confidence and renewed energy to continue with the study.

The lead biostatistician prepares a progress report that addresses all the aspects of recruitment, enrollment, retention, protocol adherence, and data quality that are study- and site-specific. Blinded tables of all data collected are also presented to point to the areas of deficiencies and strengths in data collection.

The site investigator will then discuss strategies to improve any aspect of the study such as enrollment, retention, or compliance. Sites can learn from each other and share solutions on various challenges they addressed and problems they solved. Sites that are performing well should be featured and should present in areas where they are excelling.

It is not uncommon to have new study sites participate at the yearly meeting to boost enrollment and other participating sites drop out due to poor performance.

Closing Meeting

The closing meeting takes place after the study ends, and the data is analyzed. The unblinded data and final results are presented to all the participating investigators. It is not uncommon for this meeting to be omitted for budgetary reason. It is, however, good practice to bring all the investigators and research coordinators together, thank them for their efforts, and present the results of the study to them.

It is not uncommon during this meeting for site investigators to come up with research questions that can potentially be answered by additional research analysis and be the basis for secondary manuscripts from the study or for new ideas to emerge that can be the basis of future studies.

Summary

A study planning meeting prior to protocol submission will help the principal investigator in collaboration with experts in the field to discuss all study details and will give the proposal a better chance at being funded. Once funded, a study initiation meeting is essential to discuss all the aspects of the study protocol with all investigators, research coordinators, and other study personnel. This first meeting sets the tone and expectation for the duration of the study. Yearly meetings are highly desirable to present overall progress, address pitfalls, and feature best practices. A closing meeting is not essential but if budgeted will allow for the presentation of the final results to the participating investigators and for secondary analysis to be identified and assigned to interested investigators.

Chapter 38
Site Visits

Kamal M.F. Itani

Introduction

Every large prospective randomized trial with multiple study sites should plan and budget for multiple site visits. Site visits will ensure that the proper sites are selected to participate in a trial through a pre-study qualification site visit. Once selected and approved to conduct a study, another site visit called initiation site visit will ensure that the study personnel are familiar with all aspects of the study and that the site has established the proper infrastructure to conduct the study as specified by the protocol. During the conduct of the trial, several monitoring site visits can take place to verify that the rights and well-being of the enrolled subjects are protected, that the data is accurate, complete, and verifiable, and to ensure that the site personnel are following all aspects of the protocol, good clinical practice, and are in compliance with all regulatory requirements. A closing site visit can also be performed for drug or equipment accountability purposes and to review all regulatory documents and record retention guidelines. Each of these visits will be described in details. In addition, site visits for cause will also be presented in this chapter.

In federally funded trials, most site visits are conducted by members of the executive committee or other experts within the field recruited for that purpose and as needed. In trials sponsored by industry, it is more likely for the sponsor to contract all site visits to a clinical research organization. The clinical research organization will usually employ study-dedicated clinical liaison specialists, auditors, and study monitors also known as Clinical Research Associates (CRA's) who will conduct site visits on a scheduled basis. Most clinical research organization will also have the ability to act as the coordinating center for large

K.M.F. Itani (✉)
Department of Surgery, VA Boston Health Care System/Boston University and Harvard Medical School, VABHCS (112A), 1400 VFW Parkway, West Roxbury, MA 02132, USA
e-mail: kitani@va.gov

© Springer International Publishing AG 2017   323
K.M.F. Itani and D.J. Reda (eds.), *Clinical Trials Design in Operative and Non Operative Invasive Procedures*, DOI 10.1007/978-3-319-53877-8_38

industry-sponsored trials. The costs associated with contracting these functions to a clinical research organization can be prohibitive in a federally funded trial but can be budgeted if necessary and justified within the trial.

This chapter will not detail the site visits performed by outside agencies such as the FDA or the Office for Human Research Protection (OHRP) but will describe how to prepare and be ready in the event such site visits were to occur.

Pre-study Qualification Site Visit

It is not uncommon for the principal investigator of a large multi-institutional prospective randomized trial to select sites based on reputation of a site in the area of investigation, the availability and reputation of site investigators, previous participation in clinical trials, and the ability to recruit study subjects. In the Veterans Administration (VA) open versus laparoscopic inguinal hernia repair trial, the VA National surgical database was used to estimate the number of open and laparoscopic operations performed at each VA site. The availability of minimally invasive surgeons interested in laparoscopic hernia surgery and yet have the equipoise to avoid influencing patients into one procedure or the other and adversely affect recruitment into the study [1] was also assessed. Although these goals are sometimes taken for granted, they are extremely important to assess prior to effectively enlisting a site into the study. The pre-study qualification also known as the "feasibility" site visit is usually conducted prior to the investigators' meeting, assesses the suitability of the investigator, staff, and site, and reviews in detail the sponsor's expectations.

For smaller or less complex studies, the pre-study qualification site visit can be substituted with a phone interview, review of qualifications of site investigators and staff, as well as through data submitted by the site to the principal investigator. The principal investigator and executive committee will then make a decision regarding the site suitability for the trial.

Initiation Site Visit

The initiation site visit is best done after the investigator's meeting. As described in the chapter on investigators' meetings (Chap. 37), key site personnel have a chance at the investigators' meeting to hear and discuss all steps related to the protocol, review the data entry sheet, and be briefed about good clinical practice. Depending on the study, a training session specific to the details of an operative or non-operative interventional procedure might take place at the investigators' meeting.

The initiation site visit will review the steps presented at the investigators' meeting. The site visitor will review the protocol and data handling guidelines with all study staff. The site visitor will also review recruitment strategies to ensure the success and progress of the study. Other items reviewed during this visit are regulatory in nature and include a review of the regulatory binder with Institutional Review Board (IRB) submissions as well as other regulatory paperwork, a discussion on good clinical practice, source documentation, roles and responsibilities of each site personnel, and adverse event reporting. When investigational products are required in the trial, the site visitor will perform an inventory of those products. Some sponsors prefer to ship the investigational products after the initiation site visit is performed to ensure that the site is certified as ready to start enrolling subjects.

In the case of operative and non-operative procedures, it is recommended that the site investigator line up some cases and perform the procedures in the presence of one of the investigators, usually a member of the executive committee. This will allow for the site visitor to confirm compliance with procedure standardization and to ensure that the proper infrastructure is in place to perform these cases. Short of a live on site review of the procedure, the site investigator can videotape the procedure and send the videotape to the principal investigator's office for review, if applicable.

Monitoring Site Visits

The purposes of the monitoring site visits are to review the progress of a clinical study, to ensure adherence to the protocol and to assure the accuracy of the data and the safety of the enrolled subjects and that the site is compliant with all regulatory requirements. The monitoring site visits can be scheduled at regular time intervals or based on pre-specified target enrollment of subjects within the study. Other criteria that can determine the frequency of a monitoring site visit are complexity of the protocol, staff experience, and site performance. The elements that will be commonly reviewed by the site visitor at each visit are described in Table 38.1. At the end of the site visit, the monitor will share the findings with the site PI and research coordinator including any corrections that need to be made and any necessary training or remedial training. Some of the most common deficiencies identified by a monitor include failure of the research staff to follow the protocol, failure to keep accurate records, problems with the informed consent form, failure to report adverse events, and failure to account for the proper disposition of research drugs or devices. The deficiencies can be addressed at the time of the site visit or as a response to formal queries sent by the sponsor. Repeat deficiencies or perceived deviation from good clinical practice in research can jeopardize the study site and the principal investigator. As a result, the study site can be withdrawn from the study and the investigator may not be considered for future studies.

Table 38.1 Elements reviewed during a monitoring site visit

1. *Regulatory binder*
All protocol versions and approvals
All investigator brochure versions
Laboratory certifications and normal ranges
All versions of FDA form 1572
Curricula vitae, licenses, and financial disclosures for all investigators, signed and dated
All sponsor correspondence
Serious adverse events
Updated delegation of responsibility/signature log as needed
2. *All IRB correspondence (within the regulatory binder)*
IRB receipt of amendments, serious adverse events, protocol deviations
Continuing reviews
3. *Original consents are in the medical records (copy available)*
4. *Source document*
All laboratory reports (reviewed and signed by PI)
X-ray and scan reports (Reviewed and signed by PI)
Physician and nurses notes
Procedure notes reviewed and signed by PI
Drug administration and compliance
Informed consent process documentation
Missing information and documentation of why it is missing
5. *Case report form*
Review completeness and accuracy Visit dates
Adverse events and attribution
Study medication stop and start dates
Concomitant medication start and stop dates
6. *Screening and enrollment logs*
7. *Research Product accountability*
Drug or device accountability form
Proper storage of drug or devices as per recommendations
Proper disposal or returned or expired research drug or device

Close-Out Visit

The close-out visit will take place when the study is complete or less commonly, if there is inadequate enrollment, protocol deviations, regulatory violations, or breech of safety. At the time of close-out, all data has been retrieved and the central database is locked. The site visitor will again review all regulatory documents, all research and device or study drug accountability record forms and will review with the site investigator the sponsor's expectations for research files retention guidelines. Retention of records is important in case of future audits or safety concerns by federal agencies with a drug or device.

Site Visit for Cause

A site visit for cause can be initiated by the trial executive committee, the sponsor or the funding agency, the site's IRB or Research and Development Committee. Reasons to conduct a for-cause site visit usually relate to poor compliance with good clinical practice guidelines, failure to follow the protocol, safety breeches, or poor compliance with the standardized operative or non-operative invasive procedure. A cluster of serious adverse events or perceived data falsification or fabrication can also result in an urgent site visit to the site in question.

Audits

An audit is performed by an independent body to assess all trial related activities and documents. The audit will usually assess a random subset of participants and will review the same parameters as with a monitoring visit and as delineated in Table 38.1.

Although an audit can be performed by the sponsor or the funding agency, the most significant are the ones performed by the FDA or the OHRP. The FDA is usually involved in an audit when the research might lead to a new drug or device application or a biologic license application. The audit can be routine or for cause. The most common reason a site or PI are selected are because the study is outside the PI's area of specialty or expertise, discrepancy of results with other sites or other similar studies, subject, or IRB complaints and unusually high enrollment compared to other sites. The audit visit is conducted with the same level of scrutiny as a monitoring site visit and might take several days.

OHRP reviews institutional compliance with the federal regulations governing the protection of human subjects in US Department of Health and Human Services sponsored research. The audit can be for cause or not for cause and will involve institutional administrators, IRB Chairperson, IRB members, and staff as well as investigators involved in human subject research.

Summary

Site visits are planned activities of any large multi-institutional prospective randomized trial. There are many types of site visits that can be planned during the conduct of a trial to ensure proper compliance with all aspects of a research protocol and regulatory requirements for the safety of research human subjects.

Reference

1. Neumayer L, Giobie-Hurder A, Jonason O, Fitzgibbons R, Dunlop D, Gibbs J, Reda D, Henderson W, The VA Cooperative Studies Investigators. Open versus laparoscopic mesh repair of inguinal hernia. N Engl J Med. 2004;350:1819–27.

Chapter 39
Data Safety Monitoring Board: Composition and Role

Marco A. Zenati and William G. Henderson

Introduction

Data safety monitoring boards (DSMBs), also referred by other names (e.g., data monitoring committees or DMCs), were first introduced in clinical research in the 1960s to monitor preliminary data in clinical trials to ensure safety of participants [1]. However, not all randomized controlled trials (RCTs) require a DSMB [2]. DSMBs should be used if the trial is multicenter and/or has a large sample size; if there is a planned interim analysis for possible early stopping for efficacy or futility; if the primary endpoints are mortality or major morbidity; if the population being studied is high risk; or if the interventions are new with little safety data available. If the investigators propose not to use a DSMB, then they should still specify in the protocol a plan to monitor patient safety, data acquisition, and study integrity.

Composition

In establishing a DSMB, the study investigators and sponsors should think carefully about all of the important aspects of the RCT and make sure that they are represented on the DSMB. For example, in a VA cooperative study of advanced

M.A. Zenati (✉)
Department of Cardiac Surgery, Harvard Medical School, Boston VA Medical Center, 301 Prospect Street, Belmont, MA 02478, USA
e-mail: Marco_Zenati@hms.harvard.edu

W.G. Henderson
Adult and Child Consortium for Outcomes Research and Delivery Science (ACCORDS) and Department of Biostatistics and Informatics, Colorado School of Public Health, University of Colorado Denver, 13199 E. Montview Blvd., Suite 300, Aurora, CO 80045, USA
e-mail: William.Henderson@ucdenver.edu

© Springer International Publishing AG 2017
K.M.F. Itani and D.J. Reda (eds.), *Clinical Trials Design in Operative and Non Operative Invasive Procedures*, DOI 10.1007/978-3-319-53877-8_39

laryngeal cancer conducted in the 1990s [3], the treatment modalities included chemotherapy, radiation therapy, and surgery. Also, functional outcomes (voice preservation and laryngectomy rehabilitation) were important secondary outcomes. So the DSMB included physicians representing each of the treatment modalities and also a speech pathologist in addition to a biostatistician. If the important outcomes in the RCT include some non-traditional ones (e.g., cost or psychometric testing), then these fields should be represented on the DSMB as well.

The DSMB includes at least three and usually no more than five voting members that are experts in the matter of the research: At least one member must be a statistician. More complex trials may have more members on the DSMB. The DSMB membership is expected for the duration of the clinical trial. If any member leaves the DSMB during the course of the trial, the sponsor will promptly appoint a replacement. The DSMB members are recommended and approved by the study sponsor. A DSMB chair, who is either selected by the sponsor or by the DSMB members with sponsor approval, is usually a clinician–researcher with a strong background in the subject matter of the trial. Voting members must consist of individuals who are impartial and independent of the study and who have no financial, scientific, or other conflict of interest (COI) with the study. DSMB members meet either in person, or via electronic mail or telephone conference at mutually agreeable times and places with a sponsor representative and a study investigator as appropriate. The meeting frequency will be at a minimum once a year. Meetings are closed to the public because discussions may address confidential patient data, and also, at least part of each meeting is closed to the study investigators who are involved in the design and conduct of the trial. A quorum will be determined (e.g., three members) in order to make the expected recommendations on the trends, incidences and overall safety results reported in the study, related safety adverse events and deaths as appropriate to the conduct of the study. Decisions and recommendations are usually made by consensus.

Masking of interim safety and efficacy outcomes during the course of the RCT is an important issue. Standard practice is to have the study investigators and sponsors masked to interim outcome results during the conduct of the RCT; only the DSMB members and the biostatistician who prepared the DSMB statistical report should see the interim outcome results during the course of the RCT.

Role

In order for the DSMB to fulfill its responsibilities, the members will follow these guidelines: (a) Members must be free of apparent COIs involving financial, scientific, or regulatory matters; (b) members will assess trial objectives and design in an unbiased way; (c) DSMB members will review safety and efficacy data and pertinent procedures in order to be confident that the data in which the decisions are based are accurate and complete; (d) all decisions of the DSMB shall be independent of all study personnel; and (e) the primary purpose of the DSMB sessions is to address safety data and critical efficacy endpoints of the research [4].

At the end of each meeting, the DSMB will make one of these recommendations: (A) *"Members recommend that the study continue without major modification."* (B) *"Members recommend that the study continue with specific modifications."* (C) *"Members recommend that all or a portion of the study be stopped due to safety or efficacy concerns."* and (D) *"Members recommend terminating the study."* These recommendations are shared with the study investigators, sponsors, and the institutional review boards (IRBs) monitoring the RCT.

Initial DSMB Meeting

Prior to or close to the beginning of data collection on the trial, the DSMB holds an initial meeting with the sponsor, the lead study investigator, and the study biostatistician. At the initial meeting, the design of the clinical trial is reviewed. It is not the purview of the DSMB to conduct a scientific review of the trial, since it has already undergone peer review and possibly review by FDA. However, it is important for the DSMB to carefully consider the study design so that it can determine what will be important to monitor during the conduct of the study.

The DSMB reviews the proposed data summaries and analyzes the study biostatistician will provide them during the study. The DSMB will also review the interim monitoring plan and safety monitoring plan. The DSMB will also review and approve the DSMB charter, which outlines its purview and rules of operation.

"Open" DSMB Sessions

In order to allow the DSMB to have adequate access to information provided by the sponsors and study investigators, a session of the DSMB members, the sponsor representative, and the study investigators (usually the study chairperson and biostatistician) will take place in an "open session." At the discretion of the DSMB, this session gives the DSMB an opportunity to query sponsor representatives and/or clinical trial investigators about issues such as patient recruitment and retention, site performance, and data quality. With this format, important interactions are facilitated through which safety and other problems affecting trial integrity can be identified and resolved. These individuals will either be present at the DSMB meeting or by telephone link. The open session will be followed by a closed session as appropriate in which the DSMB will conduct an independent, confidential evaluation.

"Closed" DSMB Sessions

Closed sessions will be conducted only by DSMB membership and the biostatistician and are held to allow discussion of confidential data from the clinical trial, including information about the safety and efficacy of interventions. The sponsor representative and study investigators who manage study patients may not participate in these meetings. At the conclusion of the closed session, the DSMB chairperson will communicate the decisions and the recommendations to the DSMB committee and to the sponsor and study investigators in writing.

Major Responsibilities of DSMB

The major responsibilities of the DSMB are as follows:

1. **Monitoring for safety**. A primary responsibility of the DSMB is to review the safety data submitted in the DSMB report to assess whether there are any increased or untoward risks to the participants in the study that may require a change in the protocol (intervention or procedures) or possible termination of part or the entire study. The level of inspection of the safety data varies from study to study and is described in the study protocol and/or DSMB monitoring plan. Also, guidance on criteria for recommending early stopping of a study is established by the DSMB and included in the study protocol and/or DSMB monitoring plan. Safety data are submitted to the DSMB on a schedule defined by the DSMB and include summaries of the proportions of participants who developed a reportable adverse event and serious adverse events in the whole study population (for open session reports) and by blinded treatment group (if requested by the DSMB for closed session reports). This is typically presented overall by diagnostic groups (e.g., MedDRA system organ class or body system). Samples of adverse event tables are included in the DSMB monitoring plan. The DSMB typically reviews summary adverse event data but not detailed information on every adverse event or serious adverse event reported. This responsibility lies with the study sponsor, who must assure prompt review of such events. Individual adverse event reports may be reviewed for adverse events of particular concern.

2. **Make recommendations on continuation of the study**. The DSMB makes recommendations to the sponsor concerning whether to continue, modify, or terminate a clinical study based on the ongoing study information and/or new external information that may make the original study unethical, the design inappropriate or the research questions no longer scientifically significant, or safety information that places research subjects at risk. Inherent to this question are considerations such as patient accrual, overall study progress, treatment efficacy, adverse events and participant safety, futility, and adequate monitoring and reporting to ensure participant safety and data integrity.

3. **To assess the performance of participating sites**. The DSMB assesses the performance of each participating site and makes appropriate recommendations regarding continuation, probationary status, or termination of sites with performance issues. The sponsor, study chairperson, and biostatistician also assess the performance of each participating site and make recommendations regarding termination of sites or initiation of new sites.
4. To review and provide recommendations regarding protocol changes, interim analysis, sample size re-estimation, and subprotocols.
5. It is not the role of the DSMB to ensure regulatory compliance.
6. It is good practice to ask the DSMB to review and comment on study manuscripts, particularly the main outcome analysis, because they are often experts in the fields of investigation and are likely able to provide important insights into the interpretation of the results. However, they need to maintain their independence from the sponsor and study investigators and should be acknowledged in the manuscript but not be co-authors.

Independence of DSMB Committees

Interaction of study investigators and sponsors with the DSMB is considered inappropriate, and breaking this "wall" is considered a threat to its independence. One of the reasons for the existence of this "wall" is to prevent the leak of preliminary findings that may prejudice the study. For instance, if it was known that the DSMB was examining a marginal increase in cardiovascular risk in a trial, then this knowledge may bias future recruitment by excluding subjects at risk for such events. Recent reports have been published that point to clear violations of the integrity of the DSMB [5]; in two recent cases, the commercial entity sponsoring the study decided to unblind aspects of the trial data rather than let the DSMB exercise their important responsibilities [6].

A DSMB reform proposal is calling for convening a DSMB under the aegis of an independent public body (e.g., the foundation for the NIH or similar body): Under this proposal, the sponsor will provide funding to the third party who would be responsible for choosing the DSMB members, supervising the panel's activities, and ensuring its integrity. To prevent sponsors from interfering with an ongoing study, the trial steering committee would report only to the DSMB [5].

References

1. Slutsky AS, Lavery JV. Data safety and monitoring boards. N Engl J Med. 2004;350:1143–7.
2. Ellenberg S, Fernandes RM, Saloojee H, Bassler D, Askie L, Vandermeer B, Offringa M, Van der Tweel I, Altman DG, van der Lee JH, StaR Child Health Group. Standard 3: data monitoring committees. Pediatrics. 2012;129:S132–7.

3. The Department of Veterans Affairs Laryngeal Cancer Study Group. Induction chemotherapy plus radiation compared with surgery plus radiation in patients with advanced laryngeal cancer. N Engl J Med. 1991;324:1685–90.
4. Hulley SB, Cummings SR, Browner WS, Grady DG, Newman TB. Designing clinical research. 4th ed. Philadelphia: Wolters Kluwer/Lippincott Williams & Wilkins; 2013.
5. Drazen JM, Wood AJJ. Don't mess with the DSMB. N Engl J Med. 2010;363:477–8.
6. Califf RM, Harrington RA, Blazing MA. Premature release of data from clinical trials of ezetimibe. N Engl J Med. 2009;361:712–7.

Chapter 40
Endpoints Committee

Leigh Neumayer and William G. Henderson

Adjudication of study endpoints is an important consideration in the planning of a clinical trial [1]. Definitions of nonfatal events are often subjective, and the purpose of adjudication is to help make the collection of these data more uniform and unbiased. This will give the consumers of the clinical trial more confidence in the clinical trial results.

The clinical trial protocol should specify the details of the adjudication process. These should include: (1) definition of the major endpoints; (2) how the events will be chosen for the adjudication process; (3) what data elements will be presented to an endpoints committee to help them carry out their responsibilities; (4) composition and responsibilities of the endpoints committee; (5) frequency and format of committee meetings; and (6) how the adjudication process will meld with the process of interim reviews of the study by the Data and Safety Monitoring Board (DSMB). If adjudication of endpoints is not planned, this should be stated in the protocol and the reasons for absence of adjudication.

In most cases, adjudication is done only for the primary outcome of the clinical trial. However, there might be some trials in which other endpoints (e.g., important safety events) are adjudicated as well. Ideally, the timing of the adjudication of events should be planned so that the DSMB makes their decisions on the basis of adjudicated events only.

L. Neumayer (✉)
Department of Surgery, University of Arizona College of Medicine-Tucson,
1501 N. Campbell Ave, PO Box 245066, Tucson, AZ 85724, USA
e-mail: lneumayer@surgery.arizona.edu

W.G. Henderson
Adult and Child Consortium for Outcomes Research and Delivery Science (ACCORDS) and Department of Biostatistics and Informatics, Colorado School of Public Health, University of Colorado Denver, 13199 E. Montview Blvd., Suite 300, Aurora, CO 80045, USA
e-mail: William.Henderson@ucdenver.edu

© Springer International Publishing AG 2017   335
K.M.F. Itani and D.J. Reda (eds.), *Clinical Trials Design in Operative and Non Operative Invasive Procedures*, DOI 10.1007/978-3-319-53877-8_40

Dechartres et al. [2] performed an interesting systematic review of the planning and reporting of endpoint committees (ECs) in randomized clinical trials (RCTs) reported in five high-impact medical journals in 2004–2005. ECs were reported in 33.4% of 314 RCTs. RCTs in the cardiovascular areas were by far the most prominent users of ECs (81.3%) compared to other areas of medicine (8.8% for infectious diseases to 28.6% for neurology). Larger, multicenter trials with DSMBs also tended to be higher users of ECs. In the vast majority of the RCTs using ECs (93.3%), suspected events as identified by local investigators were the events that were adjudicated. Of the 56 trials that reported on information provided to the EC, 32.1% provided results of tests and procedures performed, 25.0% provided the complete medical file for each case, and 23.2% used a standardized case report form. Ninety-two percent of the ECs were independent, but, surprisingly, only 54% were blinded to the treatment group of the case. The median number of members of the ECs was 3 (interquartile range 3–6). The study investigators made some important recommendations from their systematic review: (1) An EC should be used in all RCTs having a primary outcome that has subjectivity and especially if the intervention is not delivered in a blinded fashion; (2) suspected events requiring adjudication should be defined and sensible methods (e.g., local investigator identification and laboratory tests) should be used to identify suspected events; (3) information on each case provided to the EC should be defined, and this information should not include variables that could potentially unblind the adjudicators; (4) the EC should have at least three clinical experts; if the primary outcomes are in different medical areas, several ECs might be needed or the EC might need to include more people with different of expertise; (5) members of the EC should be independent and blinded to treatment arms of the cases; (6) adjudicators should be trained and the method to reach consensus should be defined before the RCT begins; and (7) a random selection of cases should be readjudicated.

An EC is modeled on the traditional DSMB but has a different scope and has different membership [3]. Given that clinical trials are usually comparing one treatment to another (drug vs placebo, one surgical technique to another, surgical therapy to medical therapy), the primary and secondary outcome measures are the lynchpins of proving or disproving the hypotheses. The purpose of the EC is to objectively determine whether the outcome has been achieved. In clinical trials, there is truly only one outcome that can be 100% free of bias and that outcome is death (the subject is either dead or alive). Every other outcome measure has the potential for bias, whether it be cause of death or some other outcome. Even outcomes that traditionally are objective such as laboratory values can be subject to bias with calibration of machines or ascertainment environment.

An EC is composed of independent experts who will centrally review and classify outcomes (whether they be primary or secondary or events of special interest) in a blinded and unbiased manner, determining whether the endpoints meet the protocol definitions/criteria. Centralized adjudication with an independent committee's review enhances the consistency, validity and integrity of clinical study outcomes.

Table 40.1 Potential measurements of hernia recurrence

Measurement	Potential bias	Design response
Physical examination	Varies from assessor to assessor, may not detect small recurrences	Two independent examiners must agree
Patient symptoms	Symptoms are not a good predictor of recurrence	Could be used as a surrogate, however would be poor measure of recurrence
Findings at reoperation	Most surgeons will be able to find a "recurrence" (for instance, a small residual indirect) when reoperating. Surgeon might have some preconceived bias in that they would not be operating if they did not believe there was a recurrence	Videotape operations for independent operators to view

The assessment of clinical outcomes is particularly subject to bias. For instance, when the outcome is hernia recurrence, there is no "gold standard" for measurement of recurrence. Options for measuring hernia recurrence (and the potential sources of bias) are listed in Table 40.1.

The risk of bias in assessment is not limited to primary outcome measures. It is also a risk of similar magnitude for any outcome or side effect that occurs in a trial. When a side effect profile is being used to determine safety of a drug or procedure, the assessment and attributions become exceedingly important. For instance in the VA inguinal hernia trial [4], the investigators wanted to capture the complications associated with type of anesthesia. During study design, they determined that hypotension in the OR requiring administration of a vasoconstrictor (phenyle-phrine) would be assessed as a significant complication with the measurement being administration of the vasoconstrictor. At the first DSMB meeting, one of the 14 sites had this "complication" occur six times (no other site had assessed even one case with this complication). Looking into the charts of these patients and the practices at the site, it was apparent that the vasoconstrictor was given prophy-lactically with a spinal anesthetic to prevent hypotension. An EC can, with minimal bias, use predefined criteria to determine whether the complication meets the criteria and if it does, then adjudicate the attribution. An EC could be used to objectively assess and attribute events such as cause of death, or whether the side effect was present and/or attributable to the treatment.

ECs should have separation from the investigators and the sponsor of the trial to minimize the perception, appearance or introduction of bias. The committee should have clearly defined, written procedures for assessing outcomes, minimizing introduction of observer bias. They should be blinded where possible to the sub-ject's assignment to a treatment group. The committee needs clearly defined pro-cedures for adjudicating outcomes without ambiguity when reviewers disagree. In addition, the EC should have a quality management system that is independent of the reviewers and sponsor (Table 40.2).

Table 40.2 Key constructs for endpoints committee

• Clearly defined roles for all groups (central reviewers, sponsor, contractors, FDA, etc.)
• Written policies and procedures for dealing with data received from study sites or central study office such as what to do about missing data or poor-quality data
• Quality control and assurance procedures for the handling of all data in any form
• Written procedures for ensuring blinded (when possible) review of the data
• Written procedures for data transfers to and from contractors and/or central reviewers
• Content and format for interim and final committee reports
• Prescribed criteria for selecting and compensating central reviewers
• Written procedures for training central reviewers in the systematic assessment of data
• Validation process for all databases used in data analysis
• Procedures for data and material storage (HIPAA compliant)
• Clear definitions for all possible outcome categories
• Defined procedures for adjudicating between central reviewers or committee members who do not agree
• If applicable, defined procedures for adjudicating between site physicians' assessment and that made by a central reviewer

Adapted from Kradjian et al. [3]. With permission from Sage Publications

An additional benefit of an EC is control of the inherent variability presented when numerous raters are asked to apply a complex set of medical endpoint criteria. Classifications can vary due to differences in individual medical training and application in clinical judgment. An EC limits the number of individuals/experts who are providing such classification thereby controlling the variability.

Members for the EC must be chosen carefully. They should be rigorously vetted to ensure subject matter (for the outcomes) expertise and ability to access data/variables (for instance, if the outcome is based on imaging, they must have access to digital systems that comply with standards and privacy regulations). The members must be able to commit to the workload, duration and timelines of their duties, operate with medically relevant adjudication competence and work with the appropriate level of independence so that the outcomes they provide are both clinically sound and not subject to bias [5]. The members of the EC should not be investigators nor serve on the study's DSMB.

ECs are still used relatively rarely in clinical trials in surgery. Some recent examples include studies on substances influencing hemostasis in vascular surgery [6] and orthopedic trials involving fracture healing assessments [7]. Web-based endpoint adjudication systems have recently been developed to make the process more efficient and timely [8, 9].

It is our recommendation that an endpoints committee be considered when the primary outcome is subjective (e.g., presence or not of a hernia recurrence) or if the outcome requires attribution (e.g., cause of death). Endpoint committees should be part of the design of a trial and be sufficiently separate from investigators and sponsor and have adequate expertise and training.

References

1. Granger CB, Vogel V, Cummings SR, Held P, Fiedorek F, Lawrence M, Neal B, Reidies H, Santarelli L, Schroyer R, Stockbridge NL, Zhao F. Do we need to adjudicate major clinical events? Clin Trials. 2008;5:56–60.
2. Dechartres A, Boutron I, Roy C, Ravaud P. Inadequate planning and reporting of adjudication committees in clinical trials: recommendation proposal. J Clin Epidemiol. 2009;62:695–702.
3. Kradjian S, Gutheil J, Baratelle A, et al. Development of a charter for an endpoint assessment and adjudication committee. Drug Inf J. 2005;39:53–61.
4. Neumayer L, Giobbie-Harder A, Jonasson O, Fitzgibbons R Jr, Dunlop D, Gibbs J, Reda D, Henderson W, for the Veterans Affairs Cooperative Studies Program 456 Investigators. Open mesh versus laparoscopic mesh repair of inguinal hernia. N Engl J Med. 2004;350:1819–27.
5. Tyner CA, Somaratne RM, Cabell CH, Turner JR. Establishment and operation of clinical endpoint committees: best practice for implementation across the biopharmaceutical industry. http://www.quintiles.com/library/white-papers/establishment-and-operation-of-clinical-endpoint-committees.Quintiles white paper, 29 Feb 2012.
6. Bergqvist D, Clement D. Adjudication of endpoints in studies on substances influencing haemostasis—an example from vascular surgery. Eur J Vasc Endovasc Surg. 2008;36:703–4.
7. Vannabouathong C, Sprague S, Bhandari M. Guidelines for fracture healing assessments in clinical trials. Part I: definitions and endpoint committees. Injury. 2011;42:314–6.
8. Nolen TL, Dimmick BF, Ostrosky-Zeichner L, Kendrick AS, Sable C, Ngai A, Wallace D. A web-based endpoint adjudication system (WebEAS) for interim analyses in clinical trials. Clin Trials. 2009;6:60–6.
9. Zhao W, Pauls K. Architecture design of a generic centralized adjudication module integrated in a web-based clinical trial management system. Clin Trials. 2016;13:223–33.

Chapter 41
Regulatory Issues with Devices in Clinical Trials

Gregory Campbell

Implantable Medical Devices

Implantable medical devices require invasive procedures, and most involve a surgical operation. There are many implantable devices across the very broad range of medicine. The annual sales for each of the eleven most implantable medical devices in the USA, according to the Wall Street Journal (July 18, 2011), range from 130,000 to 2 and a half million: (1) artificial eye lenses, (2) ear tubes, (3) coronary stents, (4) artificial knees, (5) metal screws, pins, plates, and rods (traumatic fracture), (6) intrauterine devices, (7) spinal fusion hardware, (8) breast implants, (9) heart pacemakers, (10) artificial hips, and (11) implantable cardioverter defibrillators. If a medical device company has a new investigational implantable device that it wishes to study in a clinical investigation in the USA in order to provide evidence to the U. S. Food and Drug Administration (FDA) of the device's safety and effectiveness, it will ordinarily rely on surgeons (or interventionalists) as clinical investigators to perform the procedure to implant the device. Therefore, these clinicians need to know what the regulatory requirements are for their participation in such a study and more generally about the clinical trials for these implantables. Because of the wide variety of implantable medical devices, the invasive procedure could call upon the surgical (or interventional) skill of any medical specialty: orthopedic, cardiovascular, cardiothoracic, obstetric/gynecological, ophthalmic, plastic, oral, neurological, otolaryngological (ENT), or general surgeons.

G. Campbell (✉)
GCStat Consulting LLC, 14605 Sandy Ridge Road, Silver Spring, MD 20905, USA
e-mail: GCStat@verizon.net

© Springer International Publishing AG 2017   341
K.M.F. Itani and D.J. Reda (eds.), *Clinical Trials Design in Operative and Non Operative Invasive Procedures*, DOI 10.1007/978-3-319-53877-8_41

The Regulation of Medical Devices in the USA

The Food and Drug Administration regulates medical devices in the USA. This stems from legislation passed by Congress and approved by the President to amend the Food, Drug and Cosmetic Act in 1976 to include provisions for the regulation of medical devices. These amendments set up the classification system for medical devices. A medical device is classified into one of three classes: Class 1 are general controls, Class 2 require what are called Special Controls and are "cleared" through a Premarket Notification (also called 510(k)), and Class 3 devices include life-saving or life-threatening or novel technologies. Implantable devices could be classified as Class 2 or Class 3. Most Class 3 devices require what is called a Premarket Approval (PMA) application. Clinical studies to demonstrate the safety and effectiveness of a medical device are submitted to the FDA in PMA applications; clinical study data may also be needed in a small proportion of Premarket Notifications (510(k)) submissions. In these cases, the sponsor conducts clinical studies of the investigational device.

Significant Risk Devices and IDEs

For any device that poses significant risk, the sponsor of the study is required to submit to the FDA an investigational device exemption (IDE) application and it must be approved by FDA before the clinical study conducted in the USA can proceed. The analog of this in U.S. regulation of pharmaceutical and drugs and biological therapeutic products is the Investigational New Drug (IND) application. A significant risk device is one that presents the potential for serious risk to the health, safety, or welfare of a subject. This includes most if not all implants. In addition to the potential risk associated with the new investigational device, if the implantation of the device requires a surgery, it is extremely likely that the device will be categorized as a significant risk device, since no surgery is without some risk. In some cases, the surgical operation may require anesthesia which contributes additional risk. A determination by FDA about significant risk could be appealed. In addition, a sponsor can request FDA to waive any requirement of the IDE regulations by submitting a waiver request with supporting documentation.

A significant risk device that is approved for one indication would usually require another IDE to conduct a study for either a different (or an expanded) indication. It is possible that an investigational study involving an implantable device would be exempt from the IDE regulations if it is a legally marketed device that is used in accordance with its labeling. However, if a device is used for a different indication (a different label) than one for which it is approved, then the use of that device is called "off-label." For example, if the investigation is for a different population than the one for which the product is approved, that would be a different indication. If physicians use a device off-label, they have the responsibility to be well informed about it, to base its use on firm scientific rationale and on sound medical evidence, and to maintain records of the product's use and effects. Use of a marketed device in this manner *when the intent is the "practice of medicine"* does not require the submission of an IDE or review by an institutional review board (IRB) [1]. With that caveat, the IDE regulations apply not only to sponsors which are medical product companies but also to sponsor-investigators who are individuals conducting the investigational study [2]. So for an investigation for a novel implantable or an implantable device used off-label outside the "practice of medicine," the IDE regulations apply, regardless of whether the sponsor is a device company or a sponsor-investigator. Note, however, that surgical trials on humans that do not involve an investigational medical device would not be subject to FDA's IDE regulations but investigators would still need to gain IRB approval from their institution and follow good clinical practices (GCPs).

An approved IDE allows the applicant, also called the sponsor, to proceed with the clinical study of the investigational device. The sponsor is usually the device company but it could also be a clinical investigator or an academic researcher that submits the IDE application. IDE applications are acted on by FDA within 30 days or by default they are considered approved. There are three actions that FDA can take for an IDE application: An IDE can be approved by FDA, approved with conditions or disapproved. If it is approved with conditions the sponsor is generally given 45 days to successfully address the concerns that generated the conditions but the study is allowed to proceed in the interim. FDA will not disclose the existence of an IDE or an IDE application. There are several types of IDEs: first in human, feasibility, and pivotal. Note that each of these clinical studies for a significant risk device would require an approved (or conditionally approved) IDE before the study would commence. In the case of a pivotal study, an IDE allows an investigational device to be used in a clinical study to collect data on its safety and effectiveness for a submission to FDA of one of the following four kinds of marketing applications:

1. Premarket Approval (PMA) applications are for novel technologies or life-saving or life-threatening devices, called Class III devices;
2. Premarket Notifications, also called 510(k)s, are based on the evaluation of what is called "substantial equivalence" to a marketed (predicate) product for what are called Class II devices under what are called Special Controls. Whereas FDA approves PMAs, successful Premarket Notifications are said to be "cleared" by FDA;
3. De Novo applications are like 510(k) applications but there is no predicate so what are called Special Controls for these Class II devices need to be written by FDA;
4. Humanitarian Device Exemption (HDE) is an approval for humanitarian use that is limited to 4000 devices per year due to the rarity of the condition.

Good Clinical Practices (GCPs)

The clinical investigators in an investigational study whether a study has IDE approval (if the device is significant risk) or not are required to follow GCPs including: (1) protection of human subjects, (2) IRB approval, (3) financial disclosure by clinical investigators, and (4) design controls for Quality System Regulation.

Of primary concern is the protection of the subjects or patients who are the participants in the trial. This is accomplished through the informed consent. Each of the study's clinical investigators is responsible for obtaining in writing the informed consent of each of their subjects (or patients) in the study.

Good clinical practices (GCPs) require approval of the IRBs for all the institutions involved. It is the task of each IRB to help to ensure the trial is ethical and the rights of the patients are protected at that institution. Each IRB needs to conduct its review for an IDE study before it is approved by FDA. The clinical investigator and the sponsor need to keep detailed records [including Case Report Forms (CRF)] for each subject in the study and report adverse events in a prescribed manner. In some cases, the study has a Data Monitoring Committee (DMC), also called a Data and Safety Monitoring Board (DSMB). DMCs are not required except in the rare case of the waiver of informed consent (usually due to emergency that makes informed consent impossible). The role of the DMC is twofold: to protect the patients in the trial and to preserve its scientific integrity. For more information about DMCs, see the FDA guidance document "Establishment and Operation of Clinical Trial Data Monitoring Committees."

Thirdly, financial disclosure by clinical investigators is required to avoid any conflicts of interest that could potentially create an impression that the best interests of the study subjects have been compromised.

Devices studied under an IDE are exempt from the FDA Quality System Regulation except for the design control requirements which assure that the device has been designed to perform as intended when produced for commercial distribution.

Responsibilities of Clinical Investigators for Significant Risk Device Studies

1. Investigator is responsible for obtaining informed consent of each subject under the investigator's care in the clinical study under Title 21 Code of Federal Regulations (CFR) Part 50.
2. Investigator is responsible for the use of the investigational device only for those subjects under his or her supervision in the clinical study (CFR 812.110).

3. Investigator must disclose to the sponsor sufficient accurate financial information to allow the IDE applicant (the sponsor) to submit certification under (812.110).
4. Investigator must return to the sponsor any remaining supply of the device or dispose of the device as the sponsor directs (812.110).
5. Investigator must maintain accurate and complete records relating to the investigation, including all correspondence and required reports, records of receipt, use or disposition of the investigational device records of each subject's case history and exposure to the device, the protocol and documentation for each deviation (date and reason) for each protocol deviation and any other records that FDA requires (812.140).
6. Investigator reports—The investigator must provide reports in a timely manner to the sponsor and/or the IRB for unanticipated adverse device effects, withdrawal of IRB approval progress reports, deviations for the investigational plan, failure to obtain informed consent, final report, and other reports (812.150). The sponsor has additional reporting requirements to FDA.
7. In addition, the investigator is responsible for appropriate delegation of study tasks, appropriate training of study staff, and supervision of staff including contracted personnel.
8. Lastly, the investigator is responsible for adherence to the study protocol.

The sponsor of an IDE has additional requirements compared to that of the clinical investigator. One such responsibility is the reporting of serious adverse events and adverse events to FDA within established timelines. The main sources of these reports are, of course, the reports that the investigators provide to the sponsor.

FDA has an inspection program through its Bioresearch Monitoring (BIMO) division for approved IDEs to make sure the sponsor, clinical investigators, and the IRBs are complying with the FDA regulations. This includes FDA investigators visiting the clinical sites during the study and inspecting the records.

There are many challenges for surgical trials and interventional studies involving medical devices. It is well recognized that for many procedures there are differences in the skill of the surgeons performing the procedure. In addition, this skill generally improves with experience and so there is a well-known phenomenon called the learning curve that reflects the improvement in the surgical skill with accumulating experience. The learning curve can affect the ability to measure the safety and the effectiveness of the device since both may depend on each individual's surgical skill and the learning curve. Another challenge concerns the control arm in the traditional randomized two-arm trial. One option would be that the medical device is implanted in the patients in the experimental arm but a placebo device is implanted in the other arm. This placebo surgery, also called the more derogatory phrase "sham surgery," can in some cases create an ethical dilemma, especially if the procedure involves anesthesia. A reason to consider this control is that there is a well-known placebo effect in many surgical trials. Another option would be to have as a control a group that did not receive the surgical procedure (and hence not the implant). But this suffers from another challenge, namely, the inability in many cases to blind or mask the patient and the clinical personnel from which group they have been assigned. It is almost always the case that the surgeon is not blinded or masked to this information. In a placebo controlled trial, the patients can usually be successfully masked (unless the device is visible to them), but this is not the case in a trial with a no surgery arm. It is highly recommended if at all possible that the third party evaluators of the safety and effectiveness endpoints be masked or blinded to the treatment assignment. Another challenge of surgical trials is that the endpoints can in some cases be quite long-term (on the order of several months or a couple years); the effort to continue to follow patients for such a long time can be thwarted by patient dropout, missed appointments, revocation of informed consent, and other forms of missingness in the data that can create analytical nightmares.

An approved protocol includes the outline for a statistical analysis of how to analyze the primary safety and effectiveness endpoints in the clinical study. A more detailed statistical analysis plan (SAP) is subsequently developed by the sponsor that details the precise statistical analysis outlined in the protocol before any clinical data from the study have been collected. The expectation then is that this plan is then followed in terms of the statistical analysis. Any deviations from it in the analysis will require a detailed explanation by the sponsor to the FDA.

Concluding Remarks

In conclusion, invasive procedures that implant investigational medical devices usually require an IDE to be approved by FDA before the study can commence. Further, there are a number of responsibilities that each clinical investigator must satisfy in participating in such a study. These studies can be difficult and challenging to perform.

References

1. FDA "Off-Label and Investigational use of Marketed Drugs, Biologics and Medical Devices—Information Sheet. 2016. http://www.fda.gov/RegulatoryInformation/Guidances/ucm126486. htm.
2. U.S. Code of Federal Regulations, 21 CFR 812.

Chapter 42
Trial Registration and Public Access to Data

Shachar Laks, Lawrence T. Kim and Yvonne Lucero

Part I. Why Register Clinical Trials?

Prior to the initiation of comprehensive clinical trial registries, recruitment to clinical trials would occur primarily by word of mouth, local and regional advertising, established referral patterns, and availability at local health care facilities. This practice resulted in regional, social, economic, and occasionally racial biases in patient recruitment and ultimately participation. One goal of registration is to allow potential participants equal, accessible, comprehensive, and unbiased access to available clinical trials. Registration also allows referring physicians access to information about clinical studies and thus to more accurately and methodically advise their patients of potential opportunities. Registries allow potential participants and referring physicians to get complete, unbiased information in an un-pressured environment and the ability to compare multiple clinical trials for which patients may be appropriate candidates. In this way, clinical trial registries contribute to the process of adequately informed consent.

S. Laks · L.T. Kim
Department of Surgery, University of North Carolina, 170 Manning Dr. 1150 POB,
Campus Box 7213, Chapel Hill, NC 27599, USA
e-mail: slaksmd@hotmail.com

L.T. Kim
e-mail: Lawrence_Kim@med.unc.edu

Y. Lucero (✉)
Cooperative Studies Program Coordinating Center, Hines Veterans' Affairs
Hospital/Loyola University, 5000 S. 5th Ave. (151), Hines, IL 60141, USA
e-mail: yvonne.lucero@va.gov

© Springer International Publishing AG 2017
K.M.F. Itani and D.J. Reda (eds.), *Clinical Trials Design in Operative
and Non Operative Invasive Procedures*, DOI 10.1007/978-3-319-53877-8_42

Another important benefit is the ability to ensure national and worldwide access to clinical trials. Patients are no longer limited to participating in trials available locally because they or their physicians were unaware of trials ongoing elsewhere. Registries may afford patients the choice to travel nationally or internationally to participate in clinical trials.

Registration of clinical trials is beneficial to clinical trial administrators and investigators in a variety of ways. Initially, at the time of trial design, it provides the ability to easily search for similar or competing trials. This can help minimize the possibility of duplicating an existing trial. Further, it allows for improved communication between investigators and encourages collaboration to optimize study design, accrual, and analysis.

Trial registration databases are also important tools for institutional review boards (IRBs), journal editors, and reviewers. By accessing a database, it is possible to better understand the context in which a clinical trial is undertaken as well as its significance in relation to other ongoing works. Identifying previously unpublished work would allow IRBs to anticipate potential issues such as difficulties with accrual, negative results, and excessive toxicities, among others. Journal editors and reviewers can compare submissions to an original trial design and track the revisions and edits as well as outcomes in the database [1].

Part 2. Where to Register Clinical Trials

All US federally funded clinical research (regardless of FDA oversight) must currently be registered at http://ClinicalTrials.gov. An eight-digit registry number is assigned after centralized review of the proposal, certifying that the work is indeed a clinical trial. The http://ClinicalTrials.gov results database, containing information on characteristics of study participants and outcomes, was created following the primary registry site as part of the requirements.

The World Health Organization (WHO) website maintains a global, searchable clinical trial registry that includes a multitude of regional and national databases. This list can be found on their website at http://www.who.int/ictrp/en/. Pharmaceutical and medical device companies also maintain private trial registries required for certain clinical trials. Globally, the five largest databases in descending order are: (1) http://ClinicalTrials.gov; (2) EU Clinical Trials Register (https://www.clinicaltrialsregister.eu/); (3) Japan Registries Network (JPRN—http://rctportal.niph.go.jp/en/); (4) ISRCTN (International Standard Randomized Controlled Trial Number Registry—http://isrctn.org/); (5) Australia and New Zealand Trial Registry (ANZCTR—http://www.anzctr.org.au/Default.aspx). In 2013, these five registries registered 204,349 clinical trials, of which 150,551 were registered at http://ClinicalTrials.gov (see Fig. 42.1 for data reported in 2015).

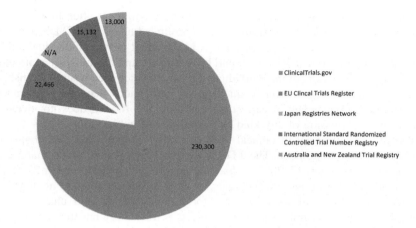

Fig. 42.1 Five largest clinical trial registries as of 2015 with number of studies listed (when available)

Part 3. Which Trials Must Be Registered, and When?

For all practical purposes, the concept of registration in the USA began in 1997, under the Food and Drug Administration Modernization Act (FDAMA), in collaboration with the National Institutes of Health (NIH), as a means of keeping track of federally and privately funded trials that involved investigational new drug applications (IND's). Moreover, the Food and Drug Administration (FDA) has mandated that all interventional studies that include drugs or devices (e.g., a trial of efficacy of antibiotic covered vascular access devices) must be registered. The guidance was amended to include more types of studies (observational and device studies) and additional information (summary of study outcomes, adverse events, etc.) in 2007. The Association of American Medical Colleges and the WHO have both released consensus policy statements that all interventional trials should be reported to a registry [2, 3]. The WHO definition of a clinical trial is "any research study that prospectively assigns human participants or groups of humans to one or more health-related interventions to evaluate the effect of health outcomes." The International Committee of Medical Journal Editors (ICMJE) adopted this definition in 2007. The ICMJE further expands on the definition of "health-related interventions" as any modification of a biomedical or health-related outcome including "drugs, surgical procedures, devices, behavioral treatments, dietary interventions, and of process of care changes."

On July 1, 2005, the ICMJE also reinforced the importance of clinical trial registration when they released their policy stating that registration is mandatory as a condition of publication for results of all interventional research studies [4]. The ICMJE allows that "purely observational studies (those in which the assignment of the medical intervention is not at the discretion of the investigator) will not require registration." All clinical trials beginning recruitment after July 1, 2008, must be registered *prior to* initiating patient enrollment under the ICMJE rules [5]. However, due to funding limitations, the ICMJE cannot provide individual advice to investigators about which trials should be registered, and thus, investigators must either contact the editors of the individual journals in which they wish to publish, or err on the side of registration in questions of ambiguous need for registration. Despite the FDA mandate of early data reporting, the ICMJE does not mandate early results submission of any kind as a condition of publication.

The FDA requirement of clinical trial registration is more limited and specific than the WHO requirement. The FDA requires registration of trials that began accrual after September 27, 2007, or had ongoing accrual after December 27, 2007, that include trials of drugs and biologics, or trials of devices that are regulated by the FDA. The FDA allows exemption for feasibility trials and phase I trials. ClinicalTrials.gov registration for these projects is mandatory but free, and listings are maintained through the National Library of Medicine. To view the complete statute, please refer to: https://www.gpo.gov/fdsys/pkg/PLAW-110publ85/pdf/PLAW-110publ85.pdf#page=82. Studies can be placed on http://ClinicalTrials.gov prior to initiation of actual study procedures, but there are also categories of trial activity to which a study can be assigned. A trial can be "not yet recruiting," "recruiting," "active-no longer recruiting" "available for expanded access" or "completed." Status cannot be "recruiting" until approved by an IRB and may require additional safety or other review. Documentation to start is only part of the information submitted to http://ClinicalTrials.gov, as listings must be updated regularly to be accurate and useful to those who access them. The number of registries to which a trial must be reported is growing, since not all registries communicate with one another, or feature links to all other sources. Likewise, many individual researchers who serve as unfunded sponsors must find time to perform the filings, as well as making sure the data themselves are correct when transferred. Unlike the WHO requirement for registration prior to accrual, the FDA allows registration up to 21 days after the accrual of the first patient [6, 7].

Since different registries have different criteria for submission, this becomes a critical concern in developing a harmonized set of rules for posting information to the research community. A unified clinical trial registry format would be of great time-saving value to investigators, as well.

Part 4. Who Should Register Clinical Trials?

The question of who is responsible for clinical trial registration is strictly defined by the FDA. It is important to clearly establish a responsible party to ensure appropriate registration and minimize redundant, incomplete, or inaccurate registrations. The FDA has defined the "responsible party" as either the sponsor of the study, or the principal investigator that has been assigned by the sponsor of the study. Thus, in either case a sponsor must be defined for each trial. Title VIII of the Food and

Drug Administration Amendments Act of 2007 (FDAAA) (PL 110-85) reads as follows:

(1) the sponsor of the clinical trial (as defined in section 50.3 of title 21, Code of Federal Regulations (or any successor regulation); **or**

(2) the principal investigator of such clinical trial, if so designated by a sponsor, grantee, contractor, or awardee, so long as the principal investigator is responsible for conducting the trial, has access to and control over the data from the clinical trial, has the right to publish the results of the trial, and has the ability to meet all of the requirements under this subsection for the submission of clinical trial information.

To understand this statute, we must define a "sponsor" per Title 21 of the Code of Federal Regulations, as it is somewhat dependent on the type of study that must be registered. The code offers two definitions of "sponsor": (1) Under 21 CFR § 50.3(e), sponsor means a person who *initiates a clinical investigation*, but who does not actually conduct the investigation, i.e., the test article is administered or dispensed to or used involving, a subject under the immediate direction of another individual. A person other than an individual (e.g., corporation or agency) that uses one or more of its own employees *to conduct* a clinical investigation it has initiated is considered to be a sponsor (not a sponsor-investigator), and the employees are considered to be investigators. (2) Under 21 CFR § 50.3(f), "sponsor-investigator" means an individual who both *initiates and actually conducts*, alone or with others, a clinical investigation, i.e., under whose immediate direction the test article is administered or dispensed to, or used involving, a subject. The term does not include any person other than an individual, e.g., corporation or agency [7].

In trials that involve Investigational New Drug Applications (IND) or Investigational Device Exemptions (IDE), the IND/IDE holder is considered the initiator of the study and thus the sponsor. In cases where **no** IND/IDE is involved, the funding of the trial is considered. If the study is funded through a grant mechanism, then the funding *recipient* is considered the initiator and thus the sponsor. If the funding occurs under a procurement agreement such as a contract, the funder is the initiator and the sponsor. In cases of **unfunded** research, the person or entity who initiated the trial by preparing and/or planning the trial, and who has appropriate authority and control over the trial to carry out the responsibilities under FDA, will be the sponsor. The consequences of establishing the identity of a sponsor is important to linking not only what studies are being done by which entities, but to document the sponsor's body of experience in a given category of medical care.

Part 5. Making Results Publicly Available

In 2013, the White House Office of Science and Technology Policy released the "Increasing Access to the Results of Federally Funded Scientific Research" memorandum. This document directed all federal agency research and federally funded scientific research to make results available and useful to the public, and directed the Agency for Healthcare Research and Quality (AHRQ) in establishing a policy for public access in *digital* format [8]. Among the objectives of this memorandum was to facilitate easy public search, analysis of and access to peer-reviewed, scholarly publications directly arising from funded research, full and free of charge access to data, ensure all data are stored and maintained in a digital form, and ensure expedited translation of research results into knowledge to improve health. There is an important distinction to be made between posting "results" of a study and the raw data gathered from which conclusions can be drawn. Results can be conveyed in a summary manner or as articles which allow the positive, negative, or equivocal answers to research questions to be placed within the public's grasp, while individual data points do not have to be enumerated as they appear on case report forms. The extent to which original data will be made publicly available continues to be debated within the biomedical and regulatory communities.

AHRQ has contracted with the National Library of Medicine (NLM) to archive publications in PubMed Central (PMC) no later than 12 months after the official date of publication. Nonetheless, Chapman et al. [9] showed that one-fifth of randomized, controlled studies are discontinued prior to planned conclusion, and one-third of the remaining trials are unpublished. This lack of publication of results is concerning to funding sources and the medical community, as it demonstrates significant waste and potential positive publication bias as well as ethical concerns that hidden results could place patients at increased risk of participating in either futile or harmful studies. In response to this issue, the National Cancer Institute (NCI) released in 2015 a policy for all NCI Interventional Clinical Trials, including research grants, cooperative agreements, and contracts to conduct Interventional Clinical Trials in all phases and disciplines (e.g., treatment, prevention, supportive care, diagnosis). This policy excludes observational studies and any NCI Interventional Trial in which no subjects are enrolled. The policy states "final trial results" must be reported within 12 months of study completion date, regardless of actual completion or early termination. Results from incomplete trials should be reported within twelve months of the date that the last subject had data collected or was examined [10]. Reporting can occur either directly to publicly accessible registries, or through publication. If publication is chosen, the article must be submitted as guided by the NIH public access policy. This policy states that all NIH funded or initiated trials published after April 7, 2008, must also submit an electronic version of their final peer-reviewed manuscript to the National Library of Medicine's PubMed Central, to be made available within 1 year of publication [11, 12]. However, a report in March, 2015, in the New England Journal of Medicine stated that of 13,327 trials terminated or completed between Jan 1, 2008, and August 31, 2012, 77.4% were drug trials, but only 13.4% had results posted by 12 months after cessation [13].

The types of information that Clinicaltrials.gov requires be placed on the site are termed the "minimum reporting data set" and include demographic/baseline participant characteristics, outcome and secondary outcome measures, adverse and serious adverse event reports, the full protocol and amendments. The deadlines for these postings run between 30 days and 12 months after the end of a study, or after the last contact between a participant and the study team. As of January 18, 2017, additional guidance applicable to all the categories mentioned above is available, and investigators are urged to include more detailed data as part of transparency and responsibility to consumers.

There are those who criticize "undue haste" in placing results on ClinicalTrials.gov, implying that posting confers a degree of "legitimacy" or finality to results that might not yet have been fully peer-reviewed, debated, or corroborated by other protocols [14].

Such reporting could also potentially pose a risk to patient privacy, and it is not the intent of the policy to release identifiable patient information, or any information that could lead to patient identification. Specifically, trials closed early due to minimal accrual, trials at the extremes of age, or trials involving rare or sensitive diagnosis, among other unique situations, place data at risk of being linked back to individual patients. Thus, the NCI policy allows for exceptions to be made for sensitive data, and the AHRQ also has a de-identified database for public release. Given the unique situations that can arise, the US government has created "Project Open Data" that serves as a guide to implementation of open data practices with valuable resources and tools. This can be accessed at http://project-open-data.cio. gov.

Requirements for data sharing have led to some members of the research community demanding that participant-level data be available for request as soon as it can be transferred to a public holding place. However, objections to providing ready access to data include re-identification of subjects, to what extent participants can prospectively govern the use of their information at the time of consent, fear of duplication of analysis, possibly with different outcomes; and issues of "data ownership." Although generally agreed that data must be sufficiently de-identified to protect study participants, as of 2016, there are no standardized procedures for posting data, how to determine who will have future access to them, for what purposes, and how data can be safely conveyed from one investigator to another, even when data use agreements (DUAs) are employed that specify transfer, storage, updates, publication, and boundaries for further use. Further, DUAs are often reviewed by legal counsel prior to implementation, adding another step to the approval process. The question is not whether or not to allow others to share the results of the work to leverage the greatest benefits from it, but how to accomplish this by the safest, fastest, and most comprehensive means.

References

1. Zarin DA, Keselman A. Registering a clinical trial in ClinicalTrials.gov. Chest. 2007;131:909–12.
2. World Health Organization [Internet]. Washington DC, Regional Offices for the Americas of the World Health Organization; ©2016 [cited 5 June 2016]. Available from: http://www.who. int/ictrp/network/criteria_summary/en/.

3. Korn D, Ehringhaus S. Principles for strengthening the integrity of clinical research. PLoS Clin Trials. 2006;1(1):e1. doi:10.1371/journal.pctr.0010001.

4. International Committee of Medical Journal Editors [Internet]. International Committee of Medical Journal Editors; © 2016 [cited 5 June 2016]. Available from: http://www.icmje.org/about-icmje/faqs/icmje-recommendations/.

5. Huser V, Cimino JJ. Evaluating adherence to the International Committee of Medical Journal Editors' policy of mandatory, timely clinical trial registration. J Am Med Inform Assoc. 2013;20:e169–74.

6. ClinicalTrials.gov [Internet]. Bethesda MD, National Institute of Health [Reviewed Nov 2015, cited 5 June 2016]. Available from: https://clinicaltrials.gov/ct2/manage-recs/fdaaa.

7. Public Law 110-85—27 Sept 2007. 110th Congress. 121 STAT.823. TITLE VIII—Clinical Trial Databases Sec. 801. Expanded clinical trial registry data bank.

8. AHRQ Public Access to Federally Funded Research [Internet]. Rockville, MD, Agency for Healthcare Research and Quality [Feb 2015, cited 5 June 2016]. Available from http://www.ahrq.gov/funding/policies/publicaccess/index.html.

9. Chapman SJ, Shelton B, Humza M, Fitzgerald JE, Harrison EM, Bhangu A. Discontinuation and non-publication of surgical randomized controlled trials: observational study. BMJ. 2014;349:g6870. doi:10.1136/bmj.g6870 (Published 9 Dec 2014).

10. The National Cancer Institute Policy Ensuring Public Availability of Results from NCI-supported Clinical Trials [Internet]. Bethesda MD, National Cancer Institute [January 2015, cited 5 June 2016]. Available from: https://grants.nih.gov/grants/guide/notice-files/NOT-CA-15-011.html.

11. NIH Public Access Policy [Internet]. Bethesda MD, U.S. Department of Health & Human Services [25 March 2016, cited 5 June 2016]. Available from: http://publicaccess.nih.gov/policy.htm.

12. Zarin DA, Tse T, Sheehan J. The proposed rule for U.S. clinical trial registration and results submission. N Engl J Med. 2015;372(2):174–80.

13. Anderson ML, Chiswell K, Peterson ED, Tasneem A, Topping J, Califf RM. Compliance with results reporting at ClinicalTrials.gov. N Engl J Med. 2015;372:1031–9.

14. Drazen JM, Morrissey S, Campion EW, Jarcho JA. A SPRINT to the finish. N Engl J Med. 2015;373:2174–5.

Part VII
Common Errors

Chapter 43
Mistakes in Clinical Trials

William G. Henderson

Overestimating Patient Intake

This is probably the most common mistake in conducting a clinical trial. It is not unusual for only a small fraction of screened patients (<20%) to be eligible and randomized in a clinical trial. Probably, up to 80% of clinical trials fail to meet recruitment targets on time. I will describe one trial as an example, and then, more generally, describe factors that affect rates of accrual to a clinical trial, and how we can realistically estimate recruitment.

VA Cooperative Study #385 was a randomized clinical trial (RCT) to compare all-cause long-term mortality in patients with medically refractory unstable angina randomized to percutaneous coronary intervention (PCI) versus coronary artery bypass grafting (CABG) [1]. Patients were treated and followed every 6 months for up to 5 years. The 5-year study included a 4-year intake period and an additional year of follow-up. The target sample size was 700 patients from 14 VA medical centers (VAMCs) to detect a difference of 82% versus 75% in 3-year survival with a power of 80%. We were able to decide on the need for 14 participating sites by analyzing a large VA registry of cardiac surgery [2]. We calculated that there would be about 2300 patients eligible for our study at 14 VA medical centers in a 4-year accrual period. We did not know what percentage of patients the physicians at each center (cardiac surgeons and interventional cardiologists) would agree to randomize and what percentage of patients would agree to be randomized, but we assumed the percentages would be 60 and 50%, respectively. This would enable the attainment

W.G. Henderson (✉)
Adult and Child Consortium for Outcomes Research and Delivery Science (ACCORDS)
and Department of Biostatistics and Informatics, Colorado School of Public Health,
University of Colorado Denver, 13199 E. Montview Blvd., Suite 300,
Aurora, CO 80045, USA
e-mail: William.Henderson@ucdenver.edu

© Springer International Publishing AG 2017
K.M.F. Itani and D.J. Reda (eds.), *Clinical Trials Design in Operative
and Non Operative Invasive Procedures*, DOI 10.1007/978-3-319-53877-8_43

of our target sample size of 700 (2300 × 0.60 × 0.50) with the 14 participating centers.

The required recruitment rate in units of numbers of patients per hospital per month was 700/(14 × 48) = 1.04. In the first 4 years of the study from 1995 to 1998, the actual recruitment rates were 0.49, 0.46, 0.74, and 0.72, respectively. Since we were closely monitoring recruitment during the accrual period, we knew that recruitment was behind schedule and made concerted efforts to improve the rate. These efforts included: (1) The study co-chairmen making personal calls to the site investigators to emphasize the importance of randomizing patients; (2) the co-chairmen site visiting the low-accruing hospitals; (3) making presentations at study meetings using angiograms of selected controversial cases; (4) replacing a few of the low-accruing sites; and (5) successfully arguing at the 3-year review of the study for funding for an additional year of patient intake. In spite of these efforts, the study eventually realized only 454 randomized patients (64.9% of the target sample size of 700) and had 80% power to detect a larger difference in 3-year survival (82% vs. 73%) than the study was originally designed to detect. During the study, we collected data on reasons for screened patients not being randomized. In the analysis of these data, we discovered that the main driving force for lower patient randomization was reluctance on the part of the physicians to randomize the patients. After 4 years of accrual, the study screened 2178 eligible patients at the 14 centers (close to the target 2300); 59% of the patients agreed to be randomized (above our assumption of 50%); but the physicians agreed to randomize only 30% of eligible patients (below our assumption of 60%).

There are many factors that affect patient accrual rates into a randomized clinical trial (see Table 43.1). The VA Cooperative Studies Program Coordinating Center (VACSPCC) in Hines, IL coordinated 44 multicenter studies in the period 1976–2002 (mostly RCTs) with widely varying accrual rates of 0.40–9.74 patients per hospital per month. Table 43.2 presents a sample of 19 of these studies (11 hypertension studies were grouped together), their accrual rates, and the factors that were related to the accrual rates observed.

Table 43.1 Factors affecting accrual rates of studies

Factor	Higher accrual	Lower accrual
Study design	Observational	Randomized
Definition of study population	Broad (few exclusion criteria)	Narrow (many exclusion criteria)
Prevalence of disease	Common disease	Rare disease
Similarity of randomized treatments	Similar (e.g., Drug A vs. Drug B)	Dissimilar (e.g., surgical vs. medical treatment)
Invasiveness of interventions	Not very invasive (e.g., drug treatment)	Very invasive (e.g., surgical treatments)
Acceptance of treatments by patients and providers (equipoise)	High equipoise	Low equipoise
Competing protocols	No	Yes

Table 43.2 Examples of studies with high to low accrual rates and factors associated with these accrual rates from 44 multicenter studies coordinated by the Hines, IL VA Cooperative Studies Program Coordinating Center, 1976–2002

Study	Accrual rate (No. of patients per hospital per month)	Factors affecting accrual rate
Processes, structures, and outcomes of cardiac surgical care	9.74	Health services observational study
Rapid access to primary care versus usual care following hospital discharge to prevent readmissions	8.62	Health services RCT, patients with common diseases (diabetes, CHF, COPD), not very invasive interventions
Laparoscopic versus open tension-free inguinal hernia repair	6.29	RCT comparison of two operative methods for a common disease
Average accrual rates for 11 hypertension studies	4.37	Many of the RCTs involved comparison of drugs for a common disease
Transurethral resection of the prostate (TURP) versus watchful waiting for patients with moderately symptomatic benign prostatic hyperplasia (BPH)	1.82	Common disease, but RCT comparing two very different treatments (one being very invasive), and narrowly defined population (moderately symptomatic)
Tight glycemic control versus usual care in Type II diabetes	1.80	RCT in a common disease, but intervention was very intensive requiring many visits and oral agents and insulin to reach target HbA1c of 6%
CARP Study (CABG or PCI vs. medical treatment prior to vascular surgery)	0.68	RCT of two very different treatments before vascular surgery; some patients in intervention group faced two major operations (CABG and vascular surgery)
CABG versus PCI in medically refractory unstable angina	0.60	RCT of two very dissimilar invasive treatments, low equipoise among treating physicians
Chemotherapy + radiation versus surgery + radiation in advanced laryngeal cancer	0.46	RCT in relatively uncommon disease, very dissimilar treatments (the usual care group lost their larynx)

CHF Congestive heart failure; *COPD* Chronic obstructive pulmonary disease; *RCT* Randomized controlled trial; *CARP study* Coronary artery revascularization prophylaxis study; *CABG* Coronary artery bypass grafting; *PCI* Percutaneous coronary intervention

In the planning of a clinical trial, how can we realistically estimate recruitment? These strategies could be tried: (1) If similar studies have been done in the past, these experiences could be used (our center conducted 11 hypertension studies in the years 1976–2002, so we could easily draw on past experiences); (2) Try to use databases to estimate the number of potentially eligible patients (this was done in VACSP #385) or use the medical centers' electronic health records, if available; (3) If no databases are available, try to conduct a pilot study for estimates of recruitment; (4) Be very conservative on estimates of percentage of patients willing to be randomized and physicians willing to randomize patients; and (5) Realize that the percentage of patients initially screened who are eventually randomized can be quite low (It was 454/2431 = 18.7% in VACSP #385).

Planning Too Complex a Clinical Trial

In the mid-1990s, the Hines VACSPCC developed a very productive collaboration with the American College of Surgeons (ACS) that included development of the ACS clinical trials course, offering the National Surgical Quality Improvement Program (NSQIP), first developed in the VA in 1991, to non-VA hospitals through the ACS, and the development of specific multicenter clinical trials in various areas of interest to surgeons. One of the areas of specific clinical trial development was the clinical management of inguinal hernias in adult men. Interventions that we were interested in testing included open hernia repair (Lichtenstein tension-free method), laparoscopic hernia repair, and watchful waiting. Other complicating factors included how to handle patients with varying levels of symptoms, acute hernia events, what outcomes were most important, and how to handle the issues of primary versus recurrent, and unilateral versus bilateral hernias. Although the investigators in the planning of this study were very experienced, in hindsight, we probably let our enthusiasm to try to answer too many questions in one clinical trial cloud our judgement in the design of the research.

The first study proposed had two primary aims and four secondary aims. The two primary aims were: (1) In patients with a primary or recurrent inguinal hernia, to compare two types of operative treatment (open tension-free and laparoscopic herniorrhaphy) (Study 1). The primary outcome was a combination of hernia recurrence at one year and/or the occurrence of perioperative life-threatening events. Secondary outcomes included operative complications, physical function, patient-centered outcomes, and cost; and (2) In patients who were asymptomatic or with minimal symptoms, to compare the two operative arms and watchful waiting (Study 2). In this part of the study, the primary outcome was physical function at one year, and secondary outcomes were operative complications, patient-centered outcomes, and cost. The four secondary aims included: (1) To determine the role of comorbidity in influencing the outcomes of treatment; (2) To determine the natural history of inguinal hernias in men who were not referred for operation (Pilot Study A); (3) To determine if the symptom scale developed for this study could be used to predict the likelihood of acute hernia events and need for operation; and (4) To conduct a pilot study of treatment of bilateral hernias using study assignments and outcome measures as in the primary aims (Pilot Study B).

The scientific peer review committee concluded that the topics of the study were important, but that the design was much too complex. In Study 1, the reviewers had concerns about combining hernia recurrence with life-threatening events into one primary outcome; whether there would be an adequate number of patients available to be randomized; the experience of the surgeons in performing laparoscopic repair; and the one-year follow-up period being too short. In Study 2, the reviewers had concerns about the adequacy of the primary outcome variable. In general, the reviewers believed that Study 1 had the stronger design but was of marginal interest; whereas Study 2 was of greater interest but had the weaker design. The final outcome of the review was disapproval.

After much deliberation, the planning committee for the study decided to split the proposal into two separate clinical trials and eliminate many of the secondary aims: (1) Open mesh versus laparoscopic mesh repair of inguinal hernia with the primary outcome being hernia recurrence rates at two years. This clinical trial was approved and funded by the VA and conducted in 14 VA medical centers from 1999 to 2003 [3]; and (2) Watchful waiting versus open tension-free repair in minimally symptomatic inguinal hernia patients with pain and the physical component score of the SF-36 as the primary outcomes. This clinical trial was approved and funded by the Agency for Healthcare Research and Quality (AHRQ) and conducted in five North American community and academic medical centers from 1999 to 2004 [4].

Trying to Collect Too Much Data

The VA PSOCS Study (Processes, Structures, and Outcomes of Care in Cardiac Surgery), although a prospective, observational cohort study and not a RCT, presents a good, and probably extreme, illustration of what can happen when investigators try to collect too much data. The objective of the study was to determine what processes and structures of cardiac surgical care are associated with 30-day and 6-month outcomes of open-heart surgery. "Processes of care" refer to procedures that are done to and for individual patients in the care of those patients; "structures of care" refer to aspects of care such as equipment used, education and training of staff and use of quality review committees. The outcomes of the study included 30-day and 6-month postoperative mortality, morbidity, and health-related quality of life. The study was conducted between 1992 and 1996 in 4969 patients from 14 VA medical centers [5].

The conceptual model for the study was that the combination of patient risk factors, processes and structures of care, and random chance lead to the outcomes of cardiac surgical care. There were 6 process hypotheses relating to the preoperative evaluation, surgical procedure, postoperative care, degree of supervision, patient/family communication, and care provider communication; and 3 structure hypotheses related to the integrating system, care provider profiles, and facilities and equipment. However, each hypothesis had multiple dimensions and sub-dimensions. There were also a multitude of patient risk factors related to the severity of the cardiac disease, comorbidity and general health status of the patient, and demographic and socioeconomic factors. There were also a multitude of short-term (30 days) and longer term (6 month) outcomes, including mortality, operative complications, patient cardiac status, patient satisfaction, and health-related quality of life. In total, there were about 1100 variables collected for each patient and 300 variables related to provider-specific and facility-specific characteristics.

There was a multitude of effects of too much data collection on the conduct of the study: excessive data collection burden on the one nurse who was funded at each of the participating sites resulting in disgruntled site nurses; poor data quality; a data analysis nightmare that included the need for extensive use of data reduction techniques prior to the final analysis of the study; and inordinate delays in the final analysis and publication of the study. During a pilot study at 5 sites before implementation of the study in all 14 participating sites, we developed a laptop distributed data entry system that somewhat alleviated the data collection burden. Although the study resulted in 22 manuscripts published in the peer-reviewed medical literature, the final results of the study were underwhelming in terms of a significant effect on the practice of cardiac surgical care and in improving patient outcomes.

How can we avoid excessive data collection in a RCT? The ideal selection of variables for inclusion in a RCT should include these data collection areas (and not much more): variables related to (1) the primary and secondary objectives of the RCT as stated in the protocol; (2) safety issues; (3) the interventions in the RCT (dose, frequency, duration, compliance, surgical techniques); (4) all endpoints or outcomes; (5) variables anticipated to have a high correlation with the outcome variables; i.e., predictor variables for the outcomes known from the literature; (6) demographics, disease stage, and other variables to characterize the sample and to use in the reporting of the first table (Table 43.1) of the RCT to look at balance of the treatment groups produced by the randomization; (7) selected comorbidities; (8) concomitant treatments; (9) death, date and cause of death; and (10) some administrative variables (e.g., missed visits, terminations, and reasons). In planning the RCT, one should resist the temptation of collecting data on variables that would be interesting to know about, but are not related to the primary and secondary objectives of the study.

Not Anticipating Problems in Following Patients

Adequate follow-up of patients in a RCT involving long-term treatment and/or follow-up is crucial to the success of the RCT. Ideally, follow-up rates should be $\geq 80\%$. There should be close and continuous monitoring not only of patient recruitment into the RCT, but also of patient follow-up rates and receipt and completeness of baseline and follow-up data collection forms.

In the VA inguinal hernia clinical trial of open mesh versus laparoscopic mesh repair, the primary outcome variable was recurrence rate at two years. When we first looked at the follow-up data at a study group meeting, we found that follow-up rates were only around 50%. This was likely due to patients not returning for follow-up visits because their inguinal hernia was satisfactorily repaired and they saw no need to come back to the clinic. The study group quickly instituted a series of ongoing actions to improve the follow-up rate of the study. These actions included: (1) The study chair and members of the study Executive Committee contacted sites with low follow-up rates; (2) The data coordinating center sent monthly reminders to sites of patients due for follow-up and/or missing their follow-up visits; (3) Alternative follow-up arrangements were made for patients who moved or lived at long distances from the recruiting VA medical center (e.g., using other VA medical centers, local clinics, or ACS fellows); (4) Travel funds and birthday cards with inclusion of phone cards were given to the patients; (5) The study chair sent letters to the patients reminding them of the importance of the study and the follow-up visits; (6) The site nurses started to telephone their patients every 3 months to keep in contact with them; and (7) Equifax searches for addresses of the lost-to-follow-up veterans were made. Some of these actions might not be allowed under current IRB regulations (e.g., VA patients seen by non-study personnel; or Equifax searches). The final result of these actions was to boost the 2-year follow-up rates in the study to 77% in the open mesh repair treatment arm and to 80% in the laparoscopic mesh repair arm of the RCT [3]. In the trial, 2164 patients were randomized, and 468 patients (21.6%) did not have a 2-year endpoint evaluation. Reasons for the missing evaluation included: 175 (37.4%) missed the 2-year visit; 92 (19.7%) withdrew consent; 78 (16.7%) died before the 2-year visit; 69 (14.7%) were lost to follow-up; and 54 (11.5%) were never cleared for the operation.

Making Errors in the Randomization Scheme

An accurate randomization procedure is critical for the scientific integrity and the validity and interpretation of a RCT. We had one RCT in which there was an error in the randomization program and threatened these aspects of the RCT.

The Department of Veterans Affairs healthcare system uses an electronic informed consent system, called iMedConsent, to help educate patients about the medical procedures and surgical operations they are to undergo, and to obtain patient informed consent prior to the interventions. As part of the iMedConsent program, we helped to develop a repeat-back module that quizzed the patients about their understanding of the operation they were told about, including the nature of the operation, risks, benefits, and alternative treatments. If the patients did not understand certain aspects of the operation, then these aspects were again explained to the patients. We conducted a multicenter RCT of this repeat-back feature to determine whether use of this feature improved patient comprehension about the operations that they were to undergo. The RCT of iMedConsent versus iMedConsent + the repeat-back feature was conducted in 2006–2008 in 575 patients from seven participating VA medical centers. Patients were stratified by VA medical center and four types of operations (carotid endarterectomy, laparoscopic cholecystectomy, radical prostatectomy, and total hip arthroplasty) and then randomized to the two treatment arms in block sizes of 2, 4, or 6. The primary outcome was patient comprehension of their operation as assessed by a patient questionnaire of 23–26 items [6].

To do the randomization, we developed a new program for use via an Internet Web site. To randomize a patient, the study nurse at each participating medical center would access the study Web site to register the patient into the trial, answer a set of questions to check eligibility and to stratify the patient, and then receive the randomization assignment. Part way through the conduct of the study, we noticed some imbalances in the number of patients being randomized to the two treatment arms within some of the strata. Upon checking on these imbalances more closely, we found an error in the randomization program—the blocking was not functioning properly. The end result was some imbalances on baseline patient characteristics between the two treatment arms at the end of the study, including age, race, gender, employment, SF-12 mental scale, and state-trait anxiety scale.

When these types of imbalances occur, it is often recommended that they be adjusted for in the final analysis of the RCT. In the final analysis of the study, we found that the repeat-back feature resulted in a small but statistically significant improvement in comprehension for all operations combined, and particularly for patients undergoing carotid endarterectomy, with p-values of 0.03 and 0.02, respectively. Fortunately, upon adjustment for the baseline variables that were imbalanced between the two treatment arms, these p-values remained statistically significant, $p = 0.05$ for all operations combined, and 0.03 for carotid endarterectomy, so that the conclusions of the study did not change in unadjusted or adjusted analyses [6]. The major lesson learned from this experience was that randomization programs for each RCT should be tested and validated prior to the first patient being randomized into the study.

Making Errors in Programming the Statistical Analyses

The statistical analyses to support the final analysis, interpretation, and publication of a RCT can be quite complex and involve thousands of lines of computer code. Thus, it would not be surprising to occasionally have errors in the computer code that could potentially alter the final analysis of a study.

In the early 1990s, we conducted a large double-blind multicenter RCT to evaluate which antihypertensive drugs were most effective in lowering patients' blood pressure. We randomized 1292 men with baseline diastolic blood pressure (DBP) of 95–109 mm Hg at 15 VA medical centers to receive placebo or one of six different antihypertensive drugs representing the different classes of antihypertensive drugs available at the time. The drug doses were titrated until DBP was <90 mm Hg, and the patients were treated and followed for one year. The primary outcome variable was success rate of lowering DBP, defined as percent of patients with DBP <90 mm Hg at the end of the titration period and <95 mm Hg at the end of one year. The average age of the patients was 59 years, and 48% were African–American. The results of the study were published in *New England Journal of Medicine* in 1993 and showed the following overall success rates: Diltiazem 59%; Atenolol 51%; Clonidine 50%; Hydrochlorothiazide 46%; Captopril 42%; Prazosin 42%; and Placebo 25% [7]. We also found that different drugs worked better in different age and racial groups: Diltiazem was best for younger and older African–American patients; Captopril was best for younger Caucasian patients; and Atenolol was best for older Caucasian patients.

At some time after the publication of the main results of the study, we were performing analyses for additional manuscripts and discovered an error in the original computer code for the main paper, one line of code had been inadvertently deleted. Correction of the error lead to higher overall success rates, but little change in the relative rankings of the different antihypertensive drugs: Diltiazem 72%; Clonidine 62%; Atenolol 60%; Hydrochlorothiazide 55%; Prazosin 54%; Captopril 50%; and Placebo 31%. We also found that Diltiazem continued to be best for younger and older African–American patients, but that Clonidine was now best for younger and older Caucasian patients, although Atenolol was a close second best for older Caucasian patients. The revised results were published both as a letter to the editor in *New England Journal of Medicine* in 1994 [8], and in the *American Journal of Hypertension* in 1995 [9].

What can be done to try to prevent analysis errors in RCTs? The errors in the computer code for the original analyses for the hypertension study were probably not discovered because the computer programs produced results that "looked reasonable" to the programmers, statisticians, and physicians working on the study. Possible solutions to prevent these occurrences might include: (1) Having the analysts incorporate more validation steps into the analysis programs; (2) Establishing an organized system of filing statistical analyses during the conduct of the study, and periodically comparing analysis output to check for consistency; and (3) Building in redundancy in the analyses by having independent analysts writing computer code for the same analyses and comparing the results. The first two solutions do not necessarily require major increases in study budgets, but the third solution definitely would. In our experience, building in redundancy in the analyses is seldom done, probably due to larger budget requirements. However, a compromise might be to do this for the most important analyses in the study, but not for all analyses.

Drawing Wrong Conclusions that are not Supported by the Study Data

The best clinical researcher will carefully review and think about the final analysis of the study, and only draw conclusions from the study that are supported by the study data. In a RCT, these conclusions should also only be related to primary and secondary objectives as stated in the RCT protocol.

We were involved in a study a few years ago, published in a highly respected medical journal, in which our enthusiasm probably got the better of us and resulted in a conclusion that was, in hindsight, not totally supported by the study data [10]. Although the study was observational and not a RCT, this kind of mistake could happen in either type of study design.

One of the objectives of the study was to compare the long-term mortality of obese patients receiving bariatric surgery to a propensity-matched control group of obese patients who did not receive bariatric surgery. Long-term mortality was examined for 847 obese veterans who had bariatric surgery in the Department of Veterans Affairs medical centers between January, 2000, and December, 2006, and 847 propensity-matched obese veterans who did not have the surgery. Median follow-up time was 6.7 years. The final hazard ratio in the propensity-matched samples from Cox regression analysis for bariatric surgery (yes vs. no) was 0.94, with a 95% confidence interval of 0.64–1.39. Our conclusion from the study was stated as, "In propensity score-adjusted analyses of older severely obese patients with high baseline mortality in Veterans Affairs medical centers, the use of bariatric surgery compared with usual care was not associated with decreased mortality during a mean 6.7 years of follow-up." The "fall-out" from this study was stories in the popular media with headlines like "Obesity surgery doesn't help older men live longer" (Associated Press story in the *Denver Post*, June 13, 2011).

A few months after publication of our article, we had a conversation with a nationally and internationally well-respected biostatistician who was a statistical consultant to the journal of publication (but who did not review our article) reminding us that we should have phrased our conclusion from the study differently. Our mistake was that our sample size for the study (847 patients in each group) was fairly small, thus our statistical power for the study was minimal and the 95% confidence interval for the hazard ratio was fairly wide (0.64–1.39), meaning that our results were consistent with up to a 36% improvement or a 39% worsening in survival from bariatric surgery. The biostatistician's main objection to our conclusion was that "Absence of evidence is not evidence of absence" [11]. In hindsight, our conclusion probably should have been written as follows: "In propensity score-adjusted analyses of older severely obese patients with high baseline mortality in the Veterans Affairs medical centers, the data are consistent with as much as a 36% improvement or a 39% worsening in survival from bariatric surgery. More definitive data are needed in the future with larger sample sizes and longer term follow-up."

Summary

This chapter has presented some examples of mistakes we have made in the design, implementation, conduct, analysis, and interpretation of over 60 research studies (mostly multicenter RCTs) in my almost 50-year career in clinical research. All studies involved supervision and decision-making by committees of very experienced physicians and biostatisticians. In most instances, we eventually recognized the mistakes and were able to take corrective actions so that the studies were eventually successful. We hope that these examples will be useful to others in the planning and conduct of future studies and RCTs.

References

1. Morrison DA, Sethi G, Sacks J, Henderson W, Grover F, Sedlis S, et al. Percutaneous coronary intervention versus coronary artery bypass graft surgery for patients with medically refractory myocardial ischemia and risk factors for adverse outcomes with bypass: a multicenter, randomized trial. J Am Coll Cardiol. 2001;38:143–9.
2. Grover FL, Johnson RR, Marshall G, Hammermeister KE, Department of Veterans Affairs cardiac surgeons. Factors predictive of operative mortality among coronary artery bypass subsets. Ann Thorac Surg. 1993;56:1296–307.
3. Neumayer L, Giobbie-Hurder A, Jonasson O, Fitzgibbons R Jr, Dunlop D, Gibbs J, et al. Open mesh versus laparoscopic mesh repair of inguinal hernia. N Engl J Med. 2004;350:1819–27.
4. Fitzgibbons RJ Jr, Giobbie-Hurder A, Gibbs JO, Dunlop DD, Reda DJ, McCarthy M Jr, et al. Watchful waiting versus repair of inguinal hernia in minimally symptomatic men. A randomized clinical trial. JAMA. 2006;295:285–92.
5. O'Brien MM, Shroyer ALW, Moritz TE, London MJ, Grunwald GK, Villanueva CB, et al. Relationship between processes of care and coronary bypass operative mortality and morbidity. Med Care. 2004;42:59–70.
6. Fink AS, Prochazka AV, Henderson WG, Bartenfeld D, Nyirenda C, Webb A, et al. Enhancement of surgical informed consent by addition of repeat back. A multicenter, randomized controlled clinical trial. Ann Surg. 2010;252:27–36.
7. Materson BJ, Reda DJ, Cushman WC, Massie BM, Freis ED, Kochar MS, et al. Single-drug therapy for hypertension in men. A comparison of six antihypertensive agents with placebo. N Engl J Med. 1993;328:914–21.
8. Materson BJ, Reda DJ. Correction: single-drug therapy for hypertension in men. N Engl J Med. 1994;330:1689.
9. Materson BJ, Reda DJ, Cushman WC, for the Department of Veterans Affairs Cooperative Study Group on Antihypertensive Agents. Department of Veterans Affairs single-drug therapy of hypertension study. Am J Hypertens. 1995;8:189–92.
10. Maciejewski ML, Livingston EH, Smith VA, Kavee AL, Kahwati LC, Henderson WG, Arterburn DE. Survival among high-risk patients after bariatric surgery. JAMA. 2011;305:2419–26.
11. Altman DG, Bland JM. Absence of evidence is not evidence of absence. BMJ. 1995;311:485.

Part VIII
Adjuncts to Clinical Trials

Chapter 44
Combined Drugs and Procedure Trials

Ankur Kalra and Deepak L. Bhatt

Fundamentals of Trial Design

Clinical trials play a vital role in medical research and drug development. The validity of a clinical trial depends on the study design and elimination of bias. The first clinical trials lacked essential characteristics such as randomization and blinding. The design of combined drug and device trials is far more complex than a typical randomized controlled trial of a drug.

All drugs or devices are tested in human beings only after they have undergone laboratory testing. Clinical development programs typically include four phases. Phase I is designed to determine the safety, efficacy, maximum tolerated dose, and toxicities in human beings. Phase II begins once initial safety has been established. It evaluates the therapeutic efficacy and safety in patients with a specified disease condition. Patients are given different doses of the drug which were found to be safe in Phase I, and efficacy and side effects are compared for ascertainment of safest dosing regimens. Phase III is the final stage before licensure of the drug. For Phase III, the study population is much larger, and the main aim is to demonstrate the safety and efficacy of the drug in the safest dose ascertained. In this phase, drugs are compared with current standard treatment(s) using randomized controlled trial designs, and patients are closely monitored for potential side effects. After this phase, the drug is approved and licensed. Phase IV is the post-marketing phase.

A. Kalra
Department of Cardiovascular Medicine, Division of Interventional Cardiology,
Harvard Medical School, Beth Israel Deaconess Medical Center,
185 Pilgrim Road, West Campus, Baker 4, Boston, MA 02215, USA
e-mail: kalramd.ankur@gmail.com

D.L. Bhatt (✉)
Brigham and Women's Hospital Heart & Vascular Center, Harvard Medical School,
75 Francis Street, Boston, MA 02115, USA
e-mail: dlbhattmd@post.harvard.edu

© Springer International Publishing AG 2017
K.M.F. Itani and D.J. Reda (eds.), *Clinical Trials Design in Operative and Non Operative Invasive Procedures*, DOI 10.1007/978-3-319-53877-8_44

During this phase, drugs are evaluated in a much larger group and subgroups of patients with the aim of establishing long-term safety and efficacy of the drug. During this phase, a drug may be combined with other standard treatments and tested accordingly [1].

Combined drug and device (or procedure) trials are often Phase III or Phase IV clinical trials. The study is designed to compare the efficacy of a drug versus a device or a procedure or the efficacy of a drug versus a combination of drug and procedure. This can be further subgrouped based on the type of procedure carried out and also the combination of drugs that can be used. There are no clear protocols on how these studies are designed currently. This chapter discusses study designs based on the following case studies and also analyzes challenges in these types of study designs [2, 3].

Case Studies

Design of the SYMPLICITY HTN-3 Trial

The SYMPLICITY HTN-3 trial was designed to evaluate the safety and effectiveness of catheter-based bilateral renal denervation for the treatment of uncontrolled hypertension [4]. The SYMPLICITY HTN-3 trial compared the safety and efficacy of a combination of medical treatment and procedural treatment versus medical treatment alone. The relationship between sympathetic renal nerve activation and high blood pressure, and the possibility of selective renal denervation in patients with resistant hypertension provided potential therapeutic opportunities for the treatment of hypertension [5]. Earlier trials before the SYMPLICITY HTN-3 were SYMPLICITY HTN-1, a first-in-man Phase I trial with limited sample size, and SYMPLICITY HTN-2, an open-label randomized trial conducted in Europe and Australia [6, 7]. Other randomized and non-randomized unblinded trials had shown a significant reduction in blood pressure following renal denervation. However, there were several limitations, i.e., small sample size, lack of blinding, and lack of a sham procedure for control, making these trials' findings unreliable.

The SYMPLICITY HTN-3 was a multicenter, prospective, 2:1 randomized, masked control and single-blinded trial (Fig. 44.1) [4]. Patients of ages 18–80 years with severe resistant hypertension were prospectively enrolled in the study. These patients had an initial systolic blood pressure of 160 mmHg or higher and were on maximally tolerated doses of three or more antihypertensive medications. These patients were asked to record their blood pressure at home and record adherence to medications for the following 2 weeks. A final confirmatory screening was performed in these patients for a systolic blood pressure of 160 mmHg or higher, compliance with their medications, and automated 24-h ambulatory blood pressure monitoring to record a systolic blood pressure of 135 mmHg or higher. This ensured that these patients had definitive severe resistant hypertension. All patients

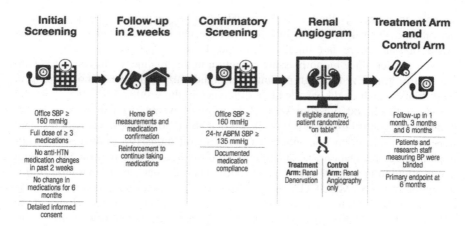

Fig. 44.1 Design of the SYMPLICITY HTN-3 trial (abbreviations: *ABPM* ambulatory blood pressure monitoring; *anti-HTN* antihypertensive; *BP* blood pressure; *SBP* systolic blood pressure)

underwent renal angiography before randomization. Patients were then randomized in a 2:1 ratio to undergo either renal denervation or sham procedure. Randomization was carried out on the table while the patient underwent renal angiography, provided the anatomy was favorable. Patients were blinded from knowing whether they underwent renal denervation or renal angiography alone (sham control). The personnel performing blood pressure monitoring were also blinded from knowing about the patient being in the treatment or control group. Renal denervation was carried out using the Medtronic Symplicity™ Catheter (Santa Rosa, CA, USA). At 6 months, patients in the control group were allowed to cross over to the treatment group to undergo the procedure if they still met the inclusion criteria. The primary efficacy endpoint was a mean change in office systolic blood pressure in the treatment group compared with the control group with a superiority margin of 5 mmHg [2, 4]. At 6 months following the procedure, the difference in the mean change in blood pressure between the treatment group and the sham group was -2.39 mmHg (95% CI, -6.89–2.12; P = 0.26 for superiority). In conclusion, the trial did not show any significant reduction in systolic blood pressure at 6 months in patients who underwent renal denervation [2]. The results of this trial were in contradiction with the results from previous non-blinded trials.

Lessons from the Renal Denervation Trials

There are numerous trials on the effects of renal denervation—140 non-randomized; 6 randomized, open-label; and 2 randomized blinded studies [8]. In many of the unblinded trials, a much larger reduction in office blood pressure was reported compared with ambulatory blood pressure. Both were measured using a sphygmomanometer, albeit with the possibility of re-measuring blood pressure in the office if the value did not fit with the expectation, as the staff measuring the blood pressure were not blinded. Unblinded randomized controlled trials also showed greater office blood pressure reduction in the treatment arm compared with the control arm. Even though patients were randomized, there was no blinding in these trials, which could have led to a difference in the results. The office staff who measured the blood pressure were still aware of whether a patient was in the treatment or control group [8]. It is known that about 50% of patients with resistant hypertension are often non-adherent to their medications [9]. Adherence to anti-hypertensive medications is difficult to confirm. Continued reinforcement with documentation in a diary, and frequent follow-ups were carried out to minimize this limitation in the SYMPLICITY HTN-3 trial. The success of an intervention can be affected by an operator learning curve in renal denervation trials. However, in SYMPLICITY HTN-3 trial, there were no significant differences in outcomes between high-volume versus low-volume operators. There was no single test which can be performed to confirm renal denervation in these trials. In SYMPLICITY HTN-3 trial, the catheter system allowed confirmation of energy delivery. Many of the renal denervation trials were based on a specific catheter system. The results from one catheter system might not be applicable to another catheter system. Also, the primary endpoint for most of the trials was clinical follow-up up to 6 months from the date of the procedure, resulting in short follow-up time and the potential for declining placebo effect over time.

Design of the STAMPEDE Trial

The Surgical Treatment and Medications Potentially Eradicate Diabetes Efficiently (STAMPEDE) trial was designed to evaluate the safety and efficacy of intensive medical therapy alone versus medical therapy plus either Roux-en-Y gastric bypass or sleeve gastrectomy in obese patients with uncontrolled type 2 diabetes [10]. Prior observational and randomized controlled trials had suggested that bariatric surgery can significantly improve glycemic control and cardiovascular risk factors in severely obese patients [11]. In the STAMPEDE trial, medical therapy was compared with a combination of medical therapy and surgical procedures.

The STAMPEDE trial was a randomized, non-blinded, single-center trial. Patients who met the inclusion criteria (age 20–60 years, a diagnosis of type 2 diabetes mellitus with a glycated hemoglobin level of greater than 7.0%, and a body mass index of 27–43 kg/m^2) were randomized in a 1:1:1 ratio between intensive medical therapy versus intensive medical therapy plus either Roux-en-Y gastric bypass or sleeve gastrectomy (Fig. 44.2). All patients received intensive medical therapy as defined by American Diabetes Association with a goal to reach a gly-cated hemoglobin level of 6.0% or less unless they became intolerant to medical treatment [12]. In this trial, patients were not blinded nor did the intensive medical treatment only group receive a sham procedure, as it was felt that a sham surgery

Fig. 44.2 Design of the
STAMPEDE trial
(abbreviations: *HgbA1C*
glycated hemoglobin)

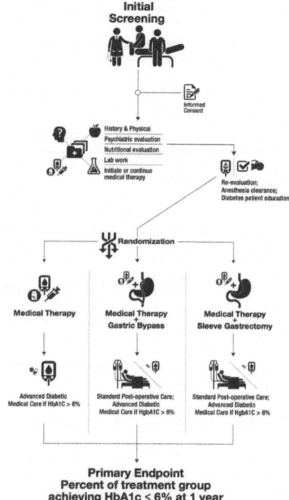

would be too risky. The primary efficacy endpoint in the STAMPEDE trial was the
proportion of patients with a glycated hemoglobin level of 6% or less at the end of
12 months. The primary endpoint was met by 12% of patients in the intensive
medical therapy group, 42% in the gastric bypass plus medical therapy group, and
37% in the sleeve gastrectomy plus medical therapy group. In conclusion, the trial
showed that in an overweight or obese patient with uncontrolled type 2 diabetes
mellitus, 12 months of medical therapy plus bariatric surgery achieved superior
glycemic control than medical therapy alone [3]. The three-year outcomes of the
study have demonstrated durable results [10].

Lessons from the Bariatric Surgery Trials

A meta-analysis by Buchwald et al. included 621 trials which studied the impact of bariatric surgery on type 2 diabetes mellitus—29 randomized controlled studies, 49 non-randomized prospective studies, 60 comparative retrospective studies, 187 uncontrolled prospective case series, 266 single-arm retrospective studies, 25 observational studies, and 2 case–control studies. Out of these, 540 studies were single-center studies, 70 were multicenter, and 11 were not reported [11]. In bariatric surgery trials, the procedure performed varied with each trial: gastric banding, gastroplasty, gastric bypass, and biliopancreatic diversion/duodenal switch, which could result in different outcomes. However, in the STAMPEDE trial, the two procedures, Roux-en-Y gastric bypass and sleeve gastrectomy, had similar outcomes [3, 10]. The majority of procedures were carried out at a single center, and the results might therefore not be applicable to all centers. There was no placebo or a sham procedure, unlike in the renal denervation trial discussed previously where renal angiography was performed as a sham procedure. The risks associated with a bariatric surgical procedure are far more compared with that of renal angiography. Compliance and loss to follow-up if patients were randomized to the control arm can be major challenges in these patients as well. This was handled in the STAMPEDE trial by mandating follow-up with an endocrinologist to try to ensure optimal medical care of diabetes. In the STAMPEDE trial, all the procedures were carried out by a single surgeon with the use of instruments from Ethicon Endo-Surgery (Somerville, NJ; Cincinnati, OH, USA). The results might vary based upon the skill level of the operator and instruments used.

Challenges in Clinical Trials Design

The challenges faced by clinical investigators in designing combined drug and device trials are multiple that together may appear insurmountable. Apart from common obstacles such as funding, approval from the Institutional Review Board, establishing a trial, agreement between sponsors and medical centers, recruitment of patients, obtaining informed consent and follow-up, challenges are often more complex and different when it comes to a combined drug and device trial or a drug versus device trial.

Drugs Versus Devices

In the USA, medical devices began to be regulated by the Medical Device Amendment Act in 1976. Medical devices are classified into three main categories: Class I, Class II, and Class III. Class I category encompasses low-risk devices such as a bandage, whereas Class III devices are moderate-to-high risk invasive devices requiring approval from Food and Drug Administration (FDA). Currently in the USA, drugs are regulated by the Center for Drug Evaluation and Research, and devices are regulated by the Center for Device and Radiological Health [13]. Only 1% of medical devices are approved by the FDA, and the approval is largely based on clinical data from small studies [14]. The primary effect of a drug is through pharmacological, immunological, or metabolic activity, unlike the primary effect of a device or a procedure. Often, it becomes difficult to compare the exact clinical outcomes when testing a drug versus a device due to differences in their mechanisms of action. This requires strict standardization of measuring clinical outcomes with standard protocols. The effect of a drug or a device is not the same in every patient. When a drug is found to have side effects, the patient has the choice to discontinue the drug and eventually the side effects may wear off. Side effects, however, are more permanent in case of a device or a procedure. Medical devices and procedures may pose more harm to patients than drugs; these need to be clearly addressed and a detailed informed consent is required from patients stating that they understand the risks associated with the procedure, and that it may be irreversible. Most trials including devices are sponsored by a single manufacturer. The results obtained from a single trial based on a single device system might not be applicable to other device systems from other manufacturers. Outcomes in procedure-based trials can be affected by the operator learning curve, with later procedures having better outcomes than procedures performed initially.

Sham Control

Blinded, randomized controlled trials in which the proposed therapy is compared with placebo are common in drug trials but uncommon in medical devices or procedures. The main reason for lack of such placebo or sham trials is that patients are subjected to the risk of a sham procedure without the actual benefit of the proposed device or procedure [15]. Some authors argue the ethical basis of performing a sham procedure or surgery. A sham trial by Freeman et al., a double-blinded trial of fetal tissue transplantation for Parkinson's disease, had patients undergo a sham procedure involving holes drilled in their foreheads, which was considered necessary for the placebo effect of the procedure [16]. There is established evidence that sham procedures can create a strong placebo effect which can mimic actual effectiveness [15]. A study carried out for migraine prophylaxis at the Institute of Medical Psychology in Munich showed that 58% of patients had a positive response to sham surgery, 38% patients had a positive response to sham acupuncture, and only 22% had a positive response to an oral pharmacological placebo drug [17]. Although sham procedures form an integral part of trials involving medical devices or procedures, the risk of the procedure needs to be compared with the benefits of the trial.

Strategies for Limiting Biases and Confounders

Combined drug and device trials are efficient methods for assessing the safety and efficacy of the device in a clinical setting. Compared with single-arm trials, randomized control trials are considered the most effective method for eliminating bias in comparing the efficacy of an intervention. As mentioned earlier, in many of the unblinded renal denervation trials, there was a possibility of bias in measurement of office blood pressure as the staff was aware of patients being in the treatment arm. This bias can be eliminated by blinding the staff who measure office blood pressure, or more generally, who make key endpoint measurements during trial follow-up [8]. This, however, cannot completely explain major differences in blood pressure readings between treatment and control arms. Patients being aware of treatment allocation could result in a placebo effect or to greater (or lesser) adherence to prescribed medical therapies. The inclusion of a sham procedure and blinding patients to treatment allocation helps in limiting these types of potential confounders [2, 15]. An operator learning curve may be a factor in evaluating the outcomes of a procedure and impact the results. Proctoring the procedure and standardizing the protocols will help in limiting this factor [2].

Conclusion

In conclusion, combined drug and device trials are effective methods in evaluating the safety and efficacy of a device or a procedure in patients. Randomization and blinding play a vital role. A control group with a sham procedure is an effective way to address the potential of the placebo effect provided the risks of the sham procedure are minimal. Multicenter trials help in recruiting a larger patient population, and the results can be applied more generally.

Acknowledgements The authors acknowledge Gerry Yumul at the Minneapolis Heart Institute Foundation for his work on the figures.

References

1. Sedgwick P. What are the four phases of clinical research trials? BMJ. 2014;348:g3727.
2. Bhatt DL, Kandzari DE, O'Neill WW, D'Agostino R, Flack JM, Katzen BT, et al. SYMPLICITY HTN-3 investigators. A controlled trial of renal denervation for resistant hypertension. N Engl J Med. 2014;370:1393–401.
3. Schauer PR, Kashyap SR, Wolski K, Brethauer SA, Kirwan JP, Pothier CE, et al. Bariatric surgery versus intensive medical therapy in obese patients with diabetes. N Engl J Med. 2012;366:1567–76.

4. Kandzari DE, Bhatt DL, Sobotka PA, O'Neill WW, Esler M, Flack JM, et al. Catheter-based renal denervation for resistant hypertension: Rationale and design of the SYMPLICITY HTN-3 trial. Clin Cardiol. 2012;35:528–35.

5. DiBona GF, Esler M. Translational medicine: the antihypertensive effect of renal denervation. Am J Physiol Regul Integr Comp Physiol. 2010;298:R245–53.

6. Krum H, Schlaich M, Whitbourn R, Sobotka PA, Sadowski J, Bartus K, et al. Catheter-based renal sympathetic denervation for resistant hypertension: a multicentre safety and proof-of-principle cohort study. Lancet. 2009;373:1275–81.

7. Esler MD, Krum H, Sobotka PA, Schlaich MP, Schmieder RE, Böhm M. Renal sympathetic denervation in patients with treatment-resistant hypertension (The Symplicity HTN-2 Trial): a randomised controlled trial. Lancet. 2010;376:1903–9.

8. Howard JP, Shun-Shin MJ, Hartley A, Bhatt DL, Krum H, Francis DP. Quantifying the 3 biases that lead to unintentional overestimation of the blood pressure–lowering effect of renal denervation. Circ Cardiovasc Qual Outcomes. 2016;9:14–22.

9. Jung O, Gechter JL, Wunder C, Paulke A, Bartel C, Geiger H, et al. Resistant hypertension? Assessment of adherence by toxicological urine analysis. J Hypertens. 2013;31:766–74.

10. Schauer P, Bhatt DL, Kashyap SR. Bariatric surgery versus intensive medical therapy for diabetes. N Engl J Med. 2014;371:682.

11. Buchwald H, Estok R, Fahrbach K, Banel D, Jensen MD, Pories WJ, et al. Weight and type 2 diabetes after bariatric surgery: systematic review and meta-analysis. Am J Med. 2009;122: 248–56.

12. Kashyap SR, Bhatt DL, Schauer PR. Bariatric surgery vs. advanced practice medical management in the treatment of type 2 diabetes mellitus: Rationale and design of the Surgical Therapy And Medications Potentially Eradicate Diabetes Efficiently trial (STAMPEDE). Diabetes Obes Metab. 2010;12:452–4.

13. Novack GD. The development of drugs vs devices. Ocul Surf. 2011;9:56–7.

14. Dhruva SS, Bero LA, Redberg RF. Strength of study evidence examined by the FDA in premarket approval of cardiovascular devices. JAMA. 2009;302:2679–85.

15. Redberg RF. Sham controls in medical device trials. N Engl J Med. 2014;371:892–3.

16. Meissner K, Fässler M, Rücker G, Kleijnen J, Hróbjartsson A, Schneider A, et al. Differential effectiveness of placebo treatments: a systematic review of migraine prophylaxis. JAMA Intern Med. 2013;173:1941–51.

17. Albin RL. Sham surgery controls: intracerebral grafting of fetal tissue for Parkinson's disease and proposed criteria for use of sham surgery controls. J Med Ethics. 2002;28:322–5.

Chapter 45
Genomics in Clinical Trials

Peter R. Nelson

Overview

In designing a clinical trial, especially one that is comparing a procedural intervention to either another intervention or a non-procedural control, you are likely focused on clinical endpoints. However, it might be important at the very beginning of the design phase to explore ways to collect mechanistic information behind the effects of that intervention. In some trials, this is not possible or feasible, but in others it may be a real missed opportunity if not considered up front. This component of your trial may not be the primary question and endpoint of the research, but it may serve as an important secondary focus. For example, to start out you may ask "What's the biology behind the resulting observations from our intervention?" or "Do differences in individual subjects' innate biology explain differential responses to our intervention?" Then you can develop the strategy from there. Again, this is the opportunity to plan to collect potentially important mechanistic data to complement the clinical observations adding a truly translational component to the study and will likely present multiple future research ideas.

Biochemical data might be available from simple standard blood testing and this avenue should be explored for ease and simplicity. More than likely you will want to incorporate novel molecular strategies and techniques to provide an in-depth level of exploration. If biopsies or tissue/organ removal is part of the intervention studied; then, tissue would be available for molecular testing and should be incorporated into your design. If you are interested in patient-level information to see how your intervention either affects or is conversely influenced by systemic

P.R. Nelson (✉)
Surgical Service, James A. Haley VA Medical Center,
13000 Bruce B. Downs Boulevard, Tampa, FL 33612, USA
e-mail: peter.nelson@va.gov

© Springer International Publishing AG 2017
K.M.F. Itani and D.J. Reda (eds.), *Clinical Trials Design in Operative
and Non Operative Invasive Procedures*, DOI 10.1007/978-3-319-53877-8_45

biological systems, then you would want to incorporate more advanced molecular techniques into your trial design. This is the basic premise of a personalized medicine approach [1].

Definitions

Genomics is broadly defined as the study of the function, structure, evolution and mapping of the entire set of deoxyribonucleic acid (DNA) within a single cell. Its development spawned from the work done in the Human Genome Project which identified and determined sequences of the 3 billion base pairs that comprise human DNA [2]. *Transcriptomics* is the term applied to moving one step further down the central dogma of molecular biology and studying the ribonucleic acid (RNA) message from actively expressed genes. This RNA-based analysis reflects influences on the genome from external factors and therefore varies between organisms and even in the same organism exposed to different environmental conditions. At the human level, this allows the study of different biological conditions and disease processes in subjects exposed to different risk factors or to intervention in a clinical trial. *Functional Genomics* is a term that describes translating the large amount of available genomic information, not at an individual gene level, but at this genome-wide level of focus, to examine changes in the resulting phenotype over time such as the response to intervention. The field of *Genomic Medicine* then studies this variation in this genome-wide functionality and how it is associated with illness and death. Although not an established field of study, one might define "*Genomic Surgery*" as incorporating an understanding of the biology behind the diseases we treat and associating small changes in genome expression or function with patient outcomes following surgery.

Tissue Genomics

If your trial involves taking biopsies, removing tumors, or even entire solid organs, then access to tissue is already inherent in your protocol. Although most commonly used to study cancer biology, these types of analyses may be broadly applicable to areas such as atherosclerosis, congenital disorders or malformations, developmental disorders, neuromuscular disorders, etc. The extraction of DNA or RNA from these tissue specimens allows direct study of differences in genomic information that might shed light into the development of and/or heterogeneity within the primary lesion, characterize the potential virulence or prognosis of the lesion, and could even direct treatment and predict tissue response to therapy. Large tissue bank data repositories have been assembled such that genomic data from samples in your trial could be screened against these datasets to identify and target novel therapies to the specific tissue characteristics of an individual lesion [3].

Gene Expression Studies

High-throughput technologies enable simultaneous examination of gene expression levels for the entire genome from a single patient sample. These human transcriptome arrays have upwards of 7 million probe sets that detect both coding and non-coding transcripts, exonic, sub-exonic, and exon-exon junction regions, and all transcript isoforms [4]. The enormity of the data generated requires complex bioinformatics which have just begun to unlock the potential of this technology but ideally requires collaboration with advanced statisticians with both expertise in the field and the computer power to run the analyses [5, 6]. With that in mind, the compelling data generated from these analyses enable you to perform comprehensive genomic profiling algorithms that can be used to develop novel predictive models of disease progression and treatment outcomes. This more advanced approach promises superior predictive ability compared to traditional clinical predictors and laboratory biochemical biomarkers, in fact, we have found the combination of clinical predictors and molecular data to be synergistic. Past attempts to base class prediction on a single biomarker have failed, so intuitively, the complexity of the data used in this proposed strategy matches the complexity of the disease processes being studied and should provide a more robust prediction model. Genomic data repositories are increasingly available for independent analysis, comparison, and validation of your results.

The bioinformatics output from genome-wide expression studies looks different to the inexperienced researcher, but the learning curve can be relatively short, at least to gain functional familiarity once you immerse yourself into these types of projects. Again, doing these analyses in collaboration with experienced statisticians is critical, however. Initial output can be in the form of a heat map or hierarchical clustering matrix (Fig. 45.1). This is the genomic spreadsheet. It shows the up- and downregulation of the genes which demonstrate significant differential expression based on your clinical parameters or response groups. It delineates which genes' expression are closely associated and begins to identify significant differences in your study cohort. Next, secondary analyses can further characterize specific functional gene pathways and allow visualization of the data in 2D, 3D or even 4D depth over time (Fig. 45.2). Finally, you can develop your class prediction models using complex (but established) probit regression algorithms to identify a manageable number of genes that in combination strongly predict your study outcome (Fig. 45.3). This generates a "standard curve" which can then be used to plot new subject data prospectively, predict clinical outcome, and therefore direct treatment.

Logistically, genome expression studies use RNA as the substrate. RNA is labile and needs to be isolated real time from fresh blood samples. Therefore, you will need access to wet laboratory capabilities and personnel experienced with advance molecular techniques in order to process the initial samples. Analysis can then be scheduled in batch format but does not provide real-time, point of care information at least at this stage. Next, you should estimate the optimal time points at which to collect blood relative to the intervention. A pre-intervention sample might be

Fig. 45.1 Gene expression cluster analysis. Genomic heat map from supervised analysis with hierarchical clustering. *Red*-shaded blocks represent varying degrees of upregulated gene expression. *Blue*-shaded blocks represent varying degrees of downregulated gene expression. Clinical outcome groupings A and B are the comparison groups in a trial. Gene clusters A and B are generated from bioinformatic analyses of the genomic data indicating differential gene expression highly associated with the clinical outcome of interest

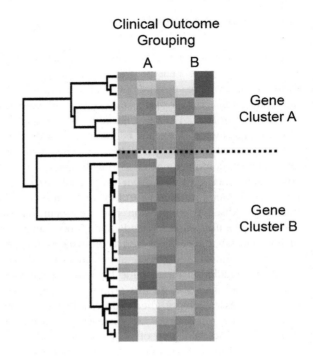

critical, and if independently predictive, may be the only time point necessary. It would be very powerful to predict late clinical outcome from a single baseline sample. In addition, time points clustered around the intervention to define the critical window to detect maximal molecular activity will define the systemic reaction to treatment. This will likely provide meaningful predictive capability early enough in the clinical course to allow adjustments in the treatment plan that would still impact outcomes. The premise to acquiring this early molecular data is that treatments delivered in reaction to this data will potentially lead to novel interventions capable of "engineering" patient outcomes. Finally, a few later time points might be informative, not as much to direct treatment, but rather to define molecular changes that might accompany late events that could be eventually used for early detection and prevention. Keep in mind, however, that these analyses are costly and the more samples planned, the bigger the budget required.

Genome-Wide Association Studies (GWAS)

GWAS, as suggested by the name, incorporate genome-wide screening to detect single-nucleotide polymorphisms (SNPs) that are "associated" with a disease process. SNPs result from a single-nucleotide substitution in the genetic code and are

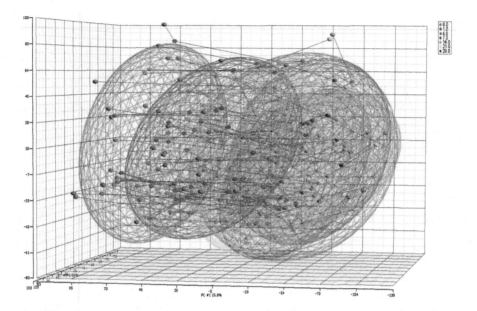

Fig. 45.2 Principal component analysis (PCA). An example of gene expression profiling that demonstrates differential expression of critical predictive genes over time. Each different colored orb represents the same gene set sampled at different time points relative to intervention

the most common type of genetic variation occurring normally throughout the human genome. It is estimated that there are upwards of 10 million SNPs, most occurring in non-coding regions of DNA. As such, SNPs may or may not be directly biologically or mechanistically related to the pathogenesis of the disease unless they occur within the coding sequence of a gene altering its function. They may, however, serve as biomarkers associated with disease incidence, prognosis, or response to therapy. SNPs may be used to identify baseline risk and relative disease susceptibility or inheritance and used to direct preventative counseling or intervention. They enable early disease detection before typical clinical presentation and therefore be used to initiate early therapeutic intervention. SNPs may be associated with the severity of disease penetration or virulence and therefore used to design different algorithms or levels of treatment intensity. These approaches can be used across a wide range of complex diseases [7].

Logistically, GWAS may be a little simpler to incorporate into your study if relevant because it utilizes DNA as the substrate which is more stable. Blood samples can be snap frozen and DNA extracted at a later time. This means that you have the option to process the samples in your own or a collaborators laboratory, or potentially to outsource the analyses if the expertise is not available locally.

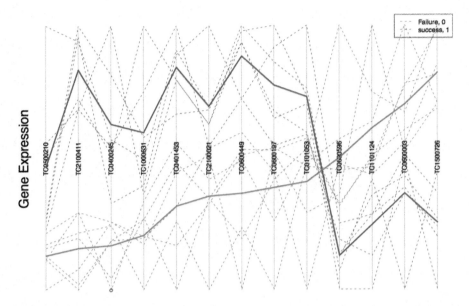

Fig. 45.3 Example of the graphic presentation of genomic profiling. Using a highly predictive set of 13 genes correlated with intervention outcome, this "standard curve" is generated to which expression data from trial subjects can then be calibrated prospectively. The *Red* curve represents mean expression values in subjects with a successful outcome. The *Blue* curve represents mean expression values for the same genes in subjects with a failed outcome. Future subjects' expression data can be plotted on the curve to predict their likely clinical outcome

As far as timing and number of samples, it is likely that just a single sample taken at study enrollment will be sufficient. This has the advantage of reducing the required time, resources, and associated costs. Current array technology allows the simultaneous genome-wide screening of hundreds of thousands of SNPs and can provide relatively rapid turnover. You might have specific SNPs known to be associated with your disease of interest and conduct a more focused candidate gene analysis, or you may be interested in searching for a novel association and screen the entire genome for any SNP that correlates with your intervention outcomes. These strategies have identified SNPs associated with a number of complex diseases such as a variety of cancers, diabetes, lipid metabolism, cardiovascular disorders, neurodegenerative disorders, and inflammatory bowel disease among others. The number of published GWAS studies has grown exponentially and new discoveries are being reported daily such that large databases are now available through the National Institutes of Health and other coordinating agencies to aid the sharing of genomic data that can be a valuable resource in the design phase of a new trial.

Pharmacogenomics

Pharmacogenomics is the study of how genome-wide differences in gene structure or function influence variability in a subject's response to drug therapy [8]. This is most commonly conducted as a specialized form of GWAS where SNPs are identified that correlate with a subject's responsivity to a certain drug or alternatively is predictive of toxicity with drug exposure. The goal is to minimize adverse drug events and is therefore twofold: (1) to avoid giving a patient a drug to which they do not respond but assume any risk with no benefit or (2) to avoid unknowingly placing a patient at higher than normal risk for adverse drug effects with exposure. Pharmacogenomic studies have identified SNPs associated with anticoagulants, antiplatelet agents, antihypertensive drugs, asthma treatments, HIV/AIDS treatments, chemotherapy, diabetes treatment, antidepressants, antipsychotics and others. In some cases, genetic testing has made it to the clinical arena, but wide spread adoption is limited indicating there is still ample opportunity for further clinical investigation and validation. The ultimate goal is to be able to customize medical therapy—drug selection, dosing, and duration—based on an individual subject's genetic information.

Innovative Technologies

The entire field of genomic study and the associated bioinformatics remains an area of great innovation. Although some of the methods described above are not necessarily new, they continue to evolve rapidly, become more user friendly, more real time, and more cost efficient. Next generation sequencing (NGS), also called high-throughput sequencing (HTS), is a relatively new methodology that provides scalable DNA sequencing from a select panel of genes of interest all the way up to the full exome depending on your needs and interest [9]. Compared to prior sequencing methods, NGS can perform whole genome sequencing much more rapidly and at relatively lower cost. It mainly provides robust SNP data with rapid turnover providing near real-time data that could have direct clinical impact in identifying disease susceptibility, prognosis, or response to treatment. The ability for NGS to provide functional gene expression information is more limited. The newest development getting a lot of attention is clustered regularly interspaced short palindromic repeats (CRISPR) analyses. This approach takes advantage of an innate adaptive immune defense system and applies it to both diagnostic and potentially therapeutic use [10]. This technology enables cutting of DNA strands at repetitive spacer sequences and applies them to sequencing methodologies. The real potential, however, is to apply this approach to target genes of interest that confer disease susceptibility or pathogenesis to cut them out of the genome and potentially replace them with normal or more favorable variants. This genetic engineering technology is obviously in an early experimental phase, but if it is applicable to your research question, you might incorporate it early in the design to take full advantage as the field evolves. The decision to incorporate any or several of these methodologies into your trial design depends on the disease of interest, what is to be learned from the genomic information, the expertise available, and the budget afforded to this line of investigation. Whatever methodology best fits your needs, stay with it throughout the study period, even if newer technology arrives to ensure completeness, consistency, and compatibility of the resulting data to maximize the likelihood of meaningful results in the end.

Personalized Medicine

The concepts explored above regarding tailoring treatment based on an individual patient's genetic makeup are the foundation for personalized medicine. It rests on the premise that using this detailed molecular information to develop more targeted, effective therapies, if not for the individual patient, at least for groups of similar patients with a specific disease process, will lead to better patient outcomes [11]. This introduces a new multidisciplinary clinical science care paradigm where clinicians, molecular biologists and biostatisticians work collaboratively to combine traditional clinical information with novel genomic data to create comprehensive care plans. Application to date has focused primarily on identification and characterization of existing disease based on the availability of subjects and blood or tissue samples. More recently, it is being applied to modifying treatment approaches either through pharmacogenomic or genome profiling studies to impact outcomes. Finally, these same technologies, applied differently, also hold promise in the screening, early detection, and primary prevention of a wide range of diseases. This may be where the greatest impact will be realized. The technology is here, and it continues to evolve. The applicability to the bedside, real-time turnaround, and improving costs all suggest that these tools will increasingly have a greater impact of healthcare delivery moving forward.

Application

By way of example, we have incorporated genomic studies into studying outcomes following lower extremity revascularization for peripheral arterial disease [12]. The premise is to identify genomic profiles or "signatures" predictive of clinical outcomes following either endovascular intervention or surgical bypass. We used a series of genomic analyses pre-intervention, immediately periprocedurally, and during short-term follow-up out to a year. We focused on genome-wide high-throughput analyses of inflammatory gene expression and correlated with clinical outcome following revascularization. A human transcriptome array and state-of-the-art bioinformatics provided the genomic data. Initial results in the endovascular treatment arm have established proof-of-principle that this type of strategy has merit [13]. Using this approach, we have demonstrated our ability to identify a limited gene set that supported our primary hypothesis that early periprocedural inflammatory changes were predictive of clinical intervention success or failure. Genes specifically involved in inflammatory cell proliferation and homing showed the most promise for future class prediction validation and application to clinical practice.

Summary

Thanks to the Human Genome Project we have a vast amount of molecular information and the accompanying complex bioinformatics tools to examine how minute changes in basic genomic signals can either lead to a primary disease process or affect a subject's response to intervention, or both. When designing a clinical trial, it is critical to stop and think whether or not an opportunity exists to incorporate this line of study into your protocol. Although the primary endpoint of your study may be a more traditional clinical endpoint in response to intervention, adding a translational aim to your study allows you to: (1) collect and bank valuable tissue or blood samples, (2) extract vital genomic data from those samples, (3) explore biochemical mechanisms underpinning the clinical observations made, (4) develop and validate robust class prediction models for clinical outcome to intervention, (5) design a personalized medicine approach for the disease of interest, (6) incorporate novel cutting edge molecular methodology into your protocol, and, importantly, (7) establish critical collaborative relationships with molecular biologists and bioinformaticists for future research direction.

References

1. Green ED, Guyer MS. Charting a course for genomic medicine from base pairs to bedside. Nature. 2011;470:204–13.
2. Lander ES, Linton LM, Birren B, et al. The international human genome sequencing consortium. Initial sequencing and analysis of the human genome. Nature. 2001;409:860–921.
3. Jones SJM, Laskin J, Li YY, et al. Evolution of an adenocarcinoma in response to selection by targeted kinase inhibitors. Genome Biol. 2010;11(8):R82.
4. Xu W, Seok J, Mindrinos MNMN, Schweitzer ACAC, Jiang H, Wilhelmy J, Clark TATA, Kapur K, Xing Y, Faham M, Storey JD, Moldawer LL, Maier RV, Tompkins RG, Wong WH, Davis RW, Xiao W. Human transcriptome array for high-throughput clinical studies. Proc Natl Acad Sci USA. 2011;108:3707–12.
5. Lee MT, Kuo FC, Whitmore GA, Sklar J. Importance of replication in microarray gene expression studies: statistical methods and evidence from repetitive cDNA hybridizations. Proc Natl Acad Sci USA. 2000;97:9834–9.

6. Romero JP, Muniategui A, De Miguel FJ, Aramburu A, Montuenga L, Pio R, et al. EventPointer: an effective identification of alternative splicing events using junction arrays. BMC Genom. 2016;17(1):467.
7. McCarthy MI, Abecasis GR, Cardon LR, Goldstein DB, Little J, Ioannidis JPA, et al. Genome-wide association studies for complex traits: consensus, uncertainty and challenges. Nat Rev Genet. 2008;9:356–69.
8. Nelson MR, Johnson T, Warren L, Hughes AR, Chissoe SL, Xu C-F, et al. The genetics of drug efficacy: opportunities and challenges. Nat Rev Genet Nat Res. 2016;17:197–206.
9. Moorcraft SY, Gonzalez D, Walker BA. Understanding next generation sequencing in oncology: a guide for oncologists. Crit Rev Oncol Hematol. 2015;96:463–74.
10. Cong L, Ran FA, Cox D, Lin S, Barretto R, Habib N, et al. Multiplex genome engineering using CRISPR/Cas systems. Science. 2013;339(6121):819–23.
11. Stratified, personalised or P4 medicine: a new direction for placing the patient at the centre of healthcare and health education. FORUM: Academy of Medical Sciences. May 2015.
12. Nelson PR, O'Malley KA, Moldawer LL, Seeger JM. Genomic and proteomic determinants of lower extremity revascularization failure: rationale and study design. J Vasc Surg. 2007;45:82A–91A.
13. Desart K, O'Malley K, Schmitt B, Hong M, Restreppo C, Lopez MC, Moldawer LL, Baker HV, Berceli SA, Nelson PR. Systemic inflammation as a predictor of clinical outcomes following lower extremity angioplasty/stenting. J Vasc Surg. 2016;64:766–78.

Chapter 46
Biomarkers as Adjuncts to Clinical Trials

George Z. Li and Jiping Wang

Introduction

Biomarkers are defined by the National Institutes of Health (NIH) as "a characteristic that is objectively measured and evaluated as an indicator of normal biological processes, pathogenic processes, or pharmacologic responses to therapeutic intervention" [1]. Under this definition, anything from serum creatinine level to the presence of a V600E mutation on the BRAF oncogene is considered biomarkers. However, currently most researchers and clinicians generally reserve the term "biomarker" for the more sophisticated measurements on this spectrum.

Scientific evidence from prospective randomized clinical trials continues to be the gold standard to guide clinical practice. Traditionally, the primary outcome measurements of clinical trials have been clinical endpoints, which reflect how a patient "feels, functions, or survives" [1, 2]. Examples of clinical endpoints include stroke, myocardial infarction, and survival. While biomarkers may not necessarily correlate with a patient's current clinical status, their ability to predict subsequent response to treatment and disease progression makes them powerful adjuncts to clinical trials. Here, we examine the various roles that biomarkers play in clinical trials, from being used to select patient populations that are most likely to benefit from an intervention to actually serving as a surrogate outcome measure in place of a clinical endpoint.

G.Z. Li
Department of Surgery, Brigham and Women's Hospital,
75 Francis St, Boston, MA 02115, USA
e-mail: gzli@partners.org

J. Wang (✉)
Department of Surgery, Division of Surgical Oncology, Brigham and Women's Hospital,
Dana-Farber Cancer Institute, 75 Francis St, Boston, MA 02115, USA
e-mail: jwang39@partners.org

© Springer International Publishing AG 2017
K.M.F. Itani and D.J. Reda (eds.), *Clinical Trials Design in Operative and Non Operative Invasive Procedures*, DOI 10.1007/978-3-319-53877-8_46

Enrichment Trial Design: Early Examples from Cancer Trials

The increasing use of biomarkers to select treatments and predict therapeutic response is best demonstrated through the evolution of clinical trials in oncology. Over time, these trials have adopted progressively more sophisticated designs as the complexity of our genetic understanding of cancer has expanded. Researchers first began to elucidate the role of genetic mutations in cancer in the mid- to late twentieth century. The key breakthroughs came in the 1980s, when several groups found that activating mutations in so-called proto-oncogenes could lead to car-cinogenesis [3, 4]. This led to the hypothesis that specific antibodies or small molecules could be designed to nullify cancer-promoting mutations, and thus, targeted therapy was born. By the 1990s, clinical trials testing several targeted drugs were underway.

One of the early successes was imatinib for chronic myeloid leukemia (CML). More than 90% of patients with CML harbor the Philadelphia chromosome (Ph), which is formed by a translocation between chromosomes 9 and 22. This translocation produces a fusion gene BCR-ABL, a proto-oncogene that encodes a constitutively active tyrosine kinase that is both necessary and sufficient for CML tumorigenesis [5, 6]. Imatinib is an oral tyrosine kinase inhibitor that competitively inhibits BCR-ABL. A landmark phase III trial published in 2003, which enrolled 1106 chronic-phase CML patients with the Ph chromosome, showed that imatinib produced dramatically more cytologic complete responses with fewer side effects compared to standard chemotherapy [7].

This trial is one of the earliest examples of an "enrichment" or "targeted design" trial in which a biomarker (the presence of Ph) is used to select patients to include in a clinical trial [8, 9]. Patients with the biomarker underwent randomization, while those without it were excluded. The goal of the enrichment trial design is to reduce sample size requirements by excluding patients who are not likely to benefit from the treatment. This, of course, requires the biomarker to be a reliable predictor of treatment response. As such, the imatinib enrichment trial was successful because 1. Ph is strongly predictive of response to imatinib and 2. Ph positivity is very common in CML patients such that enrolling enough patients was feasible.

Another early success story for enrichment trials was trastuzumab, a chimeric antibody against human epidermal growth factor receptor 2 (HER2). HER2 amplification had previously been shown in the laboratory to promote breast cancer tumorigenesis [10]. Trastuzumab had demonstrated good in vitro and in vivo efficacy against HER2-amplified breast cancer in preclinical studies [11], and a phase III trial published in 2001, which randomized 469 patients with metastatic breast cancer that over-expressed HER2 to conventional chemotherapy with or without trastuzumab, found a significant benefit in survival with the addition of trastuzumab [12]. Again, like the imatinib trial, the success of the targeted design trial for trastuzumab hinged upon the fact that HER2 amplification was relatively common and also reliably predicted response to therapy.

Adaptive Design Trials in Cancer Therapy: An Alternative to Enrichment Trials

Unlike Ph and HER2, many cancer biomarkers are not as definitively linked to tumor behavior or responsiveness to targeted therapy. An alternative trial design emerged in the late 2000s for biomarkers in which their predictive power was not fully established. These "adaptive" trials relied on interim analyses to assess biomarker association with the primary outcome, and then allowed for subsequent modifications in patient randomization based on these interim data [8]. The most basic adaptive trial design consists of two phases. In the initial "learning period," patients with positive or negative biomarkers are enrolled and randomized to either the intervention or the control treatments. Then, an interim analysis determines whether or not a futility threshold is reached for the biomarker-negative group. If futility threshold is reached, then enrollment of biomarker-negative patients stops and the trial continues as a targeted design trial. However, if futility threshold is not reached, the trial continues to enroll both biomarker-positive and biomarker-negative patients, and the final analysis would compare intervention and control therapies for both the entire trial population and the biomarker-positive subset.

An example of an adaptive trial is SWOG S0819, an ongoing phase III trial to assess the efficacy of adding cetuximab, an epidermal growth factor receptor (EGFR) inhibitor, to standard chemotherapy in patients with advanced non-small cell lung cancer (NSLC) with or without EGFR positivity on fluorescent in situ hybridization (FISH) assay [13]. In the learning phase, the trial enrolled both EGFR FISH-positive and FISH-negative patients and randomized them to standard chemotherapy with or without cetuximab. An interim evaluation will then determine futility of cetuximab in the EGFR FISH-negative group. If this is the case, the trial will continue enrolling only EGFR FISH-positive patients.

Umbrella (Platform) and Basket Trials in Cancer Therapy

With our increasing understanding of the complex genetic mechanisms in cancer, the number of cancer biomarkers has exponentially grown as well (Table 46.1). The challenge that this poses to clinical trials is that it would be difficult to test individual targeted therapies for patients with a specific cancer type harboring a specific gene mutation, as the cancer type, the gene mutation, or both may be rare. Two biomarker-based trial designs have emerged to address this challenge. One, the

Table 46.1 Examples of predictive cancer biomarkers and corresponding targeted therapies

Biomarker	Targeted therapies
BCR-ABL fusion	Imatinib [7], dasatinib [32]
HER2 amplification	Trastuzumab [12], pertuzumab [33]
CD20 expression	Rituximab [34]
KIT mutation	Imatinib [35]
EGFR mutation	Erlotinib [36], cetuximab [37]
EML4-ALK fusion	Crizotinib [38], alectinib [39]
BRAF V600E mutation	Vemurafenib [40]
DDR2 mutation	Dasatinib [41]
Mismatch repair deficiency	Pembrolizumab [42]

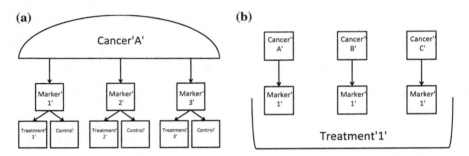

Fig. 46.1 Design schematic for **a** an umbrella trial and **b** a basket trial

"umbrella" or "platform" trial, enrolls patients of a specific cancer type but randomizes them within one of several sub-trials based on gene mutation status (Fig. 46.1a). Although patients would have the same histologic cancer type, they would be treated differently according to their biomarker signature. Another, the "basket trial," (Fig. 46.1b) enrolls patients of a specific gene mutation and randomizes them to mutation-targeted therapy that is not cancer-type specific [8]. The idea here is that patients with the same biomarkers would have similar responses to therapy even if they had different histological cancer types.

An example of an ongoing umbrella trial that began in May 2013 is FOCUS4, which enrolls patients with metastatic colorectal cancer who have completed 16 weeks of first-line chemotherapy and have responsive or stable disease on an interval CT scan [14]. Patients are screened for mutations in BRAF, PIK3CA, KRAS, and NRAS and then randomized to five biomarker-specific subgroups (the fifth group being wild type for all mutations). Each subgroup then tests a novel targeted therapy against placebo. If a targeted therapy shows promise in a biomarker-positive arm during an interim analysis, it will be tested in the wild-type arm. The advantage of an umbrella trial over an enrichment trial of a single bio-marker is that a much higher proportion of patients screened are eligible for enrollment. In addition, interim analyses allowing for subsequent alterations in patient enrollment within subgroups make umbrella trials more efficient than multiple independent clinical trials testing targeted therapies against specific mutations.

Alternatively, the basket trial enrolls patients with a specific gene mutation but is cancer-type naive. The hypothesis behind this design is that the presence of a particular biomarker may actually trump tumor type or histology in predicting treatment response. One basket trial currently enrolling is the NCI Molecular Analysis for Therapy Choice (MATCH) trial, which was launched in early 2015 [15]. The trial will have 25 treatment arms based on the presence of particular gene mutations and plans to enroll 1000 patients of any tumor type. A key advantage of this design is that it is inclusive of patients with either rare cancer types or rare mutations. However, one disadvantage of NCI-MATCH is that there are no control arms, which could either amplify or hide true treatment benefits [16].

Prognostic Versus Predictive Biomarkers

When evaluating biomarkers, one must carefully distinguish a "predictive" bio-marker from a "prognostic" biomarker. A predictive biomarker is associated with either a benefit or lack thereof from a particular therapy relative to other therapies. A prognostic biomarker, on the other hand, is associated with a clinical outcome in either the absence of therapy or with standard therapy that all patients receive (Fig. 46.2) [17].

For example, Ph positivity and HER2 amplification are excellent predictive biomarkers, because they are strongly associated with response to imatinib and trastuzumab, respectively. However, from the two clinical trials discussed above, one cannot conclude whether Ph or HER2 amplification is a good prognostic biomarker, because there were no marker-negative patients enrolled in these trials. Interestingly, in the pre-trastuzumab era, HER2 amplification was actually shown to be a negative prognostic biomarker associated with lymph node metastases and decreased survival [18, 19].

Prognostic biomarkers are widely used in surgical oncology (Table 46.2). For example, positive peritoneal washings are associated with subsequent gross intraperitoneal metastasis and poor survival in gastric carcinoma patients [20, 21]. Several studies have suggested that positive peritoneal washings are also "predic-tive" of a response to intraperitoneal heated chemotherapy [22], but this has not been formally validated in a clinical trial, and probably will not be, as it would require a negative peritoneal washing cohort to undergo the same aggressive sur-gical approach, which may be difficult to justify.

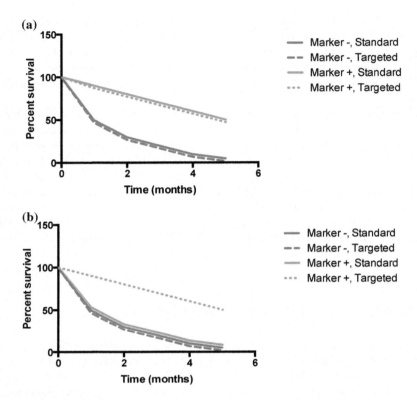

Fig. 46.2 Hypothetical survival curves demonstrating **a** a prognostic biomarker and **b** a predictive biomarker

Table 46.2 Examples of prognostic surgical biomarkers

Biomarker	Prognosis
Positive peritoneal washings in gastric carcinoma patients	Increased intraperitoneal recurrence and decreased overall survival [20]
Grossly positive surgical margins after retroperitoneal liposarcoma resection	Decreased disease-specific survival [43]
Positive sentinel lymph node in melanoma patients	Decreased overall survival [44, 45]

Biomarkers as Surrogate Endpoints: Examples from Endocrinology and Infectious Disease Trials

Traditionally, endpoints of clinical trials have been clinical outcomes, such as survival, stroke, or myocardial infarction. While biomarkers may not necessarily reflect a patient's current clinical state, their ability to predict future clinical outcomes or response to treatment potentially allows them to be used as "surrogate endpoints" for clinical trials. Furthermore, biomarker surrogate endpoints often can be observed or measured in a shorter period of time, making them particularly attractive for phase II trial endpoints [23].

However, there are several potential pitfalls that preclude them from being widely accepted as phase III trial endpoints. Notably, an intervention may have a favorable effect on a biomarker but have other off-target effects that ultimately result in a worse clinical outcome [24]. For example, the Action to Control Cardiovascular Risk in Diabetes (ACCORD) trial randomized 10, 251 patients with diabetes mellitus to receive either standard of care, which targeted a glycated hemoglobin (HbA1c) level between 7.0 and 7.9%, or intensive diabetes therapy which targeted a HbA1c level below 6.0%. Increased HbA1c levels have been shown to be strongly associated with adverse cardiovascular events, renal events, and death in patients with diabetes [25–27]. However, at the end of the ACCORD trial, the intensive diabetes therapy group actually had higher mortality even though they had lower HbA1c levels, potentially due to significantly higher rates of hypoglycemia in that group [28]. Thus, the off-target effect of hypoglycemia indicates the HbA1c biomarker would not be an appropriate surrogate outcome for mortality.

Using a biomarker as a surrogate outcome can also create false-negative results if an intervention affects a clinical outcome via a pathway independent of the biomarker [24]. In 2001, researchers conducted a phase III trial studying whether interferon gamma could reduce infections in patients with chronic granulomatous disease, an inherited NADPH oxidase deficiency that impairs phagocyte-mediated microorganism clearance. The trial found a significantly lower rate of serious infections in patients treated with interferon gamma compared to those treated with placebo. However, the two groups had identical levels of superoxide production by phagocytes, a biomarker for disease severity and predilection for infection [29]. Thus, had superoxide production been used as a surrogate endpoint in this trial, a potential treatment benefit would have been missed.

Due to these disadvantages, biomarker-based surrogate outcomes have generally not been used for phase III clinical trials in most fields. However, a few areas of research do widely use biomarker-based endpoints, especially those in which clinical endpoints are difficult to use. For example, hepatitis C (HCV) infection is often chronic and silent, so effects on survival and other clinical endpoints would be difficult to demonstrate in a clinical trial because the required length of follow-up would likely be prohibitively long. Thus, the standard outcome measure for HCV trials is sustained virologic response (SVR), which is based on quantification of HCV RNA. SVR was the primary outcome measure for two recent landmark parallel HCV trials. ASTRAL-1 and ASTRAL-3 showed that sofosbuvir plus velpatasvir produced a 99 percent SVR rate in patients with HCV genotypes 1, 2, 3, 4, 5, and 6, [30, 31] and these results have been widely accepted as proof of cure of HCV infection.

Conclusion

With our growing understanding of the molecular basis of disease, researchers and clinicians now have an increased ability to predict disease progression and response to treatment based on biomarkers. In various different medical fields, from oncology to endocrinology to infectious disease, biomarkers have emerged as adjuncts to clinical trials. In fields such as oncology, biomarkers are primarily used as predictive variables for response to various targeted agents, with the potential for "personalized" therapy based on specific genetic profiles. In fields such as infectious disease, biomarkers such as SVR for HCV are actually widely accepted as surrogate outcomes that serve as primary endpoints for phase III clinical trials.

References

1. Biomarkers Definitions Working Group. Biomarkers and surrogate endpoints: preferred definitions and conceptual framework. Clin Pharmacol Ther. 2001;69:89–95.
2. Strimbu K, Tavel JA. What are biomarkers? Curr Opin HIV AIDS. 2010;5:463–6.
3. Der CJ, Krontiris TG, Cooper GM. Transforming genes of human bladder and lung carcinoma cell lines are homologous to the ras genes of Harvey and Kirsten sarcoma viruses. Proc Natl Acad Sci U S A. 1982;79:3637–40.
4. Parada LF, Tabin CJ, Shih C, Weinberg RA. Human EJ bladder carcinoma oncogene is homologue of Harvey sarcoma virus ras gene. Nature. 1982;297:474–8.
5. Daley GQ, Van Etten RA, Baltimore D. Induction of chronic myelogenous leukemia in mice by the P210bcr/abl gene of the Philadelphia chromosome. Science. 1990;247:824–30.
6. Heisterkamp N, Jenster G, ten Hoeve J, Zovich D, Pattengale PK, Groffen J. Acute leukaemia in bcr/abl transgenic mice. Nature. 1990;344:251–3.
7. O'Brien SG, Guilhot F, Larson RA, et al. Imatinib compared with interferon and low-dose cytarabine for newly diagnosed chronic-phase chronic myeloid leukemia. N Engl J Med. 2003;348:994–1004.
8. Renfro LA, Mallick H, An MW, Sargent DJ, Mandrekar SJ. Clinical trial designs incorporating predictive biomarkers. Cancer Treat Rev. 2016;43:74–82.
9. Simon R, Maitournam A. Evaluating the efficiency of targeted designs for randomized clinical trials. Clin Cancer Res. 2004;10:6759–63.
10. Hudziak RM, Schlessinger J, Ullrich A. Increased expression of the putative growth factor receptor p185HER2 causes transformation and tumorigenesis of NIH 3T3 cells. Proc Natl Acad Sci U S A. 1987;84:7159–63.
11. Seshadri R, Firgaira FA, Horsfall DJ, McCaul K, Setlur V, Kitchen P. Clinical significance of HER-2/neu oncogene amplification in primary breast cancer. The South Australian Breast Cancer Study Group. J Clin Oncol. 1993;11:1936–42.
12. Slamon DJ, Leyland-Jones B, Shak S, et al. Use of chemotherapy plus a monoclonal antibody against HER2 for metastatic breast cancer that overexpresses HER2. N Engl J Med. 2001;344:783–92.
13. Redman MW, Crowley JJ, Herbst RS, Hirsch FR, Gandara DR. Design of a phase III clinical trial with prospective biomarker validation: SWOG S0819. Clin Cancer Res. 2012;18:4004–12.
14. Shiu KK, Maughan T, Wilson RH, Adams RA, Pugh C, Brown L, Fisher D, Wasan H, Middleton GW, Steward WP, Kaplan RS. FOCUS4: a prospective molecularly stratified, adaptive multicenter program of randomized controlled trials for patients with colorectal

cancer (CRC). In: Cannistra SA, editors. ASCO. Chicago, IL: American Society of Clinical Oncology; 2013.

15. Conley BA, Doroshow JH. Molecular analysis for therapy choice: NCI MATCH. Semin Oncol. 2014;41:297–9.

16. Mullard A. NCI-MATCH trial pushes cancer umbrella trial paradigm. Nat Rev Drug Discov. 2015;14:513–5.

17. Polley MY, Freidlin B, Korn EL, Conley BA, Abrams JS, McShane LM. Statistical and practical considerations for clinical evaluation of predictive biomarkers. J Natl Cancer Inst. 2013;105:1677–83.

18. Berger MS, Locher GW, Saurer S, et al. Correlation of c-erbB-2 gene amplification and protein expression in human breast carcinoma with nodal status and nuclear grading. Cancer Res. 1988;48:1238–43.

19. Slamon DJ, Clark GM, Wong SG, Levin WJ, Ullrich A, McGuire WL. Human breast cancer: correlation of relapse and survival with amplification of the HER-2/neu oncogene. Science. 1987;235:177–82.

20. Burke EC, Karpeh MS Jr, Conlon KC, Brennan MF. Peritoneal lavage cytology in gastric cancer: an independent predictor of outcome. Ann Surg Oncol. 1998;5:411–5.

21. Kodera Y, Yamamura Y, Shimizu Y, et al. Peritoneal washing cytology: prognostic value of positive findings in patients with gastric carcinoma undergoing a potentially curative resection. J Surg Oncol. 1999;72:60–4; discussion 4–5.

22. Coccolini F, Catena F, Glehen O, et al. Effect of intraperitoneal chemotherapy and peritoneal lavage in positive peritoneal cytology in gastric cancer. Systematic review and meta-analysis. Eur J Surg Oncol. 2016;42(9):1261–67.

23. De Gruttola VG, Clax P, DeMets DL, et al. Considerations in the evaluation of surrogate endpoints in clinical trials. Summary of a National Institutes of Health workshop. Control Clin Trials. 2001;22:485–502.

24. Fleming TR, Powers JH. Biomarkers and surrogate endpoints in clinical trials. Stat Med. 2012;31:2973–84.

25. Gerstein HC, Pogue J, Mann JF, et al. The relationship between dysglycaemia and cardiovascular and renal risk in diabetic and non-diabetic participants in the HOPE study: a prospective epidemiological analysis. Diabetologia. 2005;48:1749–55.

26. Selvin E, Marinopoulos S, Berkenblit G, et al. Meta-analysis: glycosylated hemoglobin and cardiovascular disease in diabetes mellitus. Ann Intern Med. 2004;141:421–31.

27. Stratton IM, Adler AI, Neil HA, et al. Association of glycaemia with macrovascular and microvascular complications of type 2 diabetes (UKPDS 35): prospective observational study. BMJ. 2000;321:405–12.

28. Action to Control Cardiovascular Risk in Diabetes Study Group, Gerstein HC, Miller ME, et al. Effects of intensive glucose lowering in type 2 diabetes. N Engl J Med. 2008;358:2545–59.

29. Group TICGDCS. A controlled trial of interferon gamma to prevent infection in chronic granulomatous disease. The International Chronic Granulomatous Disease Cooperative Study Group. N Engl J Med. 1991;324:509–16.

30. Feld JJ, Jacobson IM, Hezode C, et al. Sofosbuvir and velpatasvir for HCV genotype 1, 2, 4, 5, and 6 infection. N Engl J Med. 2015;373:2599–607.

31. Foster GR, Afdhal N, Roberts SK, et al. Sofosbuvir and velpatasvir for HCV genotype 2 and 3 infection. N Engl J Med. 2015;373:2608–17.

32. Shah NP, Tran C, Lee FY, Chen P, Norris D, Sawyers CL. Overriding imatinib resistance with a novel ABL kinase inhibitor. Science. 2004;305:399–401.

33. Baselga J, Cortes J, Kim SB, et al. Pertuzumab plus trastuzumab plus docetaxel for metastatic breast cancer. N Engl J Med. 2012;366:109–19.

34. Coiffier B, Lepage E, Briere J, et al. CHOP chemotherapy plus rituximab compared with CHOP alone in elderly patients with diffuse large-B-cell lymphoma. N Engl J Med. 2002;346:235–42.

35. Demetri GD, von Mehren M, Blanke CD, et al. Efficacy and safety of imatinib mesylate in advanced gastrointestinal stromal tumors. N Engl J Med. 2002;347:472–80.
36. Zhou C, Wu YL, Chen G, et al. Erlotinib versus chemotherapy as first-line treatment for patients with advanced EGFR mutation-positive non-small-cell lung cancer (OPTIMAL, CTONG-0802): a multicentre, open-label, randomised, phase 3 study. Lancet Oncol. 2011;12:735–42.
37. Pirker R, Pereira JR, von Pawel J, et al. EGFR expression as a predictor of survival for first-line chemotherapy plus cetuximab in patients with advanced non-small-cell lung cancer: analysis of data from the phase 3 FLEX study. Lancet Oncol. 2012;13:33–42.
38. Shaw AT, Kim DW, Nakagawa K, et al. Crizotinib versus chemotherapy in advanced ALK-positive lung cancer. N Engl J Med. 2013;368:2385–94.
39. Gadgeel SM, Gandhi L, Riely GJ, et al. Safety and activity of alectinib against systemic disease and brain metastases in patients with crizotinib-resistant ALK-rearranged non-small-cell lung cancer (AF-002JG): results from the dose-finding portion of a phase 1/2 study. Lancet Oncol. 2014;15:1119–28.
40. Chapman PB, Hauschild A, Robert C, et al. Improved survival with vemurafenib in melanoma with BRAF V600E mutation. N Engl J Med. 2011;364:2507–16.
41. Hammerman PS, Sos ML, Ramos AH, et al. Mutations in the DDR2 kinase gene identify a novel therapeutic target in squamous cell lung cancer. Cancer Discov. 2011;1:78–89.
42. Le DT, Uram JN, Wang H, et al. PD-1 blockade in tumors with mismatch-repair deficiency. N Engl J Med. 2015;372:2509–20.
43. Singer S, Antonescu CR, Riedel E, Brennan MF. Histologic subtype and margin of resection predict pattern of recurrence and survival for retroperitoneal liposarcoma. Ann Surg. 2003;238:358–70; discussion 70–1.
44. Balch CM, Soong SJ, Gershenwald JE, et al. Prognostic factors analysis of 17,600 melanoma patients: validation of the American Joint Committee on Cancer melanoma staging system. J Clin Oncol. 2001;19:3622–34.
45. Morton DL, Wanek L, Nizze JA, Elashoff RM, Wong JH. Improved long-term survival after lymphadenectomy of melanoma metastatic to regional nodes. Analysis of prognostic factors in 1134 patients from the John Wayne Cancer Clinic. Ann Surg. 1991;214:491–9; discussion 9–501.

Chapter 47
Patient-Centered Designs (and Outcomes)

Frances M. Weaver

There is no question that randomized clinical trials (RCTs) have led to important findings regarding the best available treatments for a variety of different diseases and conditions. Important clinical outcomes including survival and mortality, prevention of disease, improvements in key measures such as blood pressure and blood glucose, physical function, and reductions in healthcare use have been demonstrated in these trials. These trials are the basis for evidence-based medicine.

However, despite these significant impacts, there are a number of issues that have been raised regarding traditional clinical trials [1]. A well-designed clinical trial can take 10 years or more to complete. The costs associated with the conduct of these trials are often in the millions of dollars per trial. We can't afford to continue to pay for these large trials with long completion times to get the answers we need. Further, the eligibility requirements for participation in a clinical trial often exclude many of the persons who might benefit the most from the intervention [2]. RCTs emphasize internal validity. As a result, the generalizability of the findings to a more heterogeneous population of patients with the disease or condition under study is unknown. Further, the outcomes of greatest interest to patients may not be assessed as part of the trial. Outcomes that may be of particular concern to patients might include: "how did the treatment make the patient feel," or what is the patient most concerned about—"survival or quality of life?" These outcomes are referred to as patient-reported or patient-centered outcomes. Finally, while important findings are disseminated in high-visibility journals, seldom are these findings implemented into routine practice across providers, clinics, and health systems. Barriers to implementation range from lack of knowledge, inability to

F.M. Weaver (✉)
Center of Innovation for Complex Chronic Healthcare and Public Health Sciences,
Edward Hines Jr. Veterans Administration Hospital and Loyola University Chicago,
Bldg. 1, Room C203 (151H), 5000 S. 5th Avenue, Hines, IL 60304, USA
e-mail: frances.weaver@va.gov

© Springer International Publishing AG 2017
K.M.F. Itani and D.J. Reda (eds.), *Clinical Trials Design in Operative
and Non Operative Invasive Procedures*, DOI 10.1007/978-3-319-53877-8_47

obtain the treatment (e.g., medication is not on the formulary), costs of the treatment, complexity of the treatment, and system barriers.

Below are some methods and strategies that can be used to augment or modify the traditional clinical trial to address the concerns raised above and enhance patient centeredness.

Shortening the Time to Conduct a Trial

It has been estimated that the time it takes to go from conception of the research question and study design, to funding, to study initiation, data collection and analysis, to the dissemination of results of a clinical trial averages 10–15 years. Speeding up the time of a trial not only gives you answers more quickly, it is also likely to cost less to conduct the study and decreases the time to which the general population can access the intervention. A number of strategies have been shown to facilitate trial completion.

Use of Registries and Electronic Medical Records (EMRs) for Case Finding and Data Collection

One way to shorten a trial and incorporate patient data is to take advantage of existing data and resources for case finding and data collection. An example of this approach is the registry-based randomized trial [3, 4]. This design builds on the platform of a high-quality observational registry which already collects information on a defined patient cohort and uses this information to identify and enroll participants quickly. In this approach, all or most of the baseline data will have been collected already (in the registry). Furthermore, you are able to enroll larger numbers of patients that are more representative of the population. For example, a study compared the clinical effectiveness of microdecompression and laminectomy in patients with central lumbar spinal stenosis using a comprehensive registry of spine surgery patients [5]. Cases were identified and matched using propensity scores to closely approximate a randomized trial, providing the greatest balance between the two treatment groups. The results indicated that microdecompression was equivalent to laminectomy for treatment of central stenosis at one year. One caution is that there may be concerns about the quality of the data that are collected for a different purpose (accuracy, completeness), and there is a need to address the data privacy and consent issues when a registry is used.

Similarly, as most health systems have EMRs, we have the ability to find potentially eligible patients more quickly and to access their health information from the records. Development of algorithms using the EMR to identify patients who meet certain criteria (e.g., everyone who has diabetes and is age 65 and older and had a lower limb amputation; children who had ear infections before age 1 year) is becoming more common. The success of the algorithm to identify targeted patients is only as good as the data it is based on; thus, it is critical to validate the algorithms before utilizing them. These algorithms, also referred to as medical record phenotypes, are often used for observational database studies for cohort characterization and to identify eligible patients for study recruitment [6]. Algorithms are created using multiple variables to define inclusion and exclusion criteria.

There are several challenges to EMR phenotyping [7]. Complex processing of the EMR may be required based on the multi-dimensional and temporal nature of different data types (e.g., codes, notes, laboratory results). EMRs are designed for data on individual patients, so aggregation across a cohort of patients may be challenging. In addition, the number of data points in the EMR is very large and often complex if there isn't standardization of data elements across sites (e.g., laboratory tests and results). Communication between the researcher, clinician, and the data analyst may require multiple iterations, and miscommunication is a risk. On the other hand, a valid phenotype can identify a cohort of patients in the EMR quickly and facilitate case finding and recruitment. Recruitment is often time-consuming and labor intensive, and many studies fail due to poor recruitment. EMR phenotyping may offer a viable solution for many trials.

Web-Based Recruitment, Consenting, and Data Collection

With the proliferation of technology available to communicate in secure environments, there is growing use of technology for study recruitment, for informed consent, and for data collection. One of the most costly aspects of a clinical trial is the time and manpower required to identify and screen potentially eligible patients, conduct the informed consent process, and collect patient data. In a study that is patient centered, it is critical to ask questions that patients are most interested in learning the answer (e.g., how tired will the treatment make me? How will I feel emotionally afterward?) These are not data that can be obtained any other way than by asking the patient. Groups such as the Federal Drug Administration (FDA) are now making efforts to include patients' perspectives at the point of drug development [8]. In addition to testing how the drug affects the condition, developers are also prioritizing patient-centered outcomes such as symptoms, function, and quality of life. Basch outlines several key steps toward patient-centered drug development in his article [8].

Patient data can include self-reported information such as responses to standardized questionnaires and/or obtained through the use of sensor-based recordings (e.g., a pedometer or blood pressure monitor) captured from the patient and downloaded through an app to a secure location. Physiological measures such as weight, heart rate, blood pressure, and oxygen levels can be captured as frequently as the investigator thinks is necessary (e.g., daily). Activities such as walking and sleeping can be monitored, and patients can respond to questions through text messaging about symptoms and experiences at various times throughout the study.

Apple™ has created ResearchKit, an open-source framework that can be used to create apps for research [9]. The apps can be used to recruit and consent patients, deploy questionnaires and surveys for research participants to complete, and collect real-time dynamic activities and tasks. Anyone with a smartphone can participate in a study that utilizes the ResearchKit app. This makes research activities flexible and portable and increases the study reach and heterogeneity of the populations that can participate in research studies. The limitation, however, is for those individuals who do not own or have access to a smartphone. Web-based versions of many of these tools also can be made available so that those without their own resources can access them in places like public libraries and community centers.

Several observational studies are utilizing ResearchKit and other technologies for recruitment and data collection [10, 11]. The Patient-Centered Outcomes Research Initiative (PCORI) embarked on its first large randomized trial utilizing these technologies in 2016. The trial, called ADAPTABLE, is a pragmatic comparative effectiveness trial of two doses of aspirin for prevention of secondary cardiovascular events following a heart attack [12]. Patients who may be eligible and interested in participating in the study are referred to a website where they learn about the study and then participate in an online informed consent process including reviewing a video about the consent process. Patients who consent to participate are then screened for eligibility using a set of online questions. Patients who meet the eligibility requirements are randomized to the dose of aspirin that they will be asked to take daily, either low dose (81 mg) or regular dose (325 mg). Randomized patients complete baseline questionnaires online and are contacted periodically over the course of the study to return to the secure website to complete follow-up questionnaires. Their medical records will be reviewed to look for clinical outcomes including readmissions, comorbid conditions, cardiac events, and death. The ADAPTABLE trial plans to enroll, randomize, and follow 20,000 patients from multiple sites across the country.

Surgical trials also are beginning to use pragmatic approaches to facilitate the determination of study eligibility and recruitment. A study by Handoll et al. [13] used a pragmatic multicenter randomized trial comparing surgical and non-surgical treatment of adults with displaced fractures of the proximal humerus. Rather than requiring recruiting surgeons to classify the fractures as to whether or not they were displaced, eligibility was determined centrally by two experts at the clinical trials center. With this approach the investigators took practical measures to ensure that the intended fracture population reflected good standard clinical practice and maximized the relevance and applicability of the trial findings.

Comparative Effectiveness Trials

These studies, which can be randomized or observational, involve the direct comparison of existing healthcare interventions, programs, policy, and community interventions to determine which intervention works best for which patients and which pose the greatest benefits or harms. The interventions compared have been shown to be efficacious, but have not been compared to each other. In everyday practice, providers often have multiple medications to choose from to treat a patient for a particular condition, but may not have good information about whether one is better for a particular type of patient. The purpose of comparative effectiveness research is to help patients, clinicians, and others making informed decisions that will improve their health [14]. These types of studies tend to be faster to complete, include a more heterogeneous population, and focus more on patient outcomes.

Patient Engagement: Incorporating Patient Questions, Concerns, and Preferences

Patient Advisory Panels

Increasingly, research sponsors, contract research organizations, and research centers are utilizing patient advisory panels to obtain feedback and obtain insights from patients about a variety of study-related topics [15]. Topics such as what is the right study question(s), what interventions should be studied, what outcomes are important to patients, what are appropriate incentives for participation, development of education materials, how best to conduct the informed consent process are some of the topics patients can provide valuable input. However, involvement of patients and the public in RCTs, which may particularly benefit from this involvement, remains low [16]. The Center for Information and Study on Clinical Research Participation (CISCRP) has been organizing and facilitating patient panels and advisory boards for many years to look at and make suggestions for changes to study protocols, informed consent documents, study communications, study procedures and measures, and post-study communication. This feedback is provided to the researchers. In a recent effort to design a comparative effectiveness trial to address health disparities in socioeconomically disadvantaged women, researchers used a combination of a community advisory board, focus groups, and individual patient input to develop two intervention options for disadvantaged women attending women's health practices [17]. A recent letter to the editor describes a study group's efforts to engage patient and clinician stakeholders in assessing the feasibility of conducting the study, identifying barriers and facilitators to implementation, and proposing relevant outcomes [18]. The study, a pragmatic clinical trial of how to manage acute appendicitis (i.e., antibiotics vs. surgery), raised many questions with respect to quality of life and safety; thus, obtaining the input of these key stakeholders for study design and implementation was critical to the success of the trial.

Community-Based Participatory Research (CBPR)

CBPR is a collaborative approach to involve all the partners in the research process in an equitable way and recognize the unique strengths each partner brings to the table [19]. The partners include everyone who affects or is affected by the problem being studied (e.g., patients, providers, health system leadership, community programs, payers). While CBPR has been used in public health and other areas for a long time, it is a new concept for medical/clinical research [20]. This is the approach that has been embraced by the Patient-Centered Outcomes Research Institute (PCORI). PCORI, funded as part of the Affordable Care Act, was established to identify critical research questions of particular importance to patients, to conduct research more efficiently, and to disseminate findings in ways that stakeholders will find useful and valuable [21]. Patients and community partners are part of the research team, serving as investigators and collaborators in identifying questions, determining study design, identifying key outcomes (e.g., patient-reported outcomes), and playing a critical role in dissemination and implementation of findings [22]. Further details about PCORI are available in Chap. 52.

Patient-Reported Outcome Measures

RCTs in medicine typically collect physiological, physical, morbidity, mortality, and utilization outcomes. While these are important outcomes, patients often report that they are concerned about other types of outcomes such as whether the intervention will cause fatigue or pain, how the intervention will make them feel (symptoms and side effects), and how the intervention will affect their quality of life. Only patients can provide information about feelings, preferences, and things that cannot be observed, and these are often the most valuable outcomes [23]. The FDA defines a patient-reported outcome (PRO) as any report of the status of a patient's health condition that comes directly from the patient and is not interpreted by anyone else [24]. Clinical trials have increasingly included PROs in their data collection and outcome assessments [25]. Use of electronic methods, such as electronic diaries, computers, and telephones, makes data collection more efficient with fewer errors and is more portable than traditional methods [23].

Funded by the National Institutes of Health, the Patient-Reported Outcomes Measurement Information System (PROMIS®) provides a set of highly reliable and precise measures of patient-reported health status for physical, medical, and social well-being [26]. PROMIS® tools are used to allow clinicians and researchers to better understand the effects of various interventions on patients' experiences and what they are able to do. These tools have comparability (they are standardized across conditions), reliability and validity, flexibility (they can be administered in different ways and different forms), and inclusiveness (the measures encompass a highly heterogeneous population and are specific to health domains rather than diseases or conditions). PROMIS® measures are increasingly being used in research including clinical trials to augment traditional outcome measures.

The shape and implementation of RCTs are changing. The availability of technology, the increased access to and use of big data, and the demands to get answers that patients care about and to get these answers quickly are driving much of this change. While RCTs are still considered the gold standard for studies to establish the efficacy and safety of treatment modalities, incorporation of patient-reported outcome measures has become increasingly important. In addition, the ability to generalize to the larger population has fueled the need to move research more quickly down the pathway from discovery to testing to implementation.

References

1. Tricoci P, Allen M, Kramer J, Califf R, Smith S. Scientific evidence underlying the ACC/AHA clinical practice guidelines. J Am Med Assoc. 2009;301:831–41.
2. Booth CM, Tannock IF. Randomized controlled trials and population-based observational research: partners in the evolution of medical evidence. Brit J Cancer. 2014;. doi:10.1038/bjc:2013:725.
3. Fröbert O, Lagerqvist B, Gudnason T, Thuesen L, Svensson R, Olivercona GK, James SK. Thrombus aspiration in ST-Elevation myocardial infarction in Scandinavia (TASTE trial). A multicenter, prospective, randomized, controlled clinical registry trial based on the Swedish angiography and angioplasty registry (SCAAR) platform. Study design and rationale. Am Heart J. 2010;160(6):1042–8.
4. Laurer MS, D'Agostino RB. The randomized registry trial—the next disruptive technology in clinical research? New Engl J Med. 2013;369:1579–81.
5. Nerland SU, Jakola AS, Solheim O, Weber C, Rao V, Lenne G, Solberg TK, Salvesen O, Carlsen SM, Nygaard OP, Gulati S. Minimally invasive decompression versus open laminectomy for central stenosis of the lumber spine: pragmatic comparative effectiveness study. BMJ. 2015;350:h1603. doi:10.1136/bmj.h1603.
6. Rubbo B, Fitzpatrick NK, Denaxas S, Daskalopoulou M, Patel RS. UK Biobank follow-up and outcomes working group, Hemingway H. Use of electronic health records to ascertain, validate and phenotype acute myocardial infarction: A systematic review and recommendations. Int J Cardiol. 2015;187:705–11.
7. Xu J, Rasmussen LV, Shaw PL, Jiang G, Kiefer RC, Mo H, Pacheco JA, Speltz P, Zhu Q, Denny JC, Pathank J, Thompson WK, Montague E. Review and evaluation of electronic health records-driven phenotype algorithm authoring tools for clinical and translational research. J Am Med Inform Assn. 2015;22:1251–60.
8. Basch E. Toward patient-centered drug development in oncology. New Engl J Med. 2013;369 (5):397–400.
9. Apple™. http://www.apple.com/researchkit/ 2016. Accessed 23 June 2016.
10. Bot BM, Suver C, Neto EC, Kellen M, Klein A, Bare C, Doerr M, Pratap A, Wilbanks J, Dorsey ER, Friend SH, Trister AD. The mPower study, Parkinson disease mobile data collected using ResearchKit. Sci Data. 2016;. doi:10.1038/sdata.

11. The Health eHeart Study™. https://www.health-eheartstudy.org/ 2016. Accessed 23 June 2016.
12. Hernandez AP, Fleurence RL, Rothman RL. The ADAPTABLE trial and PCORnet: shining light on a new research paradigm. Ann Intern Med. 2009;635.
13. Handoll HHG, Brealey SD, Jefferson L, Keding A, Brooksbank AJ, Johnstone AJ, Candal-Couto JJ, Rangan A. Defining the fracture population in a pragmatic multicenter randomized controlled trial. Bone Joint Res. 2016;5(10):481–9.
14. National Academies Press (NAP). Initial national priorities for comparative effectiveness research. Institute of Medicine of the National Academies. www.nap.edu 2009.
15. The Center for Information and Study on Clinical Research Participation. https://www.ciscrp. org/our-programs/patient-advisory-board-panels/2016. Accessed 24 June 2016.
16. Gamble C, Dudley L, Allam A, Bell P, Goodare H, Preseton J, Walker A, Williamson P, Young B. Patient and public involvement in the early stages of clinical trial development: a systematic cohort investigation. BMJ Open. 2014;4(7):e005234.
17. Poleshuck E, Wittink M, Crean H, Gellasch T, Sandler M, Bell E, Juskiewicz J, Cerulli C. Using patient engagement in the design and rationale of a trial for women with depression in obstetrics and gynecology practices. Contemp ClinTrials. 2015;43:83–92.
18. Ehler AP, Davidson GH, Bizzell BJ, Guiden MK, Elliott Skopin E, Flum DR, Lavalle DC. Engaging stakeholders in surgical research: the design of a pragmatic clinical trial to study management of acute appendicitis. JAMA Survey. 2016;151(6):580–2.
19. Israel BA, Schulz AJ, Parker EA, Becker AE. Review of community-based research: assessing partnership approaches to improve public health. Ann Rev Publ Health. 1998;19:173–202.
20. Horowitz CR, Robinson M, Seifer S. Community-based participatory research from the margin to the mainstream: are researchers prepared? Circulation. 2009;119:2633–42.
21. Newhouse R, Barksdale DJ, Miller JA. The patient-centered outcomes research institute. Research done differently. Nurs Res. 2015;64(1):72–7.
22. Woolf SH, Zimmerman E, Haley A, Krist AH. Authentic engagement of patients and communities can transform research, practice and policy. Health Aff. 2016;35(4):590–4.
23. Deshpande PR, Rajan S, Sudeepthi BP, Abdul Nazir CP. Patient-reported outcomes: a new era in clinical research. Perspect Clin Res. 2011;2(4):137–41.
24. US Department of Health and Human Services Food and Drug Administration, Center for Drug Evaluation Research, Center for biologics, Evaluation and Research, Center for Devices and Radiological Health. (2009) Guidance for Industry. http://www.fda.gov/downloads/ Drugs/Guidances/UCM193282.pdf. Accessed 14 May 2016.
25. Wehrlen L, Krumlauf M, Ness E, Maloof D, Bevans M. Systematic collection of patient reported outcome research data: A checklist for clinical research professionals. Contemp ClinTrials. 2016;48:21–9.
26. HealthMeasures. www.nihpromis.org. Accessed 14 June 2016.

Chapter 48
Economic Evaluations

Denise M. Hynes and Leigh Neumayer

Introduction

Economic evaluation of new and improved procedures is a critical issue in clinical trials research. While clinical outcome measures may remain the primary focus of clinical trials, the results are typically viewed in light of the value gained [1–8]. The demonstration of safety and efficacy alone is not sufficient to inform stakeholders of implementation strategies and social context, while economic evaluation can provide a quantitative context for clinical outcomes relative to costs incurred. Standards for economic evaluation have long been advocated, if not consistently applied in study designs [7–13]. Results can vary substantially depending upon the assumptions made, the cost attribution methods used, and the analytic approaches applied. While economic evaluation within clinical trials is useful, explicit definitions and methods used in published reports have become essential.

The US Department of Veterans Affairs (VA), the largest managed care system in the USA, has included economic evaluation within its research programs for more than two decades. Notably, the VA Cooperative Studies Program (CSP), which oversees clinical trials conducted in the VA and the Health Services Research and Development Service, which oversees health services-focused studies have led efforts that have advanced economic evaluation methods [13–21]. This chapter describes experiences from the VA in evaluating economic aspects in

D.M. Hynes (✉)
Health Services Research and Development Service, Edward Hines Jr VA Hospital and Department of Medicine, University of Illinois at Chicago,
5000 S 5th Avenue (151V), Building 18, Room 206, Hines, IL 60141, USA
e-mail: denise.hynes@va.gov

L. Neumayer
Department of Surgery, University of Arizona college of Medicine,
1501 N. Campbell Ave, Tucson, AZ 85724, USA
e-mail: lneumayer@surgery.arizona.edu

© Springer International Publishing AG 2017
K.M.F. Itani and D.J. Reda (eds.), *Clinical Trials Design in Operative and Non Operative Invasive Procedures*, DOI 10.1007/978-3-319-53877-8_48

clinical trials. First is an overview of general economic principles and definitions of concepts pertinent to all trials. Next, we present experiences from two clinical trials to illustrate economic evaluation strategies. These examples were selected to demonstrate the nuances of economic measurement and the different approaches used to attribute value to the resources used. For each study, we present a brief overview, the economic perspective, the methods used to estimate intervention and procedure costs, the economic outcome measures, and a summary of key results. We conclude with a summary of the lessons learned and recommendations for future research.

Overview of Economic Evaluation Principles in Clinical Trials

Improving standardization of methods used in economic evaluation in health and medicine has been a focus in the USA since 1993, with the convening of the first panel on cost-effectiveness in health and medicine [1]. The Panel published its findings in a series of journal articles [2–4] and in a book [1]. In 2011, planning for an update of the 1996 Panel recommendations began, and the updated framework was published in 2016 [12]. Although the focus for both the 1996 and the 2016 Panels has been on improving the quality and comparability of cost-effectiveness analysis methods, the principles can be applied to other types of economic evaluations (i.e., cost identification analysis, cost–benefit analysis). The principles outlined here are based in large part upon this framework.

Perspective and Objectives

The perspective of an economic evaluation refers to the specific stakeholders for whom economic impact is measured. The scope may include health care and non-health care costs. Costs associated with specific interventions in clinical trials may be considered from the perspective of the patient (e.g., health insurance co-payments, lost work time, and travel for health care visits); employer (lost employee productivity and increased insurance premiums); third party or health care system, such as an insurer or a health care system (e.g., payments/expenses for outpatient care, tests, surgical procedures, hospital stays, and pharmaceuticals); or society (all costs, and with emphasis on avoided costs or benefits and shifts from one segment of society to another). While the health care system perspective may be more easily quantified, owing to increased availability of public and private health system payment data, the societal perspective is generally preferred because it allows evaluation of explicit trade-offs among competing alternatives [1, 10–12]. Regardless of which perspective is chosen, it must be defined a priori in order to define and collect appropriate data.

The objective of cost analysis depends upon how costs are presumed to relate to the clinical outcome measure. Cost minimization is appropriate when a clinical treatment is known or is presumed to be as effective as the comparison treatment and the focus is on comparing the relative costs [22, 23]. Cost-effectiveness analysis (CEA) and cost–benefit analysis (CBA) are used when there is uncertainty about the clinical advantage of an intervention relative to its economic impacts. CEA and CBA focus on the incremental, or marginal costs of an intervention relative to its marginal effectiveness or utility. There has also been renewed interest in value of information (VOI) analysis, a variant of CEA that calculates the expected (average) gain in welfare that can occur by multiplying the probability of an outcome by the gain in welfare that would arise from that outcome [24–26].

CEA requires measurement of both costs and effectiveness (e.g., survival, quality of life, pain avoided, days of hospitalization avoided [1, 12, 27–31]). Quality-adjusted life year (QALY) is a preferred effectiveness measure that combines life expectancy and quality of life [1, 12]. To compute a QALY, each year of life is weighted by values representing the preferences for the health states that occurred during that year. The preference weights (or utilities) assume values between 0 (representing death) and 1 (representing perfect health). Reduced pain and the ability to return to normal activities for example may be favorable influences on quality of life and valued by patients; complications and symptom recurrence, on the other hand, may have a negative impact on quality of life. To conduct the cost-effectiveness analysis, the difference in costs ($\Delta\sum C = \sum C_{T0} - \sum C_{T1}$) and the difference in QALY ($\Delta\sum QALY = \sum QALY_{T0} - \sum QALY_{T1}$) can be calculated. The ratio of net mean costs ($\Delta Cost$) and net effectiveness ($\Delta QALY$) yields the incremental cost-effectiveness ratio (ICER = $\Delta Cost/\Delta QALY$), the costs of an additional year of life in perfect health. The ICER is presented on a cost-effectiveness plane (Fig. 48.1). The x-axis shows the difference in effectiveness between the new treatment and the comparator (i.e., existing treatment), and the y-axis shows the difference in cost. Each of the four quadrants represents where cost-effectiveness is dominant in favor of the new treatment (upper left) or existing treatment (lower left) or uncertainty where effectiveness is improved, but relative to costs it is unclear whether the new treatment is a good value (upper right and lower left). In these uncertainty situations for assessing treatments, a trade-off is said to exist between effectiveness and costs, and the use of cost-effectiveness analysis to quantify these trade-offs can be especially informative. For each case, the ratio of costs to effectiveness is plotted and statistical distribution is used to estimate the line, i.e., the ICER. In Fig. 48.1, the ICER value plotted is the common standard of $50,000 per QALY [32]. Figure 48.2 is an example showing the ICER plotted in relation to the common standard. This ICER can then be used to compare health care treatments using an "acceptability curve," which indicates the probability that the intervention is cost-effective given a range of values that a decision maker might be willing to pay for the outcomes [29, 30] (see Fig. 48.3). In general, calculating this probability uses statistical bootstrap methods to examine the distribution of the cost-effectiveness ratio across regions of the cost-effectiveness plane and provides a means for quantifying the robustness of the cost-effectiveness analysis results

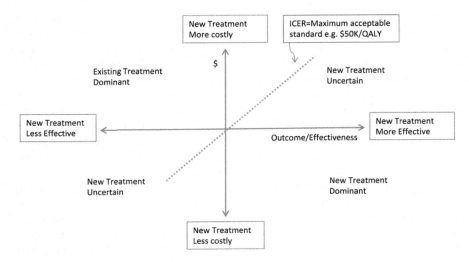

Fig. 48.1 Cost-effectiveness plane

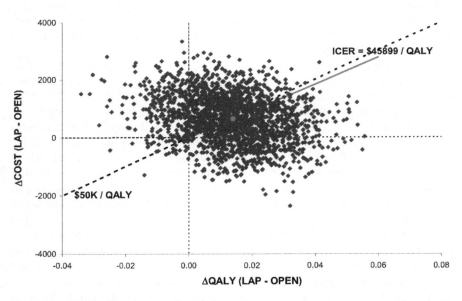

Fig. 48.2 Cost-effectiveness plane for laparoscopic (LAP) versus open hernia repair (OPEN) [Reprinted from [52]. With permission from Elsevier]

across the four quadrants of the cost-effectiveness plane, showing the relationship between differences in costs and effectiveness [33]. The bootstrap distribution then is used to derive an acceptability curve showing the probability that the cost-effectiveness ratio is below various maximum amounts (ceiling ratios) that a

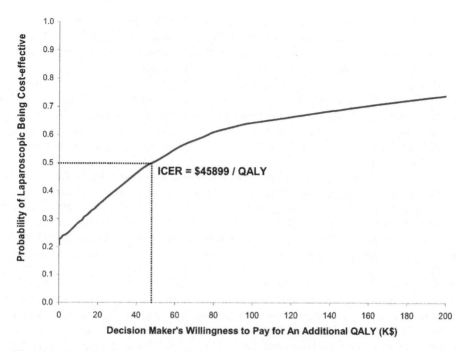

Fig. 48.3 Cost-effectiveness acceptability curve for laparoscopic (LAP) versus open hernia repair (OPEN) [Reprinted from [52]. With permission from Elsevier]

decision maker is willing to pay per effectiveness measure. Willingness-to-pay levels can be arbitrary and may vary with the specific treatments under consideration and social context, although $50,000/QALY has most commonly been used as a reference threshold. In summary, it is important to appreciate that economic evaluation involves two components in quantifying uncertainty: where a new treatment is located on the cost-effectiveness plane, and how much a decision maker is willing to pay for health gains.

Types of Costs Included in the Analyses

Costs associated with a treatment or intervention have traditionally fallen into two main categories [1, 7, 8, 12]: direct costs and productivity costs. Direct costs include health care-related (e.g., drugs, tests, supplies, health care, and personnel and medical facilities), and non-health care-related costs (e.g., transportation to and from the clinic or informal care costs) in the provision of a health care intervention. Few economic evaluations in trials include non-health care costs, thought to be due primarily to the difficulty in quantifying opportunity costs in some settings [34] and lack of agreement among economists on methods [35, 36]. However, the omission of opportunity costs may lead to significant biases in results especially in studies of chronic conditions and terminal care, unless there is strong a priori evidence that those costs are not likely to differ across arms of the study.

Productivity costs are those costs that are not directly attributable to the treatment but may be the result of the condition or of the treatment. They fall into two main categories. Morbidity costs are those associated with lost or impaired ability to work or to engage in leisure activities caused by illness. Mortality costs are those associated with lost or impaired ability to work or to engage in leisure activities caused by death.

In general, the health care system perspective includes direct health care costs, including the cost of the intervention itself and follow-up treatment costs. The societal cost perspective usually includes direct (both health care-related and non-health care-related) and productivity costs. The 2016 Panel recommendations redefined the types of costs to be included in these perspectives, such that both the health care perspective and the societal perspective include current and future medical costs and patient's out-of-pocket costs, whereas the societal perspective should include health care sector, informal costs, and non-health care costs [12]. The Panel had also recommended in 2006 that studies include a reference case, defined as a set of standard methodological practices that all CEA studies should follow. In 2016, the Panel updated this recommendation preferring that both a health care perspective and a societal perspective reference case be reported. As the goal of these recommendations is to improve the quality and comparability of costs analyses, a clear case can be made for inclusion of explicit descriptions of concepts and cost types included in any economic evaluation to ensure the methods are accessible and transparent [1, 10–12].

Inflation Adjustment and Discounting

Economic evaluations must consider temporal dimensions that impact the value of money. Cost inflation and discounting are commonly addressed in multiyear studies. Inflation implies that the value of a dollar is not constant over time, such that a dollar in 2017 does not equal the value of a dollar in 2007. Costs measured over multiple years must be converted to a common year metric, such as 2017 dollars. In the USA, the US Consumer Price Index for medical care is typically applied for this purpose [37]. Once standardized, costs can also be rescaled to any other year by multiplying by a constant.

Discounting refers to the "time preference for money," which is separate from inflation adjustment and refers to estimating the present value of a payment or a stream of payments that is to be received in the future. Future costs and health gains are commonly weighted in relation to the time at which they occur, future costs and effects receiving less weight than present ones. Increasingly, it is argued that the rate for future non-monetary health effects should be below that for future costs, to account for the growing value of health effects. Health economists commonly use a discount rate of 3–6% for costs and 1.5% for effects, although the rates used have varied over time [1, 8, 10, 11]. Differential discounting, that is, using different discount rates for costs and effects, is thought to be more appropriate when non-monetary outcomes like QALYs are also used [38].

Attributing Value to Health Care Use

From the societal perspective, it is desirable to estimate true economic cost by identifying the value of the resources in their next best alternative. Whereas market prices are presumed to reflect this alternative, true prices are more difficult to calculate in the health care market and may be subject to market distortions (such as insurance) and financing mechanisms [39]. In practice, costs are usually approximated using representative payment systems such as US Medicare reimbursement rates or UK National Health Service payments. In non-priced settings such as the VA, attributing value to specific types of health care use has used approximations from other health sectors, such as attributing Medicare prices or estimating price based on cost accounting. In our prior research, we have used a combination of approaches due to incomplete cost accounting information to distinguish costs for specific care settings such as hospital stays or outpatient settings for surgery or dialysis [21, 40, 41]. Sensitivity analysis is desirable to examine the impact of alternative cost attributions, data sources, and outliers on the results [1, 8–12, 42]. The 2016 Panel also recommended a formal impact inventory for health outcome and costs effects as a means to delineate the differences for the two reference cases and to highlight the components most affected by the condition [12].

The next section highlights how we approached these issues in our economic evaluation for two clinical trials (see Table 48.1); one focused on an operative procedure comparing surgical techniques for hernia repair and another focused on comparing a surgical and non-surgical technique for treating coronary artery blockages in high-risk patients.

Cost-Effectiveness of Open Versus Closed Laparoscopic Hernia Repair

Overview. The Hernia Repair study was a randomized controlled trial comparing open (OPEN) tension-free versus laparoscopic (LAP) hernia repair (both techniques repaired the hernias with mesh) at 14 VA medical centers, with 2-year follow-up for each patient [43]. Between January 1999 and November 2001, 2164 men with inguinal hernia were randomized. The primary outcome was hernia recurrence at

Table 48.1 Comparison of study features of two economic evaluations in large clinical trials

Study features	Laparoscopic and open hernia repair [52]	Angina With Extremely Serious Operative Mortality Evaluation (AWESOME) [55]
Perspective	Health care system	Health care system
Objectives	To compare cost-effectiveness of LAP with OPEN hernia repair in men	To compare cost-effectiveness of CABG surgery to PCI for revascularization of high-risk patients
Main economic measure	Cumulative costs and QALY at 2 years; ICER over 2 years	Cumulative costs and QALY; ICER at 3 and 5 years
Types of costs included	Direct health care costs including costs on the day of the initial hernia operation (patient information, initial hernia operation characteristics, VA hospital stays, and outpatient visits), and subsequent inpatient or outpatient care, including any subsequent operations, and medications at the VA over a 2-year period Exclusions: non-VA health care use due to use rate less than 1% of total health care use; costs of informal care supplied by family members or time lost from work or usual activities	Direct health care costs during the trial and four years post including VA and non-VA hospital stays and outpatient visits, and VA medications over five years Exclusions: costs of informal care supplied by family members or time lost from work or usual activities
Inflation adjustment and discounting	Inflation adjusted to 2003 US dollars using the CPI Costs and life years discounted at 3% per year, starting with the date of randomization	Inflation adjusted to 2004 US dollars using the CPI Costs and life years discounted at 3% per year starting with the date of randomization
Attributing value to intervention and health care use	For the initial hernia operation, operation costs were calculated for an average operation, based on operating room use and overhead, personnel, operation time, anesthesia, medications, surgical supplies, and equipment used Operating room use and overhead were estimated from VA cost accounting reports Personnel time was estimated using wage rates from VA wage reports Surgical supply costs were estimated based on supply data collected for each initial hernia	For hospital stays, physician services within a hospital stay, and outpatient visits, costs were estimated using Medicare reimbursement rates Costs for prescriptions were estimated based on VA prescription cost data

(continued)

Table 48.1 (continued)

Study features	Laparoscopic and open hernia repair [52]	Angina With Extremely Serious Operative Mortality Evaluation (AWESOME) [55]
	operation and supply vendor prices, resulting in an average differential cost per LAP procedure of $263.54 Costs on the day of initial hernia operation, other than operating room costs, and subsequent hospital stay and outpatient costs over 2 years were estimated using VA national inpatient, outpatient and average costs datasets	
Other methods	Precision of ICER assessed by bootstrap methods using 2000 re-samplings	Precision of ICER assessed by bootstrap method, using 1000 re-samplings with replacement

LAP laparoscopic hernia surgery; *OPEN* open hernia surgery with mesh; *AWESOME* Angina With Extremely Serious Operative Mortality Evaluation; *CABG* coronary artery bypass graft; *CPI* consumer price index; *PCI* percutaneous coronary intervention; *QALY* quality-adjusted life years; *ICER* incremental cost-effectiveness ratio

two years. Secondary outcomes included complications and patient-centered outcomes, including health-related quality of life. Earlier studies reported higher operating room costs for LAP compared with OPEN repairs; yet, some studies lacked specific cost data or cost-effectiveness measures needed to evaluate relative benefits and costs, and follow-up beyond 1 year [44–51]. With increased use of LAP, it was felt that an updated cost-effectiveness analysis was needed.

The economic evaluation was a cost-effectiveness analysis focused on surgical and postoperative costs, quality-adjusted life years (QALY), and incremental cost per QALY gained or the incremental cost-effectiveness ratio (ICER) at two years [52]. At the time of the study, shorter operation times and greater use of outpatient surgical centers was becoming more common practice. The economic evaluation therefore focused on the 1395 patients (708 OPEN and 687 LAP) with outpatient hernia operations.

Economic Perspective and Objectives

The economic evaluation for this study used a health care system perspective that focused on the direct health care costs incurred. We hypothesized that health care costs associated with the open procedure would be more cost-effective than the laparoscopic procedure. After carefully weighing the likely minimal impact of patient time lost from usual activities (i.e., productivity costs) versus the additional burden of data collection, we limited the study to direct health care costs, where the majority of costs for these procedures was anticipated. Thus, we sought to measure and compare costs and quality of life between the treatment groups. The primary economic outcomes in this study included the cost of the procedures, hospital stay, and any hospital readmissions due to the procedure. We considered results for specific predefined clinically relevant subgroups (unilateral and bilateral operations).

Types of Costs Included

We focused on direct health care costs including costs on the day of the initial hernia operation (patient information, initial hernia operation characteristics, VA hospital stays, and outpatient visits), and subsequent hospital stays or outpatient care, including any subsequent operations, and medications at the VA over a 2-year period. We only accounted for physician services as provided in the hospital stays and outpatient visits; therefore, consultations thought to be infrequent in this study were not included. We excluded non-VA care and informal care since rates of use were low in this population and for this treatment.

Attributing Value to the New Treatment and Health Care Use

For effectiveness, we used QALYs estimated from HRQOL data collected directly from patients over two years. We relied extensively on national administrative, clinical and economic databases available in the VA (see references in Table 48.1). Unique in this study was ascertainment of detailed costs in the surgical suites, which relied on salary and accounting data at each facility. In addition, we accounted for the additional surgical supplies and equipment costs for laparoscopy equipment. We calculated an average cost per procedure that was used in total cost calculation.

To estimate costs of hospital stays and outpatient visits, we relied on an adaptation of the Medicare reimbursement rates, applied to the VA, and VA-specific prescription pricing. We did not account separately for physician services outside of that covered under these hospital stays and outpatient reimbursement rates.

Economic Evaluation Results

Over 2 years, LAP cost an average of $638 (2003 US dollars) more than OPEN. QALYs at 2 years were similar (Fig. 48.2) with 21% of the bootstrap distribution falling in the dominant quadrant of the cost-effectiveness plane for LAP (lower cost and greater effectiveness, meaning that the probability that LAP was less costly and more effective (dominant) than OPEN was 21%. As shown in the acceptability curve (Fig. 48.3), the probability that LAP was cost-effective at the $50,000 per QALY level (slightly more costly but more effective) was 51%. For unilateral primary and unilateral recurrent hernia repair (Fig. 48.4), the probabilities that LAP was cost-effective at the $50,000 per QALY level were 64 and 81%, respectively. For bilateral hernia repair, OPEN was dominant (less costly and more effective), whereas, for unilateral recurrent hernia patients, LAP was dominant. Thus, while LAP was determined to be not cost-effective for all hernia surgeries, for specific subgroups, a dominant choice in terms of value was found.

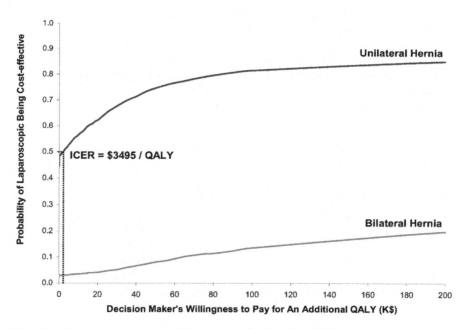

Fig. 48.4 Cost-effectiveness acceptability curve for LAP versus OPEN hernia repair for unilateral and bilateral subgroups [Reprinted from [52]. With permission from Elsevier]

Cost-Effectiveness of Coronary Artery Bypass Grafts Versus Percutaneous Coronary Intervention for Revascularization of High-Risk Patients (AWESOME) Study

Overview

The Angina With Extremely Serious Operative Mortality Evaluation [AWESOME] trial was a multicenter, randomized, controlled trial that compared PCI with CABG for the urgent revascularization of medically refractory, high-risk myocardial ischemia patients at 16 VA medical centers [53, 54]. Between February 1995 and February 2000, 454 patients with medically refractory myocardial ischemia at high risk of adverse outcomes were randomized. Primary outcomes were the survival of high-risk patients who underwent coronary revascularization with either PCI or CABG. Secondary outcomes included health care use after the initial procedure. The study was completed in 2000; however, the availability of national datasets enabled expansion of the economic evaluation through 2004, with no additional burden to subjects. In this high-risk population, the goal was to reduce mortality and adverse outcomes requiring hospitalization; therefore, the economic evaluation focused on the subsequent health care use and costs.

Economic Perspective and Objectives

The economic evaluation focused on the cumulative costs at 3 and 5 years to ascertain whether short-term differences persisted over time [55]. Costs were estimated from a health care system perspective and limited to direct health care costs. Effectiveness was measured in years of survival after randomization. We calculated years of survival as the number of years between randomization and either the date of death or the end of follow-up (September 2004). Using cost-effectiveness analysis, we calculated the cost per years of life saved.

Types of Costs Included

We focused on direct health care use costs during the trial and four years post including VA and non-VA hospital stays and outpatient visits, and VA medications. Inclusion of non-VA care and specific physician services was important in this study in anticipation of complex services provided post-procedure, and potential differentials in the treatment arms and the medically refractory high-risk population enrolled. National VA data included hospital stays and outpatient visits, VA contract care, and medications dispensed. Medicare claims data were used for

Medicare-enrolled patients to ascertain non-VA health care, including physician services [13–19, 56–58]. Informal health care supplied by family members was considered of minimal impact, burdensome to collect, and was not included.

Attributing Value to the Intervention and Health Care Use

For effectiveness, we used years of survival and relied on national mortality data available in the VA. Unlike the Hernia study, the AWESOME study focused on post-intervention health care use experience, and therefore did not account for costs of the specific interventions. On the other hand, like the Hernia study, we relied on VA national administrative and economic databases to value hospital stays and outpatient visits, which used an adaptation of the Medicare reimbursement rates applied to VA. Unique in this study is that we included additional valuation for the physician services, which comprises referrals and consultation occurring during hospital stays and the outpatient visits.

Economic Evaluation Results

After 3 years, average total costs were $63,896 for PCI versus $84,364 for CABG patients, a difference of $20,468 (2004 US dollars). Survival at 3 years was statistically similar (0.82 for PCI vs. 0.79 for CABG patients). PCI was dominant (less costly and more effective) at 3 years in 92.6% of the bootstrap replications. After 5 years, average total costs were $81,790 for PCI versus $100 522 for CABG patients, a difference of $18 732 (95% CI $9873–$27 831), whereas survival at 5 years was 0.75 for PCI patients versus 0.70 for CABG patients. Bootstrap replications showing the differences in costs and life years of survival on the cost-effectiveness plane (Fig. 48.5) at 5 years of follow-up, revealed that PCI remained dominant in 89.4% of the bootstrap replications.

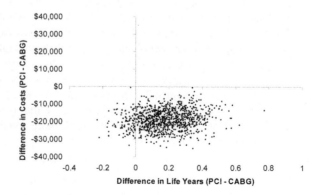

Fig. 48.5 Cost-effectiveness plane for PCI versus CABG at 5 years. Bootstrap replications showing the differences in costs and life years of survival on the cost-effectiveness plane between patients randomized to PCI or CABG at 5 years of follow-up [Reprinted from [55]. With permission from Wolters Kluwer Health]

Lessons Learned

The two clinical trials described here, although different in their scope and focus, highlight some key lessons in conducting economic evaluation within clinical trials. First, the perspective of the analysis as well as the clinical context informs the scope of the costs to be included. The two studies described here focused on direct costs of the intervention under study. The scope of the costs in the AWESOME study was broader than that in the Hernia Repair study, and was based on what was known about the clinical context of the high-risk cardiac study population. In both studies, however, it was felt that the burden of data collection to ascertain indirect costs outweighed the potential impact on overall costs.

Second, the cost attribution methods selected should be consistent with the goals of the investigation. The studies described here used similar approaches to attribute value to the health care resources itemized, relying on Medicare-adapted methods applied to the VA resources. The Hernia Repair study used a combination of sources to estimate the cost of the new treatment (i.e., LAP), including vendor equipment prices, equipment depreciation estimates, and hospital experiences for surgical supply costs and staffing of the surgical suites. This approach contrasts with the AWESOME study, in which the two surgical treatment costs were not the focus, but rather the postoperative experience. Therefore, non-VA health care costs were included.

Third, the effectiveness measure for the economic evaluation must be consistent with the study design. In the Hernia Repair study, QALYs were considered a highly relevant outcome as it may be directly impacted by pain and days away from usual activity, and therefore the CEA focused on costs per QALY. Whereas the AWESOME study focused on improving survival of high-risk cardiac patients, the CEA focused on cost per years of life saved.

Fourth, economic evaluations within clinical trials must weigh the practical burden of data collection and measurement precision with the potential yield with respect to the overall economic outcome measure. In the Hernia Repair study, it was felt that a focus on outpatient surgeries with detailed accounting of the procedural costs was most relevant given treatment trends; yet, the productivity losses from days of work were considered less important to devote data collection resources. In the AWESOME study, it was determined that the likely use of additional sub-specialists and consults for physician services both within the VA and in non-VA settings was worthy of data collection because it was expected that these services would account for some significant portion of the overall costs.

Finally, defining concepts and metrics used is critical to enable interpretation of results, as well as comparisons across studies, as in each of these clinical trials. While we did not use a formal impact inventory in our economic evaluation in these two trials, as is now advocated, we acknowledge that presenting the information in a standard format can make the information more readily accessible for comparisons with other studies.

Recommendations for Future Research

Economic evaluation approaches within randomized clinical trials need to be consistent with the study perspective and objectives. Economic evaluations can provide important information to ascertain value relative to clinical effectiveness of specific interventions; yet, methods need to be clearly explained to inform decision making. Further, if 2016 Panel recommendations [12], calling for two reference case analyses and an impact inventory, are followed when conducting economic evaluations within clinical trials, transparency will be improved. With increased availability of integrated electronic health records, billing, and insurance claims data, the burden of data collection may decrease. With increased transparency regarding methods and improved availability of economic and clinical information, economic evaluations within clinical trials will be increasingly expected and, ultimately, will be useful to decision makers.

References

1. Gold MR, Siegel JE, Russell LB, Weinstein MC, editors. Cost effectiveness in health and medicine. New York, NY: Oxford University Press; 1996.
2. Russell LB, Gold MR, Siegel JE, Daniels N, Weinstein MC. Panel on cost-effectiveness in health and medicine. The role of cost-effectiveness analysis in health and medicine. JAMA. 1996;276(14):1172–7.
3. Siegel JE, Weinstein MC, Russell LB, Gold MR. Panel on cost-effectiveness in health and medicine. Recommendations for reporting cost-effectiveness analyses. JAMA. 1996;276 (16):1339–41.
4. Weinstein MC, Siegel JE, Gold MR, Kamlet MS, Russell LB. Recommendations of the panel on cost-effectiveness in health and medicine. JAMA. 1996;276(15):1253–8.
5. Elixhauser A, Halpern M, Schmier J, Luce B. Health care CBA and CEA from 1991 to 1996: an updated bibliography. Med Care. 1998;36:MS1.
6. Power E, Eisneberg J. Are we ready to use cost effectiveness analysis in health care decision making? A health services research challenge for clinicians, patients, health care systems, and public policy. Med Care. 1998;36:MS10.
7. Hlatky MA, Boothroyd DB, Johnstone IM. Economic evaluation in long-term clinical trials. Statis Med. 2002;21:2879–88. doi:10.1002/sim.1292.
8. National Institute for Clinical Excellence. Guide to the methods of technology appraisal. London, UK: NICE; 2004. Accessed 7 Aug 2016 at https://www.gov.uk/government/uploads/system/uploads/attachment_data/file/191504/NICE_guide_to_the_methods_of_technology_appraisal.pdf.
9. Drummond M, Sculpher M. Common methodological flaws in economic evaluations. Medical Care. 2005;43(7:Suppl):II5–II14.
10. Husereau D, Drummond M, Petrou S, et al. Consolidated Health Economic Evaluation Reporting Standards (CHEERS) statement. Int J Technol Assess Health Care. 2013;29(2): 117–22.
11. Husereau D, Drummond M, Petrou S, et al. ISPOR task force report. Consolidated Health Economic Evaluation Reporting Standards (CHEERS)—Explanation and elaboration: a report of the ISPOR health economic evaluation publication guidelines good reporting practices task force. Value Health. 2013;16:231–50.

12. Sanders GD, Neumann PJ, Basu A, Brock DW, Feeny D, Krahn M, Kuntz KM, Meltzer DO, Owens DK, Prosser LA, Salomon JA, Sculpher MJ, Trikalinos TA, Russell LB, Siegel JE, Ganiats TG. Recommendations for conduct, methodological practices, and reporting of cost effectiveness analyses. Second panel on cost effectiveness in health and medicine. JAMA. 2016;316(10):1093–103. doi:10.1001/jama.2016.12195.
13. Hynes DM, Reda D, Henderson W, Hurder A, Abdellatif M, Weinberger M, Oddone E, Wasson J. Measuring costs in multi-site randomized controlled trials: Lessons from the VA cooperative studies. Med Care. 1999;37:AS27–36 (PMID: 10217382).
14. Barnett PG. See comment in PubMed commons below. Review of methods to determine VA health care costs. Med Care. 1999;37(4 Suppl VA):AS9–17 (PMID: 10217380).
15. Smith MW, Barnett PG, Phibbs CS, Wagner TH. Microcost methods of determining VA healthcare costs. Menlo Park, CA: Health Economics Resource Center; 2010.
16. Phibbs CS, Bhandari A, Yu W, Barnett PG. Estimating the costs of VA ambulatory care. Med Care Res Rev. 2003;60:54S–73S.
17. Wagner TH, Chen S, Barnett PG. Using average cost methods to estimate encounter-level costs for medical-surgical stays in the VA. Med Care Res Rev. 2003;60:15S–36S.
18. Yu W, Wagner TH, Chen S, Barnett PG. Average cost of VA rehabilitation, mental health, and long-term hospital stays. Med Care Res Rev. 2003;60:40S–53S.
19. Barnett PG. Determination of VA health care costs. Med Care Res Rev. 2003;60:124S–41S.
20. Wagner TH, Lo AC, Peduzzi P, et al. An economic analysis of robot-assisted therapy for long-term upper-limb impairment after stroke. Stroke. 2011;42(9):2630–2.
21. Hynes DM, Stroupe KT, Fischer MJ, Reda DJ, Manning W, Browning MM, Huo Z, Saban K, Kaufman JS, ESRD Cost Study Group. Comparing VA and private sector healthcare costs for ESRD. Med Care. 2012;50(2):161–70 (PMID: 21945972).
22. Briggs AH, O'Brien BJ. The death of cost-minimization analysis? Health Econ. 2001;10: 179–84.
23. Briggs AH, O'Brien BJ, Blackhouse G. Thinking outside that box: recent advances in the analysis and presentation of uncertainty in cost effectiveness studies. Annu Rev Public Health. 2002;23:377–401.
24. Claxton K, Posnett J. An economic approach to clinical trial design and research priority-setting. Health Econ. 1996;5(6):513–24 [PubMed: 9003938].
25. Hornberger J. A cost-benefit analysis of a cardiovascular disease prevention trial using folate supplementation as an example. Am J Public Health. 1998;88(1):61–7 [PubMed: 9584035].
26. Meltzer D. Addressing uncertainty in medical cost-effectiveness analysis: implications of expected utility maximization for methods to perform sensitivity analysis and the use of cost-effectiveness analysis to set priorities for medical research. J Health Econ. 2001;20(1): 109–29 [PubMed: 11148867].
27. Manca A, Hawkins N, Sculpher M. Estimating mean QALYs in trial-based cost effectiveness analysis: the importance of controlling for baseline utility. Health Econ. 2005;14:487–96.
28. Laupacis A, Feeny DH, Detsky AS, Tugwell PX. How attractive does a new technology have to be to warrant adoption and utilization? Tentative guidelines for using clinical and economic evaluations. Can Med Assoc J. 1992;146:473–81.
29. Briggs A, Gray A. Using cost effectiveness information. BMJ. 2000;320:246.
30. Petrou S, Gray A. Economic evaluation alongside randomised controlled trials: design, conduct, analysis, and reporting. BMJ. 2011;342:1756–833.
31. Petrou S, Gray A. Economic evaluation using decision analytical modelling: design, conduct, analysis, and reporting. BMJ. 2011;342:d1766.
32. Neumann PJ, Cohen, JT, Weinstein, MC. Updating cost-effectiveness—the curious resilience of the $50,000-per-QALY threshold. N Engl J Med. 2014;371:796–7.
33. O'Brien BJ, Briggs AH. Analysis of uncertainty in health care cost effectiveness studies: an introduction to statistical issues and methods. Stat Methods Med Res. 2002;11:455–68.
34. van den Berg B, Brouwer W, van Exel J, Koopmanschap M, van den Bos GAM, Rutten F. Economic valuation of informal care: lessons from the application of the opportunity costs and proxy good methods. Soc Sci Med. 2006;62:835–45.

35. Stone DF. Clarifying (opportunity) costs. Am Economist. 2015;60(1):20–5.
36. Potter J, Sanders S. Do economists recognize an opportunity cost when they see one? A dismal performance or an arbitrary concept? South Econ J. 2012;79(2):248–56. doi:10.4284/0038-4038-2011.218.
37. US Bureau of Labor and Statistics, Consumer Price Index. http://stats.bls.gov/cpi. Accessed 24 Aug 2016.
38. Brouwer WBF, Niessen LW, Postma MJ, Rutten FFH. Need for differential discounting of costs and health effects in cost effectiveness analyses. BMJ. 2005;331:446.
39. Lave JR, Pashos CL, Anderson GF, Brailer D, Bubolz T, Conrad D, Freund DA, et al. Costing medical care: using medicare administrative data. Med Care. 1994;32(Suppl 7):JS77.
40. Chapko MK, Ehreth JL, Hedrick S. Methods of determining the cost of healthcare in the Department of Veterans Affairs Medical Centers and other nonpriced settings. Eval Health Prof. 1991;14(3):282.
41. Beattie MC, Swindle RW, Tomko LA, Greenbaum MA, Recine B. Department of veterans affairs databases resource guide. Volume IV: costing of health care in veterans affairs medical centers: nationwide cost accounting and medical cost distribution systems. Version 2.0. Sept 1994.
42. Weichle T, Hynes DM, Durazo-Arvizo R, Zhang Q. Impact of alternative approaches to assess outlying and influential observations on health care costs. Springer Plus. 2013;2:614 (PMID: 24303338; PMCID: PMC3843184).
43. Neumayer L, Giobbie-Hurder A, Jonasson O, et al. Open mesh versus laparoscopic mesh repair of inguinal hernia. N Engl J Med. 2004;350:1819–27.
44. Medical Research Council Laparoscopic Groin Hernia Trial Group. Cost-utility analysis of open versus laparoscopic groin hernia repair: results from a multicentre randomized clinical trial. Br J Surg. 2001;88:653–61.
45. National Institute for Clinical Excellence. Appraisal consultation document: Laparoscopic surgery for inguinal hernia repair. Available at http://www.nice.org.uk/page.aspx?o_108145 Accessed 1 Aug 2005.
46. Jönsson B. Costs and benefits of laparoscopic surgery—a review of the literature. Eur J Surg. 2005;S585:48–56.
47. Johansson B, Hallerbäck B, Glise H, et al. Laparoscopic mesh versus open preperitoneal mesh versus conventional technique for inguinal hernia repair. A randomized multicenter trial (SCUR Hernia Repair Study). Ann Surg. 1999;230:225–31.
48. Wellwood J, Schulpher MJ, Stoker D, et al. Randomised controlled trial of laparoscopic versus open mesh repair for inguinal hernia: outcome and cost. BMJ. 1998;317:103–10.
49. Kald A, Anderberg B, Carlsson P, et al. Surgical outcome and cost-minimisation-analyses of laparoscopic and open hernia repair: a randomised prospective trial with one year follow up. Eur J Surg. 1997;163:505–10.
50. Liem MSL, Haisema JAM, van der Graaf Y, et al. Cost effectiveness of extraperitoneal laparoscopic inguinal hernia repair: a randomized comparison with conventional herniorrhaphy. Ann Surg. 1997;226:676–88.
51. Lawrence K, McWhinnie D, Goodwin A, et al. An economic evaluation of laparoscopic versus open inguinal hernia repair. J Public Health Med. 1996;18:41–8.
52. Hynes DM, Stroupe K, Luo P, Hurder AH, Neumayer L. Cost effectiveness of laparoscopic versus open tension-free hernia repair: results from the Veterans Affairs Cooperative Study. J Am Coll Surg. 2006;203:447–57 PMID: 17000387.
53. Morrison DA, Sethi G, Sacks J, Grover F, Sedlis S, Esposito R, Ramanathan KB, Weiman D, Krucoff M, Duhaylongsod F, Raya T, Pett S, Vernon S, Birjiniuk V, Booth D, Robinson C, Talley JD, Antckli T, Murphy E, Floten H, Curcovic V, Lucke JC, Lewis D, Barbiere C, Henderson W. For the Department of Veterans Affairs Cooperative Study #385, Angina With Extremely Serious Operative Mortality Evaluation (AWESOME) investigators. A multicenter, randomized trial of percutaneous coronary intervention versus bypass surgery in high-risk unstable angina patients. Control Clin Trials. 1999;20:601–19.

54. Morrison DA, Sethi G, Sacks J, Henderson W, Grover F, Sedlis S, Esposito R, Ramanathan K, Weiman D, Saucedo J, Antakli T, Paramesh V, Pett S, Vernon S, Birjiniuk V, Welt F, Krucoff M, Wolfe W, Lucke JC, Mediratta S, Booth D, Barbiere C, Lewis D. For the Department of Veterans Affairs Cooperative Study #385, Angina With Extremely Serious Operative Mortality Evaluation (AWESOME) investigators. Percutaneous coronary intervention versus coronary artery bypass graft surgery for patients with medically refractory myocardial ischemia and risk factors for adverse outcomes with bypass: a multicenter, randomized trial. J Am Coll Cardiol. 2001;38:143–9.
55. Stroupe K, Morrison DA, Hlatky MA, Barnett PG, Cao L, Lyttle C, Hynes DM, Henderson WG. For the Investigators of VA CSP #385 (AWESOME). Cost-Effectiveness of coronary artery bypass grafts versus percutaneous coronary intervention for revascularization of high-risk patients. Circulation. 2006;114:1251–57 (PMID: 16966588).
56. VIReC Research User Guide. FY2002 VHA medical SAS inpatient datasets. Hines, Ill: Edward J Hines, Jr VA Hospital, Veterans Affairs Information Resource Center; 2003.
57. VIReC Research User Guide. FY2002 VHA medical SAS outpatient datasets. Hines, Ill: Edward J Hines, Jr VA Hospital, Veterans Affairs Information Resource Center; 2003.
58. VIReC Research User Guide. VHA pharmacy prescription data. Hines, Ill: Edward J Hines, Jr VA Hospital, Veterans Affairs Information Resource Center; 2003.

Chapter 49
Telemedicine and Mobile Technology

Thomas H. Shoultz and Heather L. Evans

Telemedicine and mobile health (mHealth) represent modern and evolving forms of information and communication technologies (ICTs) whose applications aim to enhance and support the delivery of health care. The American Telemedicine Association defines telemedicine as "the use of medical information exchanged from one site to another via electronic communications to improve a patient's clinical health status" [1]. This modality has been acknowledged in more recent years to be a valid medium for delivery of health care in many clinical circumstances. The emerging component of eHealth propelled by mobile devices and technology is now known as mobile health or mHealth technology. mHealth-supporting hardware includes smartphones, tablets, gaming consoles, and wearables. The more common wearables are non-medical in design, including activity trackers worn on the wrist or implanted in shoes, and interface with cellular phone apps, computer software, and global positioning satellites (GPS). While medical wearables such as Holter monitors have been utilized with success for decades, this branch of mobile health technology has now grown to include other devices such as wireless uterine contraction monitors. The use of health-related mobile apps is growing exponentially, with such apps expected to be downloaded greater than 1.5 billion times by 2017 [2]. mHealth's employment in health care has been studied with various approaches, and a body of literature has emerged regarding advantages and limitations of telemedicine and mHealth. In order to construct clinical trials of telemedicine and mHealth technologies, the unique characteristics

T.H. Shoultz
Department of Surgery, Harborview Medical Center, University of Washington, 325 9th Ave, Box #359796, Seattle, WA 98104, USA
e-mail: tshoultz@uw.edu

H.L. Evans (✉)
Department of Surgery, University of Washington, P.O. Box 359796, Seattle, WA 98104-2499, USA
e-mail: hlevans@uw.edu

© Springer International Publishing AG 2017
K.M.F. Itani and D.J. Reda (eds.), *Clinical Trials Design in Operative and Non Operative Invasive Procedures*, DOI 10.1007/978-3-319-53877-8_49

427

of these ICTs, along with their accompanying challenges and benefits, must undergo thoughtful consideration.

Incorporating telemedicine and mHealth into health care has largely been fostered by the rapid expansion of smartphone ownership; two-thirds of Americans owned smartphones by 2015. Pew Research Center studies reveal not only increasing usage in emerging economies, but also for 19% of Americans dubbed "smartphone dependent" users who do not have broadband access at home [3]. These users rely on their devices not only for communication, but also to research health topics, utilize public transportation, and seek employment through online postings and applications. With the penetration of mHealth hardware into broader segments of society comes an associated exponential increase in the amount and breadth of personal health data collected from individual users. Wearable devices and their associated apps are able to detect, process, and log tremendous amounts of individual exercise activity and geographic information for users in local and online, or cloud-based, data storage.

The increased use of mobile technology in daily life has led to a new type of patient-generated health data (PGHD) that is more granular for medical interpretation and also actionable for medical decision making. In the USA, use of PGHD in clinical practice is incentivized under the Stage 3 Meaningful Use objectives from the Centers for Medicare and Medicaid Services. Common PGHD can assume the format of multiple types of media, from simple numerical and descriptive data to images and webcam-type interviews for clinical "visits." In considering PGHD in clinical trials, recall that no study is better than the quality of its data. In a 2015 study by Boissin et al. [4] aimed solely at assessing data quality, images captured by three common smartphones were evaluated in the context of their potential for use in medical teleconsultation. Through analysis of web-based surveys of "blinded" image assessors, the authors concluded that all three smartphones scored as well as a digital camera with regard to image quality, such that images captured by smartphones are useful for clinical practice. The potentially actionable nature of patient data is further supported by a 2016 study by Sanger et al. [5], in which supervised machine learning and serial clinical factor analysis were implemented in developing a prognostic model aimed at predicting surgical site infection (SSI). In this prospectively identified cohort of surgical patients, the Naive Bayes classifier using serial post-op clinical factors had a high negative predictive value for SSI, without additional benefit of known baseline risk factors. This concept bridges the gap between the abundance of PGHD and the ability to meaningfully utilize them. Significant PGHD may soon be derived from novel technologies such as biosensors and geolocation devices, offering further clinical and epidemiologic avenues of investigation in patients undergoing procedures.

The implementation challenges of telemedicine and mHealth stem largely from the duality of their intent to provide communication services to both patient and provider. This is in contrast to ICTs such as EHR, which are largely provider-centered. Addressing and reconciling the needs and concerns of patients and providers have been the focus of several studies which identify common themes and barriers to the implementation which must be optimized. In a systematic review by Gagnon et al. [6], mHealth adoption by healthcare professionals at the individual, organizational, and contextual levels included perceived usefulness and ease of use, design and technical concerns, cost, time, privacy and security issues, familiarity with the technology, risk-benefit assessment, and interaction with others such as colleagues and patients. From a patient perspective, similar concerns are shared by those who have been interviewed regarding their concerns and frustrations with post-discharge care after surgery. Interview-based, qualitative and mixed-method feasibility studies are often needed to assess the exact concerns of a potential study population and its attitudes toward mHealth prior to initiation of a trial involving mHealth as the intervention [7]. In a multidisciplinary effort to understand the tensions between patients and providers, Sanger and colleagues interviewed patients and physicians at University of Washington and affiliated hospitals to understand the dynamics of post-surgical wound care in order to construct a framework of design implications for a mobile postoperative wound monitoring app. The study derived themes of patient and provider concerns which are generalizable and applicable when considering the implementation of mHealth in a clinical trial [8].

Accessibility should be a primary consideration, as patients may not have a device or access to a device that supports the proposed mHealth application or telemedicine capacity. In such instances, it may be necessary to have devices which can be loaned to patients. Usability should be targeted to a patient population with a broad range of technical aptitude. Basic functions with simple wording, obvious alerts, and clear navigation are necessary for patients who may be impaired from post-procedural narcotic medications. Patients express a concern that PGHD, particularly images, should be directly and privately transmitted to intended recipients; such issues of security and privacy are shared by patients and providers [9].

A patient-centered approach enhances the implementation of telemedicine and mHealth technologies. This design implication must allow the patient to feel that the technology is genuinely useful for care and not overly burdensome or overwhelming [10]. An adequate amount of useful information must be delivered up front while offering resources for more information, if desired. Questions posed to the user must be interpreted as tailored communication with existing care providers and not just a survey. For patients undergoing procedures, gaps in pre-procedural instructions or discharge instructions may be filled with mHealth data in the form of pictures or tutorials. These easy-to-access components could facilitate a bowel prep regimen or remind a user how to pack a post-surgical wound.

As telemedicine and mHealth represent potential surrogates for the traditional in-office or emergency department visits, the same objectives must be met with these communication technologies while ensuring users that concerns are addressed with at least equal reliability and efficiency. Users want to be able to choose a communication format—text, email, or phone call—based on the context of their condition and the level of concern. The ability to send serial images may actually help alleviate anxiety by providing information which the user may not otherwise be able to articulate. Response times which are commensurate with the situational severity are important to users. Because many use the phone call as the "gold standard" for prompt and reliable communication, the expectation for mHealth applications is to provide transparent processing of communication efforts in a fashion which acknowledges the level of urgency. If these basic needs of effective communication cannot be reliably provided, little incentive exists to utilize mHealth applications preferentially over telephone calls or Emergency Department visits. Algorithmic and automated feedback is most likely to play a role in triage, when patients either need reassurance or to be made aware of a need to seek medical attention. Patient interviews have reflected the opinion that recommendations from mHealth apps would be helpful for preventing unnecessary ED visits, and conversely, for prompting earlier in-office evaluation, particularly when recommendations are substantiated by images that patients have reported [8].

The potential for mHealth and telemedicine to enhance traditional randomized controlled clinical trials has been implied by a number of studies. A feasibility study of telemedicine in 28 older male VA patients who underwent bariatric surgery demonstrated excellent (96.6%) follow-up and no difference in surgical outcomes compared to non-VA patients [11]. In a multicenter clinical trial known as the EFFECT study, patients with implantable cardioverter defibrillators (ICDs) who were randomized to internet-based remote monitoring and interrogation had lower rates of death and cardiovascular hospitalization compared to those undergoing traditional in-office follow-up visits [12]. At the same time, clinical trial research organizations have increasingly adopted electronic data methods and cloud storage for data acquisition, validation, and management. The emerging focus on patient-reported outcomes (PRO) has created a market for mobile apps to capture PGHD and integrate it into clinical trial management. One aim of such services is to obtain more thorough and consistent patient feedback, allowing long-term follow-up of large study populations in longitudinal studies. Such approaches to data gathering may be particularly beneficial in trials in which primary outcomes are defined by subjective data such as dysphagia and reflux in patients undergoing foregut surgery. A recent randomized controlled trial demonstrated mode equivalence and acceptability of tablet computer-, interactive voice response system-, and paper-based administration of cancer treatment-related symptomatic adverse events [13]. As the number of validated instruments for evaluating PROs grows, so too does the opportunity for mobile versions of such surveys to reach the patient on their own device, at their own convenience, potentially increasing response rates and data fidelity. The use of patient reminders via text messaging has been demonstrated to increase medication adherence in chronic disease, and text communications are now being explored as a means to increase patient recruitment and sustained participation in clinical trials [14]. Finally, the incorporation of wearable sensor data, such as that derived from glucose or pulse oximetry monitors, can substantially increase the amount of objective serial data recorded for clinical trials, due to ease of use and direct wireless transmission of data from device to database.

References

1. What is Telemedicine? American Telemedicine Association. http://thesource.americantelemed.org/resources/telemedicine-glossary. Accessed 17 Sept 2016.
2. Things are Looking App. The economist. http://www.economist.com/news/business/21694523-mobile-health-apps-are-becoming-more-capable-and-potentially-rather-useful-things-are-looking. Published 12 Mar 2016. Accessed 1 Aug 2016.
3. Smith A. U.S. Smartphone use in 2015. Pew Research Center. http://www.pewinternet.org/2015/04/01/us-smartphone-use-in-2015/. Published 1 Apr 2015. Accessed 1 Aug 2016.
4. Boissin Constance, Fleming Julian, Wallis Lee, Hasselberg Marie, Laflamme Lucie. Can we trust the use of smartphone cameras in clinical practice? Laypeople assessment of their image quality. Telemedicine E-Health. 2015;21(11):887–92. doi:10.1089/tmj.2014.0221.
5. Sanger PC, van Ramshorst GH, Mercan E, Huang S, Hartzler AL, Armstrong CA, Lordon RJ, Lober WB, Evans HL. A prognostic model of surgical site infection using daily clinical wound assessment. J Am Coll Surg. 2016;223(2):259–70.e2. doi:10.1016/j.jamcollsurg.2016.04.046.
6. Gagnon Marie-Pierre, Ngangue Patrice, Payne-Gagnon Julie, Desmartis Marie. M-Health adoption by healthcare professionals: A systematic review. J Am Med Inform Assoc. 2016;23(1):212–20. doi:10.1093/jamia/ocv052.
7. Semple JL, Sharpe S, Murnaghan ML, Theodoropoulos J, Metcalfe KA. Using a mobile app for monitoring post-operative quality of recovery of patients at home: a feasibility study. JMIR mHealth uHealth. 2015;3(1):e18. doi:10.2196/mhealth.3929.
8. Sanger PC, Hartzler A, Han SM, Armstrong CA, Stewart MR, Lordon RJ, Lober WB, Evans HL. Patient perspectives on post-discharge surgical site infections: towards a patient-centered mobile health solution. PLoS ONE. 2014;9(12):e114016. doi:10.1371/journal.pone.0114016 (Edited by Salvatore Gruttadauria).
9. Sanger P, Hartzler A, Lober WB, Evans H, Pratt W. Design considerations for post-acute care mHealth: patient perspectives. Washington DC [accepted for Nov 2014]; 2014.
10. Sanger PC, Hartzler A, Lordon RJ, Armstrong CA, Lober WB, Evans HL, Pratt W. A patient-centered system in a provider-centered world: challenges of incorporating post-discharge wound data into practice. J Am Med Inform Assoc JAMIA. 2016;23(3):514–25. doi:10.1093/jamia/ocv183.
11. Sudan R, Salter M, Lynch T, Jacobs DO. Bariatric surgery using a network and teleconferencing to serve remote patients in the Veterans Administration Health Care System: feasibility and results. Am J Surg. 2011;202(1):71–6.
12. De Simone A, Luzi L, et al. Remote monitoring improves outcome after ICD implantation: the clinical efficacy in the management of heart failure (EFFECT) study. Europace. 2015;17(8):1267–75.
13. Bennett AV, et al. Mode equivalence and acceptability of tablet computer-, interactive voice response system-, and paper-based administration of the U.S. National Cancer Institute's Patient-Reported Outcomes version of the Common Terminology Criteria for Adverse Events (PRO-CTCAE). Health Qual Life Outcomes. 2016;14(1):1–12.
14. Thakkar J, et al. Mobile telephone text messaging for medication adherence in chronic disease: a meta-analysis. JAMA Intern Med. 2016;176(3):340–9.

Part IX
Budgeting

Chapter 50
Budgeting for a Clinical Trial

Eric L. Lazar

Introduction

In order to seek funding for a clinical trial or any scientific research, one must reliably estimate in advance the reasonable cost to conduct the research. The budget process is often unfamiliar to if not outright avoided by some clinical scientists. Despite how mundane budget consideration may seem, one can not ask for financial backing (see Chap. 51 to follow) without having an accounting of how the funds will realistically be used to accomplish the stated goals and objectives. Essentially, the budget is a financial document that promises how you intend (and ultimately should) use the money. In this section, we will review the important elements and considerations for preparing a reasonable budget under two different circumstances—budgeting for a proposed project and reviewing a budget given to you in consideration of a capitation agreement to participate as a site in a clinical trial. The key determinants to the overall size of your budget will be sample size, the need to render non-routine clinical care, the overall time line of your proposed work, and the number of sites participating in a trial. As each of these grow, so grows the budget.

The writing of a scientific proposal, the construction of a budget, and its attendant request for funding is an iterative process. You might find, for example, that a sample size calculated based on an expected difference in a population proportion requires 3000 subjects in each arm of a study. This may define to a large extent a budget that cannot be reasonably funded. Armed with that information, the sample size can be recalculated based on an objective continuous numerical outcome which reduces the needed sample size to 250 subjects in each arm. This would represent substantial savings and results in a doable project. Those providing

E.L. Lazar (✉)
Department of Surgery, Morristown Medical Center, Atlantic Health System,
100 Madison Avenue, Morristown, NJ 07962, USA
e-mail: eric.lazar@atlantichealth.org

© Springer International Publishing AG 2017   435
K.M.F. Itani and D.J. Reda (eds.), *Clinical Trials Design in Operative and Non Operative Invasive Procedures*, DOI 10.1007/978-3-319-53877-8_50

the funding for your budget want to know that the project can be completed—that it is feasible and you will make delivery of results that are clinically meaningful and useful. In this way, the scientific details of your proposal are tightly linked to the budget and your request for funding.

Budget Basics

In general, the budget process starts with simply "walking through" your protocol and giving consideration to each element and person involved and then assigning a practical and realistic value to that activity or effort. You should refrain from "padding" costs because for the most part there are normative values for many costs that will guide your projected expenses. The first consideration should be given to determining the full life cycle of the project. From your protocol, you know how many subjects you need to recruit and how long your accrual process is expected to be. In addition, however, time is added upfront for start-up training and other pre-enrollment activities. Similarly, after accrual ends, data analysis and writing will add time to the overall project. It is important to consider the entire time horizon because certain salaries need to be budgeted for the entire project, whereas others will be limited to lesser portions of the project life. Starting with investigators and other personnel, it is best to think in terms of portions of full-time employee equivalents (FTEs). If you anticipate that being the principal investigator will occupy 20% of your time per year over the projected life of a five-year project, for example, you will account for that (0.20) times your salary per year in the five-year budget. The next question to address is 20% of what salary base? As a clinician, you might earn a certain salary that draws substantially from your clinical fees and productivity. This figure is irrelevant for budget purposes when conducting funded clinical trials or other research. The NIH publishes a salary cap summary (https:// grants.nih.gov/grants/policy/salcap_summary.htm) which is widely used to standardize maximum reimbursements for salary support for grants. Different granting agencies will have different standards, but the principle is the same–one is not going to get rich doing clinical research! For the purposes of salary support, physician researchers are generally considered similar to federal executive level II employees and for 2016, the pay for that level is $185,100. The base salary for others in the project can simply be their known institutional salary or one can search median salaries from the Bureau of Labor Statistics which would have to be adjusted for your region of the country and local cost of living. In no case, however, are salaries approved above the salary cap described above.

For your research, the FTE requirements may vary from year to year for different individuals. For example, a biostatistician may be needed at 40% FTE for the first year during planning stages, then 10% for the next three years, and lastly 50% in the final year during data analysis and preparation for publication. One should create a spread sheet that indicates time in yearly increments across the top and the different personnel and base salary on the margin to detail the personnel budget (see Table 50.1). Such a table is valuable because adjustments in any element such as salary or proportion of an FTE are readily reflected in the total.

Bear in mind that if the trial runs longer than expected in order to obtain accrual goals, the costs for the personnel budget line will also grow. Perhaps one of the most important roles among the many of a principal investigator is to insure that accrual is happening at the right pace and taking measures to improve enrollment if accrual is behind. Failing to achieve accrual goals makes meaningful analysis of any data impossible and stretching out a trial 50 or 100% of its planned time in order to achieve the required sample size will balloon the budget. Both of these events reflect poorly on the PI and can impact the future ability of that investigator to effectively compete for funds.

After personnel, one can consider "events" during the research that have real costs. An example would be a pre-trial meeting at which all personnel from all sites meet for a day or more of training in data definitions, data collection, protocol policies, and procedures relevant to the project. In a single site project, this would have very little associated costs. If the PI and nurse coordinator need to travel to several sites to train participating centers, however, their travel, meals and lodging represent real costs that must be accounted for in the budgeting process. It may be more efficient for all participating centers to come to the main site or another centrally located center to meet, and reimbursement for travel and conference center fees will need to be considered. If the protocol specifies a DSMB meeting at some point in the trial (and it should for multicenter trials), then the costs of hosting such a meeting and the associated honoraria that acknowledges the expertise of the DSMB board members need to be budgeted.

The next part of budgeting is consideration of the cost of clinical care. This requires some thought and a discussion with your office of grants and contracts and finance department. If your trial involves medical procedures that are well established and indicated for therapeutic care, the patient's insurance should (and will) cover the costs of care. For example, if you are doing a randomized trial of gastric

Table 50.1 Personnel budget

Position	Base	Year 1	Year 2	Year 3	Year 4	Year 5	Total 5Y FTE	Total
Principal investigator	$185,100.00	0.20	0.20	0.20	0.20	0.20	1.00	$185,100.00
Nurse coordinator	$92,000.00	1.00	1.00	1.00	1.00	1.00	5.00	$460,000.00
Data coordinator	$57,000.00	0.50	1.00	1.00	1.00	0.50	4.00	$228,000.00
Biostatistician	$130,000.00	0.40	0.10	0.10	0.10	0.40	1.10	$143,000.00
Administrative support	$45,000.00	0.20	0.20	0.20	0.20	0.20	1.00	$45,000.00
								$1,061,100.00

sleeve versus bypass for morbid obesity and the patient meets criteria for surgery, their clinical care including surgical procedures will be covered by the insurer. The trial should incur costs only related to tests and visits that are not part of the routine care that is already being rendered. For example, if the trial inclusion criteria mandate a series of screening tests or the outcome measures require follow-up blood tests and visits that are not routinely required for clinical care, those tests, visits, and procedures will need to be budgeted. In the world of hospital pricing and cost structure, the costs for these items are often not easily identified which is why one negotiates an applicable rate with the hospital finance department. Of course, when those costs are identified, one multiplies that figure times the required sample size and adds that figure to the budget.

If the care rendered in one or the other arm of your study is not currently the standard of care, it is unlikely that an insurer will cover the procedure or any of the associated hospital costs including anesthesia, pathology, radiology, or any other related care. These costs will then need to be added into the budget which can dramatically increase the budget. Sometimes, the distinction between what is coverable by insurance and what is not can be difficult and this is why the hospital finance office will need to be involved for this level of budgeting detail. When the research involves an investigational device or implant, the manufacturer will bear the uninsured costs if it is an industry sponsored project, a fact which must be disclosed to the patient and in the publication of any results. If, however, the investigator is using grant funding, the costs of nonstandard treatments, devices, implants, and all related care will fall to the budget of the investigator and as noted can substantially increase the costs of the project.

The "walking through" process must be thorough and detailed, particularly when it comes to elucidating those costs that are not part of routine clinical care. For example, if tissue samples must be preserved as part of the trial for the purposes of further analysis, tissue banking or simply documentation, the storage and ultimate disposal costs must be added. Depending on the specific details and nature of the trial, the clinical care section of the budget can be most significant.

Next, the product or fruit of research is data. Data cost money to collect, store, organize, protect, and analyze. Accordingly, in designing your trial, you should collect only the data that you need to establish appropriate inclusion criteria and to reach your outcome conclusions. Many are tempted, while going to the expense and effort of a trial, to grab as much data as is possible. This does have the added benefit of providing a fertile ground for subsequent data exploration and studying unanticipated relationships. On the other hand, collecting "extra" data can increase the error rate in completing data capture forms and results in increased expense in managing the data. If a data coordinating center is used to randomize the subjects and to collect and store data, the cost of that facility is budgeted. If computers, servers, or other equipment is required to manage data on site, those are budgeted in accordance with the proportion of cost related to the proportion of use attributed to the proposed trial. Twenty data points on fifty patients can be managed on the existing computer of the principal investigator. Seventy data points on 2000 patients are entirely another matter. Again, sometimes the assistance of your hospital finance and information technology specialists can help frame the issue. It may be, and sometimes is the case, that existing security and storage space is available at your clinical facility and that the costs of using those resources might be captured in what are termed indirect costs. Indirect costs are those costs which are not captured as specific items in your budget but which accrue as a part of "doing business" in a clinical facility. You make phone calls related to the trial, use computers, utilize light and heat, write on sticky notes, and you take up space. In addition, fringe benefits for the previously mentioned salaries cannot be taken for granted. All of these costs are termed indirect costs and are added on by your home institution as a percent of the final award given to fund the research. Knowing how your institution accounts for such items helps in deciding whether or not an item must be specifically budgeted as an expense for the trial.

Capitation

We have largely been describing the budgeting process for investigator initiated trials in which the principal investigator designs and executes a trial at the home institution and applies to one or more granting sources to fund such an endeavor. Often, however, multiple institutions or sites are required to guarantee accrual and the costs at each center are budgeted for and part of the grant application(s), but the funds are dispensed to the site and the site investigator as part of a capitation or per capita agreement. Essentially, the costs of conducting the trial at a site are determined as discussed above and divided by the number of subjects expected to be enrolled to get a dollar amount per subject for those costs incurred by a site. One generally does not attribute costs to the site for costs that are not incurred at the site such as the data collection center or the DSMB costs. Rather, one includes the costs for clinical care and personnel costs that are site specific. Once that amount is determined, let us say $1750.00 per subject, an agreement between the primary investigator and the grants and contracts office of the site facility is signed. It is important to commit to such a capitation amount only after you and your finance department verify that you can complete the agreed upon elements of the trial for those costs. The capitation amount is not likely to represent a profit center for your site but should fairly cover the costs incurred to the facility through the use of its laboratories, personnel, and other resources. If the associated costs are actually less than the capitation amount, a small profit may be realized. On the other hand, accepting an amount that does not cover the expenses will represent a steady loss for your center. Accordingly, it is important that you understand the budget process, so you can evaluate a capitation amount with an educated eye.

Capitation is also the usual method that industry uses to pay the site and site investigators for their efforts to conduct research. Industry-driven research relies on the reputation and patient population of the clinician. The surgeon must act in the best interest of the patient when approached to participate, not the company's bottom line. Accordingly, a clinician should not agree to participate in a trial primarily designed to advance the financial or marketing interests of a company but rather to bring an expected and otherwise unavailable benefit to his or her patients. Often the company will pay the costs of the investigational item and a capitation fee. The terms of any agreement should be clear to the patient as part of full and open disclosure and informed consent. For the purposes of this chapter, however, it is important to know that the capitation amount will cover the expenses incurred, so even if you are not acting as the principal investigator creating the budget, you nonetheless understand the cost structure of the project as it applies to your site.

Summary

Budgets for clinical trials frequently run into the millions of dollars. You can see from the brief example of a small five staff-person study in Table 50.1 that the personnel costs alone are over a million dollars. In addition to the fixed costs of personnel, there are variable per subject costs that can mount quickly for large or complex trials. A systematic walk-through of the proposed training, procedures, imaging, follow-up visits, tests, IT needs, analysis, travel, and all needed personnel for data entry and control, follow-up coordination and leadership results in a systematic accounting of costs likely to be incurred. These costs can be demonstrated on a few tables of a spread sheet for submission as part of the funding application. A site investigator must be comfortable evaluating a capitation offer to make sure that the needed services and personnel resources are covered by the offer for each research subject.

Part X
Funding

Chapter 51
Funding a Clinical Trial

Eric L. Lazar

Introduction

The conduct of clinical research is a resource intensive endeavor funded by grants from the federal government, private foundations, and philanthropy. In addition, the pharmaceutical and device manufacturing industries often fund research to demonstrate the efficacy of their products. Stewardship of these funds is a solemn responsibility and will impact the clinical investigator's suitability for future funding. Applications for grants and other funds involve presenting a sound scientific rationale and plan for the research, insuring ethical and safe treatment of the subjects, and construction of a realistic, prudent budget that justifies the investment (see Chap. 50). The budget and funding request are not afterthoughts but central to the planning of serious research endeavor. In this section, we will enumerate the different types of funding opportunities and review the way in which one goes about applying for such funds. Further, we will discuss the obligations and responsibilities that are incurred when one accepts a research grant.

While we often envision obtaining that big grant to cover the costs of the proposed research, it is increasingly common that multiple sources of revenue are used to fund a line of inquiry. As costs have steadily increased and funding levels flat or even shrinking over the last several years, it may be necessary to apply to more than one funding source to cover expected costs. It is crucial to have planned the budget in accordance with the principles discussed in the previous chapter (Chap. 50) so that you know the amount for which you are asking. Knowing the giving history of the funding agency that you are working with will help you predict whether or not you need more than one funding source.

E.L. Lazar (✉)
Department of Surgery, Atlantic Health System, Morristown Medical Center,
100 Madison Avenue, Morristown, NJ 07962, USA
e-mail: eric.lazar@atlantichealth.org

© Springer International Publishing AG 2017
K.M.F. Itani and D.J. Reda (eds.), *Clinical Trials Design in Operative and Non Operative Invasive Procedures*, DOI 10.1007/978-3-319-53877-8_51

At a fundamental level, a request for funding such as a grant application is really a business plan. A scientifically sound and well-designed protocol is developed which holds the promise of delivering impactful, clinically relevant findings that will alter or validate current practice. Funding research is an investment in knowledge and the knowledge gained, the deliverable, should result in changes in the delivery of health care that were worth the investment. This rather simple rubric helps frame any grant proposal. The entity investing, be it the federal government, a private foundation, or a professional organization, needs to see that there is a return on investment. The dividend is the knowledge. Here again, a sound plan, the prospectus, helps earn the funding and so the processes are invariably linked. The scientific plan has to have merit and the support of the scientific community in order to be valid but it must also be intellectually accessible to those deciding on whether to fund the endeavor. To facilitate the latter, it is important to review the publically available information about the granting agency and understand how their mission and values can be fulfilled by funding your work.

The single largest source of grants for biomedical research is the United States Government. Traditionally, we think of the NIH as the source of funds for research and as a branch of the Department of Health and Human Services (DHSS), it is the major player. There are, however, other sources of funding from within the DHHS including the Agency for Healthcare Research Quality (AHRQ) and from outside the DHHS such as the Department of Defense which sponsors some healthcare-related research. Other cabinet level sources of funding for healthcare research include the Department of Veterans Affairs which funds numerous clinical trials, the United States Department of Agriculture, and the Department of Energy. In addition to the federal government, state health departments fund research of importance to that state and should not be forgotten.

It is important to understand the NIH application process because to some degree or another, the process is used by funding sources in both the government and for private philanthropies, university based funds, professional associations, and even industry. The goal of this chapter was to familiarize the learner with the variety of potential sources for funding including but not limited to the NIH, introduce the fundamentals of writing the grant, enumerate the responsibilities that are incurred when accepting money for research, and to emphasize how the scientific protocol, the funding application, and the budget are interrelated, not separate parallel tasks.

Sources of Funding

As noted, the NIH has well-organized funding mechanisms in place, has an interest in surgical trials, and has an interest in new investigators. The NIH not only funds research projects based on the scientific merit of the research but also invests in developing research talent by means of several training grants. Despite the size of the NIH and the massive amounts of money involved, the staff is generally friendly and helpful and they want to steer good projects to the right funding.

The NIH mission is to foster research that extends healthy life and reduce the burden of illness and disability. Projects that are aligned with that mission are eligible for grants drawn from a $30 billion budget which has been relatively stable over the last several years. About 80% of that budget ($24.8 billion) is directed to extramural research, work done outside the NIH by investigators throughout the nation. These grants are administered through the NIH's 19 institutes and 8 research centers. The granting mechanisms relevant to most investigators are the R and K pathways. In brief, the R series are Research Awards based on a specific research proposal. The holy grail of NIH grants is the coveted R-01 but there are other Research Awards in the R series including the R-03 which is a small project grant (seed money) and the R-29 which is the award for First Independent Support and Transition Award. The K series are Career Development Awards and are based not only on a research theme but also have a program of training and learning built into further the skills and stature of the awardee. The level of funding is based less on a budget for a research project per se and rather on salary support in exchange for a substantial time commitment to the research and learning program. For young clinical scientists, the relevant awards are the K-08 and the K-23 which are the Mentored Clinical Scientist and Mentored Patient-Oriented Research Awards. The NIH has an excellent guide to help one decide what the best type of award is for a given situation. The NIH website (nih.gov) has an award wizard that is essentially an app that you follow through a series of questions that results in a list of awards appropriate to your situation: http://grants.nih.gov/training/kwizard/index.htm. The successful application to the NIH or any funding opportunity is on mission, of high scientific caliber and merit, focused and doable, and the principal investigator has a track record for success or the potential for success based on the environment provided by the applicant's institution.

As noted above, other DHHS agencies fund biomedical research. The Agency for Healthcare Research Quality has a smaller budget compared to the NIH at about $440 million and funds research into making health care safer, more accessible, affordable, and equitable. Another very large patron of healthcare research is the Department of Veterans Affairs (DVA). The funding of clinical trials by the DVA follows a rigorous, well-organized application process that is highly regarded and a model for many funding agencies. Clearly, funded trials must benefit the care of veterans and are usually conducted within the VA healthcare system. Many important surgical trials have come from the VA, such as surgical treatment of asymptomatic hernia and laparoscopic versus open herniorrhaphy.

The Patient Centered Outcomes Research Institute (PCORI) is a relatively new player to funding clinical research, having been created by Congress through the Patient Protection and Affordable Care Act of 2010. Though chartered by congress, PCORI is an independent, nongovernmental agency funded primarily by a trust fund that receives contributions from the Centers for Medicare and Medicaid Services (CMS), private insurers, and general US Treasury funds. The mission of PCORI is to fund research into evidence-based healthcare delivery improvements and takes into account patient-centered outcomes. Priority for funding goes to research that helps inform decision making for all stakeholders in the healthcare enterprise—patients foremost but caregivers and insurers as well. Their website (www.pcori.org) details many requests for proposals and catalogs previously funded projects.

In addition to the NIH and other government departments that grant research money, the hospital, medical school, or university that is home to an investigator will have an assortment of endowed sources for seed money for pilot projects including the NIH training and fellowship programs previously mentioned. In addition, many departments of surgery are fostering endowed assistant professorships in order to fund research. Your grants and contracts office will have information on the availability of these programs at your institution.

Private foundations are eager to sponsor research that is aligned with their mission and values and so often it is a matter of framing your area of interest in the context of a published mission statement of a foundation. Checking their website to see what their research priorities are for the upcoming cycle can help you frame a project that merits consideration. By way of creative example to demonstrate how you can help a funding agency see your work through their mission, consider the following. Perhaps you are planning a trial regarding surgical treatments for Crohn's and outcomes for fertility. You may have hoped for NIH money but the Crohn's and Colitis Foundation is an obvious target. Further, since you are working on fertility issues, there may be a women's health foundation or even a maternal fetal medicine funding source available since the work directly impacts those areas. Very little retooling of a basically good idea can make your project attractive to many funding agencies.

Examples of foundations that fund clinical research and researchers are the Doris Duke Charitable Foundation, the Robert Wood Johnson Foundation, the Bill and Melinda Gates Foundation, the Rockefeller Foundation, the Ford Foundation, the Pew Charitable Trust, and the Albert and Mary Lasker Foundation among many others. The application process will vary from foundation to foundation but all will require the same basic preparation if sometimes somewhat less intense than an NIH grant.

The next major sources of funding are the numerous voluntary health organizations. These include the American Cancer Society, the American Heart Association, the American Lung Association, the Susan B. Komen Foundation, the Crohn's and Colitis Foundation of America, and the March of Dimes, again, among many others. Almost every organ, every disease, every process (like infectious or inflammatory or degenerative), and every sufferer type has an association that raises money to further their goals which almost always include money for research. Any group with a colored ribbon is raising money, a significant portion of which is earmarked for research. Not every project will match every organization but certainly it is worth seeing whether your planned research shares common aims with the health organization. Like the philanthropic groups above, you should review the grants that have been awarded by these organizations to get an idea of where your work falls in the spectrum of likely work to be funded by that agency. Creative thinking is a plus when deciding where to apply as well as how to appeal to your patron.

Professional societies provide funds for research and depending upon your personal membership and eligibility, a source of funding can be the American College of Surgeons or the American Pediatric Surgery Association or the American Urological Society. The American Association of _____ (you fill in the blank) may have funds for relevant research. Most organizations and societies fund research considering the researcher rather than the research itself. Organizations might favor a native son of some state or a minority or a woman investigator and sponsor meaningful research of a much boarder scope then let us say the Cystic Fibrosis Foundation.

Lastly, there is industry funding. This is a complex endeavor, and there are many caveats of which you should be aware. There are ethical concerns that must be brought into focus. There is no question that industry sponsored investigation has a role in funding some types of research but the principal investigator must secure certain and specific assurances regarding publication of results, ownership of the data, and the general direction of the research program. Before accepting such monies, the investigator must understand the terms of disclosure of the outcome of the research. For example, as a condition of receiving the money, most companies embargo the results of any research until a time and manner of their choosing. Let us say that a new hernia patch that you are helping evaluate deteriorates and fails in thirty days. The manufacturer is likely not to rush to publish that finding but you may feel it is important to the community at large to share those results. Unfortunately, to do what you believe to be the "right" thing may violate a nondisclosure clause and subject you and your institution to civil penalties. The point here is that part of the responsibility in accepting funds to do research is to understand all of the expectations (getting the work done properly, according to specification) and obligations therein incurred.

Applying for the Grant

As we have emphasized to this point, funding agencies want to provide their money for the right cause. They have raised funds through taxes, very large and very small donations, bequests, fundraising activities, endowments, and membership dues among many other mechanisms. In addition, if they are run properly, most private foundations have grown their funds using the standard tools and instruments available on the world markets. They are not storing money for a rainy day and parsimoniously dispensing it only when absolutely necessary. They want and need to be seen as vital entities carrying out their mission and that involves substantial support of people like you who seek to improve and deliver health care. If they are successful in how they spend their money, they will be successful in raising more. The application process starts with impressing them that they are investing in someone who can deliver on promises, is highly ethical and productive, and well regarded in the medical community. Even very preliminary conversations with development officers or grant managers in a target agency are auditions. Your manner and the impressions you leave are extremely important.

Next, obtain and read the application. Deadlines and procedures matter—if they have a cycle for applying with published deadlines, those are to be taken literally. If there is a page or more commonly now a word limit for the introduction and background, it should be followed. Even a paragraph more is too much. If they ask for a budget in an importable spread sheet, then that is how it must be provided. The point is, in the very details of doing the application, you are showing your patron that you are attentive to details and that you take your work and their money seriously. If you are unclear about any aspect of the application, there is staff to help you. It is better to call and clarify than assume wrong. This is true of the behemoth NIH as it is of any other funding resource. There are grant officers available who are professional, master's degree level staff who are interested in your work, and are there to help you be successful.

The usual application starts with an introduction and background information. This is the space where you demonstrate how your work is on mission for the funding agency. You need to explain the public's interest in solving the problem that you are working on. Share the scope of the problem, the type of person suffering from the problem, the cost to the community if the issue remains unaddressed, and so forth. The language that you use must be accessible and paint a clear picture. Those reading your work are not likely experts in your specific area and so clarity is the primary objective. You need to connect on a meaningful level in this space so that before any details are discussed, you have hooked those reviewing your work.

A substantial section will be devoted to you as an investigator. Your credentials, your work to date, what funds you have been previously granted, and the outcome of those efforts are all detailed if available. One needs to try to make the most of former accomplishments but new investigators need not feel inadequate for simply being new. Emphasizing mentors and others whose work you have helped, your stewardship of other important administrative responsibilities, and the support of those with a track record are meaningful indicators of your mettle as an applicant. In addition, many funding agencies want to shepherd new investigators and seek the opportunity to reward the right candidate.

The actual details of the clinical trial protocol which have undoubtedly been the focus of most of your efforts will need to be written in clear form addressing as many details as possible without cluttering. Protocols are enhanced if pilot data are used to formulate suppositions or demonstrate feasibility. If the average reader is piqued by a question, the answer should soon follow. It is difficult for the author who has become so involved with the writing to see the holes or leaps of logic that can be obvious to the first time reader so it is imperative that you ask as many people as you can to read your work and accept their critiques with open enthusiasm. They will find those holes and leaps so that you can connect the dots. In the end, the protocol should be able to be read once by a reviewer from the funding agency and who will have few if any questions of what is happening throughout the course of the trial, what the outcome measures are, how the data will be analyzed, and what conclusions can be reasonably drawn from the information gained. A project's viability is greatly enhanced from the granting agency's point of view when any of the possible outcomes will have importance for clinical care in the future. For example, your outcome might be that a new approach is far better and more cost-effective than what we currently do or given proper comparison groups and the right data points having been obtained, you might provide previously lacking proof of efficacy for the standard of care. In either case, the outcome of your work is essentially a win-win rather than a win-bust situation. The former is more attractive to a funding source.

References should be complete and acknowledge those works upon which you have built yours. At the NIH, preassembled review panels may include those in your field who have direct knowledge of their work as a precursor to yours and acknowledgment fosters collegiality. At smaller funding agencies, your proposal may be sent out for expert scientific review and that reviewer might have contributed to the field in a similar manner. It is human nature to expect that one's work is referenced if appropriate and this can place your proposal in a better light.

Grant Notification: It is rare to obtain full funding on the first attempt. If not funded, it may be that your work is not congruent with the current funding priorities of the agency or it may be due to specific elements of your project that are concerning to the fund managers. The NIH provides a critique and has a process for offering a resubmission. That feedback is very valuable and should be taken to construct a list of action items to improve your project. Resubmission is encouraged so long as the premise of the work is sound and it is details that are holding up approval. The take home here is that rejection for funding is not uncommon, is not personal, and should be viewed as an opportunity to "re-message" your work.

When your proposal is funded, the amount may be what your budget specified or it may be less depending on the priority of the project among the granting source's other priorities. In general, however, when a grant is awarded, it may come as a lump sum or more commonly in yearly increments over the life of your grant. You should familiarize yourself with the specific details because your expenses are likely not to be spread evenly over the life of the project but rather front loaded. The payment is made to your institution which then pays for expenses and salaries as they arise. Usually a grant is placed in a cost center specific to that grant. It is important from a regulatory point of view that you and your grants and contracts office keep an accurate accounting of your expenses in case of review and those expenses should be consistent with the budget you submitted. Of course, there are always variances and changes and unexpected issues that arise, but in the main, it is your responsibility to stay on budget or you will need to rely on supplemental sources from your institution to address shortfalls. There is generally no opportunity to call upon the granting agency for additional funds beyond those promised.

We have, with the exception of a brief mention of industry sponsored research, largely addressed investigator initiated research—your idea, your study. There are other funding opportunities from the NIH, PCORI, and AHRQ among others where there is a specific request for protocols (RFP) to investigate a prespecified problem. Generally, well established investigators are positioned to respond to such RFPs, and it is difficult to obtain this sort of funding as a new investigator but it is advised that you join listservs that apprise you of such announcements because on occasion such a request aligns nicely with your needs and capabilities and should not be ignored. Be aware that deadlines and prespecified requirements are generally not flexible and so you may not be able to apply to each RFP. On the chance that you can, however, this is another source of funds available. These generally arise from efforts of the funding agency to address a specific mission-centered priority for the year. The priority may be centered on the patient population, a disease, or a process such as inflammatory mediation of the acute response.

We cannot overemphasize that the most important thing that you can do to insure future funding is to successfully complete your work so it now becomes part of your investigator portfolio as a successful investment on the part of whoever gifted you funds. Nothing predicts the potential for success better than a history of success.

Summary

It would be enough of a challenge to design and execute a clinical trial that provides important data dictating a change in practice that enhances patient outcomes. Obtaining funding for such an endeavor in some ways involves a distinct skillset and business acumen that is not part of the traditional scientific and clinical training that characterizes the backgrounds of most PIs. Submitting a grant for review for funding involves preparation of an outstanding project that is succinctly described and has scientific merit of clinical importance. It also involves imagination when deciding to what agency or organization to apply. You are seeking a patron and a partner and you are entering into a long-term relationship. It is important that you use the funds to which you have been gifted to accomplish your stated goals. It is equally important that the granting agency be able to use you and your work as a "poster-child" to demonstrate the positive influence of their work. If it is industry that is supporting your work, your integrity demands that you accept funds to do work that adds to our knowledge about a clinical problem rather than focus on a new marketable indication for a device. Does the implementation of a new technology enhance our ability to more effectively render care or is it merely a new revenue stream for a corporate sponsor?

While affairs of money sometimes appear mundane at best and sordid at worst, money does enable us to achieve our scientific and clinical goals and understanding how money is successfully planned for, procured, managed, and effectively used is, for better or worse, part of the research enterprise.

Chapter 52
Writing Your Grant for the Patient-Centered Outcomes Research Institute (PCORI)

Frances M. Weaver, Talar W. Markossian and Jennifer E. Layden

What Is PCORI?

The Patient-Centered Outcomes Research Institute (PCORI) was authorized as part of the Patient Protection and Affordable Care Act (ACA) in 2010. It is an independent, nonprofit, nongovernment organization located in Washington, DC. PCORI's charge is to fund comparative effectiveness research (CER) that generates evidence that patients, clinicians, and other stakeholders can use to make informed decisions. A requirement of PCORI is that all activities and projects funded by PCORI involve the input and engagement of patients and other stakeholders.

PCORI has established a set of national priorities for research that is cross-cutting and where additional research is needed to provide information for patients and others to make informed decisions [1]. The five priorities include the following: assessment of prevention, diagnosis, and treatment options; improving healthcare systems; communication and dissemination research; addressing disparities; and accelerating patient-centered outcomes research and methodological research. In addition to investigator-initiated projects, PCORI generates and prioritizes research topics based on input from patients and other stakeholders.

F.M. Weaver (✉)
Center of Innovation for Complex Chronic Healthcare & Public Health Sciences,
Edward Hines Jr. Veterans Administration Hospital & Loyola University,
Chicago, Bldg. 1, Room C203 (151H), 5000 S. 5th Avenue,
Hines, IL 60304, USA
e-mail: frances.weaver@va.gov

T.W. Markossian · J.E. Layden
Public Health Sciences, Loyola University Chicago, 2160 South First Ave,
CTRE 554, Maywood, IL 60153, USA
e-mail: tmarkossian@luc.edu

J.E. Layden
e-mail: jen.layden@icloud.com

© Springer International Publishing AG 2017
K.M.F. Itani and D.J. Reda (eds.), *Clinical Trials Design in Operative and Non Operative Invasive Procedures*, DOI 10.1007/978-3-319-53877-8_52

Traditional clinical research has produced important findings that have positively affected people's lives. However, there are a number of shortcomings of traditional clinical trials: they often take years to complete, they are costly, they have strict enrollment criteria which limits the generalizability to a more heterogeneous (and more representative) population, and they often do not answer the questions that patients and other stakeholders are most concerned about [2, 3]. PCORI's motto is "research done differently." By involving patients, clinicians and other stakeholders to identify questions of importance, taking advantage of existing data sources (e.g., the electronic medical record), and promoting comparative effectiveness research, PCORI strives to get answers to important questions more quickly.

PCORnet

In 2013, PCORI utilized a portion of their funds to create a national data network for research called PCORnet. This network was established to foster a range of observational and experimental comparative effectiveness research by providing a mechanism to collect patient and clinical data from the electronic medical record from a variety of healthcare settings including hospitals, physician's offices, and clinics [4]. A set of standardized, interoperable formats was developed to create a common data model which would allow for data sharing across the network using a variety of methods to maintain confidentiality and prevent identification of patients. Two sets of networks were created, one based on system-based networks from hospitals, health plans, and practice-based networks called clinical data research networks (CDRNs), and the other network was operated and governed by groups of patients and their partners called patient-powered research networks (PPRNs). There are 13 CDRNs and 21 PPRNs. CDRNs represent health systems such as Kaiser Permanente, regions such as the Great Plains collaborative, and concentrated areas such as the healthcare systems serving the Chicago area. The PPRNs include networks focused on topics such as arthritis, Crohn's and colitis, sleep apnea, rare genetic disorders, and gay/lesbian/bisexual/transgendered (GLBT) health. Logistic and technical support is provided through a coordinating center co-lead by Harvard Pilgrim Health Care Institute and Duke University. PCORnet was designed to make it faster, easier, and less costly to conduct comparative effectiveness research by utilizing the power of large amounts of health data and patient partnerships.

Two national observational studies and one CER are currently underway and supported by PCORI. These studies will work with the CDRNs. One study will examine the long-term outcomes including mortality and weight gain in persons undergoing one of three common bariatric procedures, and a second study is looking at the effects of antibiotic use in young children on subsequent growth including weight. A CER will compare low-dose and regular-dose aspirin in persons who have had a heart attack for secondary prevention of future cardio-vascular events. It is anticipated that the PCORnet structure will be sustained through other sources of funding as researchers develop proposals that would utilize the data and resources of the CDRNs and PPRNs.

Governance

PCORI is governed by a Board of Governors. The 21-member board, led by a chairperson and a vice chairperson, appointed by the Comptroller General of the USA, includes the Directors of the National Institutes of Health (NIH) and the Agency for Healthcare Research and Quality (AHRQ) or their designees and 17 other members. Other members include patients and healthcare consumers, physicians and providers, private payers, persons representing pharmaceutical, device and diagnostic manufacturers/developers, one individual who represents quality improvement or independent health services researchers; and two individuals who represent the federal government. The Board members embody a broad range of perspectives and have scientific expertise collectively in research including epidemiology, decision sciences, health economics, and statistics. The Board of Governors meets monthly, and the meetings are open to the public through teleconference/webinar. Transparency is a key element of PCORI.

What Types of Research Does PCORI Fund?

PCORI funds research designed to improve patient care and outcomes through comparative effectiveness research (CER). CER "compares the benefits and harms of alternative methods to prevent, diagnose, treat, and monitor a clinical condition or to improve the delivery of care" [5]. Studies may include pragmatic clinical trials, large simple trials, or large-scale observational studies. PCORI offers several types of funding announcements that fall into the following major categories: (a) Broad PCORI funding announcements, which seek patient-centered CER that fit into major PCORI priority areas; (b) targeted announcements, which are one-time opportunities for identified high priority areas; (c) pragmatic clinical studies announcements that fund pragmatic or large simple clinical trials, or large observations trials; and (d) engagement program awards, which facilitate the involvement of patients and other stakeholders into the research process. There also are opportunities for projects that improve CER methods and funding for dissemination and implementation results and products from PCORI-funded projects in real-world settings. Priorities for targeted announcements are identified by patients and other stakeholders.

In addition to research funding, PCORI offers a variety of other funding opportunities. For example, there are awards to encourage engagement of patients and other stakeholders in CER. The Eugene Washington PCORI Engagement Awards program provides a platform to expand the role of all stakeholders in research by encouraging patients and other stakeholders to become integral members of the research process. This program also supports meetings and conferences that align with PCORI's mission and strategic plan. The Pipeline to Proposal awards encourages patients and other stakeholders to partner with researchers to study issues that are most critical to them. These announcements are available on the PCORI website [6].

Key Components of a PCORI Grant Submission

PCORI has three funding cycles annually, and all applications must be in response to a PCORI funding announcement (PFA). There are two major steps in the application process. The process starts with a Letter of Intent (LOI) in response to one of the PFAs. Each PFA has a specific LOI, specifying the essential elements and formatting criteria. This is a short form (3–4 pages), typically including sections highlighting the importance of the proposed study, objectives and study aims, methodological approach, patient engagement elements, prior relevant work, anticipated impact, and projected budget. To submit the LOI, applicants must register on the PCORI online system, which is found on the PCORI website, and complete additional information in addition to uploading the completed template.

The LOI review is a competitive process, and not all LOIs will be invited to submit a full application. For those invited to submit a full proposal, there are several essential components and required templates that must be submitted as part of the full application. There is a research plan template, a peoples and places template, milestone template, budget template, and leadership plan template. Details on what is included in these templates are provided in Table 52.1. Applicants must pay careful attention to required elements specified in the intended PFA's research plan and other templates. Documents can be found on the PCORI funding opportunities website [7].

PCORI has devoted substantial effort to developing and improving the science and methods of patient-centered outcomes research and has developed a comprehensive report on methodology standards [8], which include 5 cross-cutting areas, and 6 study design-specific standards [1]. Proposed studies are required to adhere to these standards, and applicants are strongly encouraged to become familiar with these well before drafting the proposal. When writing the proposal, applicants should include, in parentheses, the abbreviations for the specific standards that are being addressed.

Table 52.1 Elements of a PCORI application

Research plan template	Background
	Significance
	Intended patient population
	Recruitment plans
	Study design and methodological approach
	Engagement plan (describe how patients and other stakeholders will participate as partners in various phases of the project)
	Research team environment
	Dissemination & implementation potential
	Replication, reproducibility and data sharing
	Plans
	Protection of human subject plans
	Consortium contractual arrangements
	References
People and places template	Includes biosketches, project sites, and resources
Milestones template	Provide projects goals and outcomes to be accomplished during the proposed project
Budget template	Detailed budget per year, budget summary, and justification
Leadership template	Description of roles and responsibilities

Stakeholder Engagement

Patient and healthcare community engagement are integral criteria of all supported research. All applications for PCORI funding must include an engagement plan, in which they describe how patients, caregivers, clinicians, and other healthcare stakeholders were involved from topic selection through design, conduct of research, and dissemination of results. PCORI has created an engagement rubric that provides guidance on the infrastructure development for patient and family engagement in outcomes research [9]. This rubric provides guidance to researchers and others, helps to determine milestones and track progress, and is tied to the methodology standards and review criteria that associated with PCORI grant development and review. Specific engagement principles include reciprocal relationships (between research and patient partners), co-learning, partnership, trust, transparency, and honesty (e.g., patients are part of the major decisions made). Early lessons from engaging patients and other stakeholders in PCORI supported pilot projects are shared in Forsythe et al. [10].

Review Process

Once an LOI is accepted and a full application submitted, PCORI staff review applications for administrative compliance. At this stage, PCORI staff can withdraw an application that is not compliant, submitted after the deadline, or that is not responsive to the PFA. Subsequently, there is a preliminary review of the full applications by panel members. Panel members follow specific merit review criteria to evaluate the proposal's adherence to the PCORI methodology standard and the appropriateness of human subject's protections. This stage is followed by an in-person panel discussion of a select group of full applications. The decision of which applications to discuss at the in-person panel is determined by PCORI staff, and it is based on the preliminary review scores and program priorities. At the in-person panel, which is led by a chair and a merit review officer, this select group of applications are thoroughly discussed and re-scored. After this stage, PCORI staff recommends a slate of proposals to a selection committee. The preliminary reviews, discussion notes, final application scores, and portfolio balance are all considered when proposing the slate of applications. The Selection Committee, which is made up of members of PCORI's Methodology Committee and a subset of the Board of Governors, makes final recommendations and a slate of proposals to recommend for funding, which is ultimately presented to the Board of Governors, at a publicly open meeting. The Board of Governors ultimately approves the funding of proposals.

Applicants receive their summary statements approximately two weeks before the Board of Governor's meeting. For those discussed at the in-person panel, this will include all preliminary reviews, a summary of the in-person discussions, and the final average score quartile in comparison with other discussed applications. Applicants that were not discussed will only receive the preliminary review comments. Proposals that are being recommended for funding at a Board of Governor's Meeting will get notification of this one day prior to the meeting.

Progress/Success of the Program to Date

PCORI is supported through a trust fund covering the period 2012–2018. It is not known whether additional funds for PCORI will be made available after 2018. There is the belief that other agencies such as the NIH, the FDA, and private industry will step in and provide resources for PCORnet in the future [11]. Many are concerned that PCORI has not done enough comparative effectiveness research and focused too much on building the infrastructure and methodologies for patient-centered outcomes research. To date, PCORI has spent about half (51%) of its funding on CER and has not made the impact on the healthcare system that was envisioned when it was funded [12]. Several PCORI grants will be completed in the next few years, and the expectation is that they will demonstrate the value of CER and patient engagement. Regardless, the concepts of patient engagement and patient-centered research have been embraced across research programs and funding agencies [11, 13]. PCORI has already had an impact on how we do research today.

References

1. Newhouse R, Barksdale DJ, Miller JA. The patient-centered outcomes research institute. Nurs Res. 2015;64(1):72–7.
2. Booth CM, Tannock F. Randomised controlled trials and population-based observational research: partners in the evolution of medical evidence. Brit J Cancer. 2014;110:551–5.
3. Tricoci P, Allen M, Kramer J, Califf R, Smith S. Scientific evidence underlying the ACC/AHA clinical practice guidelines. J Am Med Assoc. 2009;301:831–41.
4. Fleurence RL, Curtis LH, Califf RM, Platt R, Selby JV, Brown JS. Launching PCORnet, a national patient-centered clinical research network. J Am Med Inform Assoc. 2012;21:578–5825.
5. Institute of Medicine (US). Initial national priorities for comparative effectiveness research. Washington, DC: National Academies Press; 2009.
6. Patient-Centered Outcomes Research Institute. http://www.pcori.org. Accessed 25 July 2016.
7. Patient-Centered Outcomes Research Institute. PCORI funding opportunities. http://www.pcori.org/funding-opportunities. Accessed 25 July 2016.
8. Patient-Centered Outcomes Research Institute. PCORI methodology standards. http://www.pcori.org/research-results/research-methodology/pcori-methodology-standards. Accessed 25 July 2016.
9. Patient-Centered Outcomes Research Institute. What we mean by engagement: engagement in research. http://www.pcori.org/funding-opportunities/what-we-mean-engagement. Accessed 26 June 2016.
10. Forsythe LP, Ellis LE, Edmundson L, Sabharwal R, Rein A, Konopka K, Frank L. Patient and stakeholder engagement in the PCORI pilot projects: description and lessons learned. J Gen Int Med. 2015;31(1):13–21.
11. Vaida B. Patient-centered outcomes research: early evidence from a burgeoning field. Health Affair. 2016;35(4):595–602.
12. Emanuel Z, Spiro T, Huelskoetter T. Re-evaluating the patient-centered outcomes research institute. https://www.americanprogress.org/issues/healthcare/report/2016/05/21/138242/. Accessed 2 June 2016.
13. Selby JV, Forsythe L, Sox HC. Stakeholder-driven comparative effectiveness research: an update from PCORI. JAMA-J Am Med Assoc. 2015;314(21):2235–6.

Chapter 53
Designing Clinical Trials for Quality and Impact: The Department of Veterans Affairs Approach to Developing a Cooperative Study

Grant D. Huang and Domenic J. Reda

Disclaimer: The views expressed in this article are those of the authors and do not necessarily represent the views of the US Department of Veterans Affairs or US Government.

In overseeing the largest integrated healthcare system in the nation, the US Department of Veterans Affairs (VA) has a unique role in advancing evidence-based practice through its clinical trials. With an extensive network of care delivery sites, clinician investigators who also provide care and treatment, and roughly nine million veterans enrolled to receive care [1], VA also supports a national clinical research infrastructure dedicated to designing and conducting multisite clinical trials through its Cooperative Studies Program (CSP). CSP provides VA with a particular ability to conduct a range of trials from early phase studies to comparative effectiveness research to randomized evaluations of facility-administered interventions that address the prevalent diseases and conditions among veterans. Using a quality-driven approach in the conceptualization, design, and execution of its research, CSP studies all have a central focus aimed at changing clinical practice to advance the health and care of veterans and the public.

G.D. Huang (✉)
U.S. Department of Veterans Affairs, Office of Research and Development,
Cooperative Studies Program Central Office, 810 Vermont Ave, NW,
Mail Stop 10P9CS, Washington, DC 20420, USA
e-mail: grant.huang@va.gov

D.J. Reda
Department of Veterans Affairs, Cooperative Studies Program
Coordinating Center (151K), Hines VA Hospital, Building 1,
Room B240, Hines, IL 60141, USA
e-mail: Domenic.Reda@va.gov

© Springer International Publishing AG 2017
K.M.F. Itani and D.J. Reda (eds.), *Clinical Trials Design in Operative and Non Operative Invasive Procedures*, DOI 10.1007/978-3-319-53877-8_53

459

History and Background

The origin of CSP can be traced back to the 1940s, when VA (known then as the Veterans Administration prior to its current status as the Cabinet-level Department of Veterans Affairs) developed and conducted one of the earliest multicenter clinical trials. Driven by the need to care for thousands of veterans returning from World War II with tuberculosis, Drs. John Barnwell and Arthur M. Walker initiated a study to evaluate the efficacy of various drugs in the treatment of this disease, including the antibiotic streptomycin [2]. These efforts were among the first to actively partner clinicians with biostatistical expertise in study planning and design. The results of the study not only revolutionized the treatment for tuberculosis, but also led to the development of an innovative method for testing the effectiveness of new drugs within VA: the multisite cooperative study. It is noteworthy that the British, who are often credited with conducting the first modern-day randomized multisite clinical trial, were partners with VA in this endeavor.

VA later established the Central Neuropsychiatric Research Laboratory at the Perry Point (Maryland) VA medical center in 1955 for conducting cooperative studies in psychiatry. This program emphasized the design and conduct of randomized trials for the treatment of chronic schizophrenia. As the utility of this approach to clinical research gained acceptance, other cooperative groups were formed in the VA, including ones that focused on cardiac surgery and treatment of hypertension.

In 1970, Dr. Edward Freis and colleagues from the VA Cooperative Study Group on Antihypertensive Agents published a landmark study in the *Journal of the American Medical Association (JAMA)* indicating that use of antihypertensive drugs help prevent or delay serious cardiovascular events [3]. Considered as the first multisite randomized clinical trial involving cardiovascular medications [4], it led to a Nobel Prize nomination, Lasker Award, and the formal establishment of the modern-day CSP.

To enable a broader VA capability to design and coordinate multicenter clinical trials, the first CSP Coordinating Centers were set up at Perry Point, MD and West Haven, CT (1972). These centers were supported by the CSP Clinical Research Pharmacy Coordinating Center (CRPCC) which was subsequently created in Washington, DC (1973) to specialize in evaluating novel therapies or new uses of standard treatments. Additional CSP Coordinating Centers were established at the Hines VA medical center in 1974, followed by one at the Palo Alto VA Health Care System (1978), and a fifth in 2003 at the Boston VA medical center. During this time, the CSPCRPCC also relocated to the VA medical center in Albuquerque, NM in 1977. Centers that specialized in population-based epidemiologic research were funded starting in the late 1990s and eventually became the foundation for a larger genetic epidemiology research capability. These centers located at the Boston, Durham, Palo Alto, Seattle, and West Haven VA medical centers work with CSP's DNA Bank at the Palo Alto VA medical center, Biospecimen Repository at the Boston VA medical center and Pharmacogenomics Analysis Laboratory established at the Little Rock VA medical center.

More recently, in 2012, CSP funded selected sites to be primary locations for helping with more efficiently conducting its trials and facilitating greater quality by providing site-level insights into study design and conduct, especially in the area of recruitment. This network of sites, referred to as the Network of Dedicated Enrollment Sites (NODES), is a consortium of VA medical centers that have teams in place dedicated to enabling greater consistency across multiple CSP studies at the facility to enhance overall performance, compliance, and management.

From its outset, CSP has provided a unique national resource that funds multisite clinical trials while augmenting efforts through dedicated biostatistical, data management, project management, pharmacy, budgetary and administrative support for the planning, conduct and analysis of its research. Its emphasis on quality-based standards and adoption of Lean principles has further advanced the ability to develop best practices and innovations that help VA investigators and collaborators to conduct definitive studies that seek to broadly inform clinical practice. Within the larger context of the VA healthcare system, CSP is centrally directed to better enable a perspective on the priorities of clinical questions raised by its health care providers and of utmost importance to VA stakeholders. However, given its resources and capabilities, it can also leverage efforts with other federal and industry partners who share mutual interests.

Submitting A Letter of Intent (Planning Request)

As part of the VA Office of Research and Development, CSP is a division within this intramural funding entity that primarily supports investigator initiated ideas studying veteran-relevant topics within the agency. The CSP process begins with a Letter of Intent (LOI) that is submitted to CSP Central Office by an eligible VA investigator. This LOI is a request for planning support to initiate a multisite clinical trial. The LOI must include the key elements for a clinical trial that are commonly seen in other applications for funding including the clinical question and relevance, hypotheses, interventions, proposed primary outcome(s), and others summarized in Table 53.1. However, from the outset, CSP more heavily focuses on whether the clinical question has potential for changing practice with a rigorously designed trial, the particular relevance to veterans, and if prerequisite information and data are available to proceed with study planning.

After an administrative review by CSP Central Office for appropriateness, the LOI is sent for external review of the scientific/clinical merit and feasibility by independent experts in the field. Based on LOI reviews and recommendations, a decision to dedicate resources toward study planning is made by CSP Central Office. If the LOI is approved for planning, a CSP Coordinating Center (CSPCC) is assigned to assist the study proponent in developing a full proposal for scientific peer review. Directors of the CSPCCs can be contacted prior to this stage to provide

Table 53.1 Components of a VA cooperative study planning request

Objectives of the proposed research
Importance of the study to VA and its patients
Justification for a multisite study and the feasibility of conducting it within VA
Summary of preliminary research and data to support a large-scale evaluation
Proposed study design
Anticipated size of the study
Estimate of study budget
Documentation of qualifications, such as the principal proponent's curriculum vitae and letters of support from the proponent's institutional leadership

some limited methodological support and a review for completeness and clarity before submission of the planning request. In general, earlier input into study design from various stakeholders is encouraged to avoid common pitfalls later [5, 6].

Development and Review of the Study Proposal

After assignment to a CSPCC, the CSPCC Director assigns a study biostatistician and a project manager to the project. The Clinical Research Pharmacy Coordinating Center assigns a research pharmacist if a drug or device is involved. NODES sites may also be included to help with providing site-level insights on any methodologies and/or clinical workflow proposed. The principal proponent and the assigned CSP staff collaborate to form a planning committee that will include other clinical researchers and/or subject matter experts in the area of investigation. Funding support is not provided to the principal proponent during the planning phase as such salary support is part of their overall service and duties to VA. Rather, CSP provides the support of the CSPCC and CRPCC as well as travel funding for face-to-face meetings of the planning committee. Typically, two planning meetings over a 3- to 6-month period are required to develop a full proposal.

Upon completion, the full proposal is submitted for peer review to the Cooperative Studies Scientific Evaluation Committee (CSSEC). This diverse, independent panel of clinicians, research methodologists, and statisticians all have expertise in clinical trials and are charged with evaluating the clinical question, proposed methods, and taking a broader perspective on the proposal's ability to change clinical practice. The review of the proposal is a face-to-face defense which involves an initial blinded set of written critiques as the initial basis for discussions. The principal proponent, study biostatistician, and CSPCC Director meet with CSSEC to respond to points raised in the written reviews. CSP Central Office also participates in the review process to obtain fuller insights into committee questions and concerns. One unique aspect of this process is the need to provide a compelling case and well-designed proposal before a group of experts representing various medical and biostatistical/methodological specialties. Given the committee's experiences and awareness of challenges that are encountered in numerous clinical trials, study teams must more thoroughly consider and address such issues in their submission to be successful. It is presumed that basic requirements for study design and methodology were addressed during planning. Therefore, while such topics are reviewed, others including clinical equipoise, feasibility, appropriateness of outcome measures, ethics, safety and study operations are common targets in review discussions. Such areas are particularly of interest in pragmatic trial proposals. Furthermore, the potential impact of the clinical question is viewed from multiple medical disciplines which help with evaluations on its potential utility for a large healthcare system and not just those more immediately affected by results as often is the case in other scientific review processes that are discipline/specialty specific. After a closed executive session to deliberate on the responsiveness and any additional proposed elements that arose in discussion, CSSEC votes to approve or disapprove the study; approval indicates that the study has met standards for clinical and methodological rigor and should proceed with further consideration by the program. Subsequently, a priority score is assigned to reflect the committee's recommendation to: accept the study as proposed; accept the study with minor revisions; revise and resubmit for further consideration; or, not consider the proposal further. While approval by CSSEC may be given, as a recommendation, it does not ensure funding. Funding will be based, in part, on the priority score assigned and CSP budgetary considerations. A key point to note is that as the funder, CSP Central Office directly solicits and if warranted, discusses any concerns with CSSEC and factors any points into the final decision-making process. The interactive nature of the review also allows proponents to directly hear and understand any concerns or suggestions if a recommendation for revision is made before further consideration of funding.

Study Budget

Veterans Affairs (VA) research funding policies differ from those at the National Institutes of Health (NIH) and other federal sources of funding given the nature of its appropriations from Congress. VA receives separate appropriations for clinical care which include clinical personnel (i.e., study proponents and site investigators) and research activities and related support. Funding for study personnel support can be provided by CSP, such as for a national coordinator at the Study Chair's office and for study coordinators to assist each site principal investigator in the conduct of the trial. The study budget can support the costs of any core laboratories, purchase of the study treatments (such as study drugs and devices) that are not part of standard care, monitoring of the trial and travel to study investigator meetings.

The CSP funding mechanism is not intended to primarily support early phase investigations nor ancillary substudies. VA has other research programs within its Office of Research and Development to support those efforts that may later feed into a CSP clinical trial. Regarding substudies, the recognition that multisite clinical trials can be complex and deserve significant attention by all involved suggest that other activities may hinder the ability to achieve primary objectives and are generally discouraged. In addition, VA investigators can compete for other sources of funding to support those activities, such as NIH and the Department of Defense (DoD).

Funding Sources to Supplement VA CSP Support

VA has a long history of collaboration with other groups with shared interests and has mechanisms to enable and leverage activities into effective partnerships. CSP has partnered with other federal agencies such as the NIH (NINDS, NIAMS, NIDA, NIDDK, NHLBI, NIDCD) and the DoD. It has developed international collaborations with the Canadian Institutes for Health Research, United Kingdom's Medical Research Council and the George Institute (Australia). It has had many successful collaborations with private industry, including conducting registration trials to obtain US Food and Drug Administration (FDA) approval and obtaining unrestricted donations of study drug or devices, or funding to facilitate the conduct of the trial. Additionally, CSP studies can be supported through VA nonprofit research and education foundations affiliated at the CSPCC's VA facility when collaborations involve agreements with external parties to support VA research.

The mechanisms for collaborations have been established through various federal statutes for cooperative research. Collaboration with other federal entities involves developing an Inter-Agency Agreement (IAA) whose authority comes from the Economy Act of 1932 [7]. This allows for transfer of funds from one federal entity to another to support the research activity when it provides a benefit to the government. As a full-scale clinical research program, CSP provides efficiencies to other agencies interested in similar clinical questions that may otherwise require contracts or other requirements typically at greater cost. Partnerships with industry can be pursued through a Cooperative Research and Development Agreement (CRADA) between the industry partner and a VA-affiliated nonprofit research foundation. This mechanism is rooted in the Federal Technology Transfer Act of 1986 [8] and addresses matters related to intellectual property and licensing in addition to data use and publications when there is a potential industry interest in shared activities. To help ensure scientific integrity and remain free of influences that do not prioritize VA interests to veterans and the public, CSP policies promote unrestricted donations if monetary or material contributions are provided. Additionally, CSP CRADAs typically stipulate that an industry partner:

- Does not have a direct decision-making role in final study design
- Does not receive access to data, especially blinded, during the trial
- Does not have editorial control over manuscripts but may receive a copy prior to submission
- Uses data only for internal purposes at end of study (e.g., support FDA submissions); note that under federal statute, federal employees may not be involved in any subsequent activities in representing the company before another federal agency
- Allows CSP to hold the IND/IDE, but it can be transferred at end of study

One example of a collaboration that involved VA, another federal entity, and the private sector was the VA Cooperative Study of Deep Brain Stimulation versus Best Medical Therapy for treatment of Parkinson's disease [9, 10]. NINDS partnered with VA through an Inter-agency Agreement to provide funding support to expand the study to a group of academic medical centers. This allowed enhancement of the generalizability of the trial by increasing the number of women in the trial. In addition, a CRADA was developed with Medtronic, which owns the device used in the trial. This CRADA provided both an unrestricted donation for general support of the trial and targeted funds to conduct a higher level of monitoring in support of Medtronic's application for a labeling change with the FDA.

The principal proponent plays a key role in helping develop these partnerships. They may have contacts at other federal agencies or in industry who may have an interest in the trial. During the planning phase of the trial, they can be a conduit for VA to start discussions regarding potential support of the trial if VA decides to fund the trial. Once a decision to fund the study is made, CSP takes the lead on behalf of VA on development of an IAA or a CRADA while including the principal proponent in the negotiations.

Procedural Trials in the VA Cooperative Studies Program

CSP has supported a number of procedural trials since its inception. The Coronary Artery Bypass Graft trial published its initial findings in the 1970s which indicated that a smaller proportion of patients with angina pectoris and a significant lesion of the left main coronary artery who received surgery died compared to ones randomized to a medical treatment group [11]. Others studies have evaluated components of medical care related to procedures. As one of the earliest studies of its kind, Clarke and colleagues assessed the efficacy of preoperative antibiotics to reduce septic complications of colon operations [12].

The following table lists procedural trials conducted by the CSP that have had primary results published since 2000. These studies highlight a breadth of activities for which surgical or other interventions have been investigated and undergone the processes described previously (see Table 53.2).

Table 53.2 Recent cooperative studies of procedures

Study	Primary author	Year published
Outcomes 15 years after valve replacement with a mechanical versus a bioprosthetic valve [13]	Hammermeister	2000
Effect of epidural anesthesia and analgesia on perioperative outcome [14]	Park	2001
Long-term outcome of medical and surgical therapies for gastroesophageal reflux disease [15]	Spechler	2001
One-time screening for colorectal cancer with combined fecal occult blood testing and examination of the distal colon [16]	Lieberman	2001
Immediate repair compared with surveillance of small abdominal aortic aneurysms [17]	Lederle	2002
Rupture rate of large abdominal aortic aneurysms in patients refusing or unfit for elective repair [18]	Lederle	2002
A comparison of anterior chamber and posterior chamber intraocular lenses after vitreous presentation during cataract surgery [19]	Collins	2003
Long-term patency of saphenous vein and left internal mammary artery grafts after coronary artery bypass surgery [20]	Goldman	2004
Coronary artery revascularization before elective major vascular surgery [21]	McFalls	2004
Open mesh versus laparoscopic mesh repair of inguinal hernia [22]	Neumayer	2004
Reduction of iron stores and cardiovascular outcomes in patients with peripheral arterial disease [23]	Zacharski	2007
Optimal medical therapy with or without PCI for stable coronary disease [24]	Boden	2007
Chemotherapy after prostatectomy, a phase III randomized study of prostatectomy versus prostatectomy with adjuvant docetaxel for patients with high-risk, localized prostate cancer [25]	Montgomery	2008
Bilateral deep brain stimulation versus best medical therapy for patients with advanced Parkinson's disease [9]	Weaver	2009
On-pump versus off-pump coronary artery bypass surgery [26]	Shroyer	2009
Outcomes following endovascular versus open repair of abdominal aortic aneurysm [27]	Lederle	2009
Pallidal versus subthalamic deep brain stimulation for Parkinson's disease [10]	Follett	2010
Radial artery grafts versus saphenous vein grafts in coronary artery bypass surgery [28]	Goldman	2011
Radical prostatectomy versus observation for localized prostate cancer [29]	Wilt	2012
Percutaneous coronary intervention versus coronary bypass surgery in US veterans with diabetes [30]	Kamalesh	2013

Incorporating Quality into CSP Clinical Trials

While the ability to conduct definitive multisite trials has been demonstrated over its history, CSP has adopted a quality-based framework to enable continual improvement with key activities that promote efficiency, effectiveness, safety, and innovation in its research. CSP quality efforts extend beyond traditional targets in clinical trials related to human subjects protections and data integrity [31]. As the second federal agency to have received the President's Malcolm Baldrige National Quality Award, CSP sees quality as a top priority to its commitment to veterans and stakeholders in all facets of clinical research. International Organization of Standards (ISO) 9001 criteria are used to promote the ability for external validation of its quality program beyond ones set forth by FDA and other groups with a more direct focus on clinical trials. To date, it is believed that CSP is the only federal clinical research program to have all of its clinical trial coordinating centers attain ISO 9001 registration. Other activities centered on enhancing the quality of CSP clinical trials include requirements for adhering to Good Clinical Practices, a risk-based monitoring program to earlier identify potential areas of concern in the conduct of a trial, and promoting Quality by Design principles put forth by the Clinical Trials Transformation Initiative [32].

In addition to these efforts, CSP expects its study chairs and site investigators to also be part of the program's quality culture. The intent is not to have quality be seen as a set of activities to be completed. Rather, active promotion and reinforcement of procedures, practices and principles are to be a central part of everyone's responsibilities in the conduct of a VA Cooperative Study. To help with such directions, CSP Central Office discusses these points during planning and again prior to an announcement of funding for a CSP trial. CSP centers help provide details on any specific policies and procedures throughout the study and work with the study chair's office to identify optimal strategies to facilitate efforts for individuals who are not as familiar with concepts and cultural contexts. Successes can be measured not only in a safe and effective completion of a trial, but in the ability to develop and disseminate best practices for future studies.

Conclusion

CSP has a record of advancing evidence-based practice through rigorously conducted multisite clinical trials. As a mission-driven organization, its goals for doing clinical trials go beyond completing trials and publishing results. Rather, conducting clinical trials within the VA healthcare system is seen to serve an important contribution to enabling veterans and the public to have the best standards of care. Investigators seeking to evaluate procedural interventions should be aware of this larger context and can benefit from many foundational VA activities in the field. Furthermore, as part of a large federal agency, CSP recognizes a responsibility to the national clinical trials enterprise. In seeking to achieve high standards in clinical trial development, CSP also continues to pursue innovative approaches for designing and executing trials aimed generating evidence for transforming clinical practice.

References

1. National Center for Veterans Analysis and Statistics. Department of Veterans Affairs Statistics at a Glance. U.S. Department of Veterans Affairs: Washington, D.C. Accessed at https://www.va.gov/vetdata/docs/Quickfacts/Homepage_slideshow_06_04_16.pdf on 29 Dec 2016.
2. Barnwell JB, Bunn PA, Walker AM. The effect of streptomycin upon pulmonary tuberculosis: preliminary report of a Coöperative study of two hundred and twenty-three patients by the Army, Navy and veterans administration. Am Rev Tuberc. 1947;56:485–507.
3. Veterans Administration Cooperative Study Group on Antihypertensive Agents. Effects of treatment on morbidity and hypertension. II. Results in patients with diastolic blood pressure averaging 90 through 114 millimeters of mercury. JAMA. 1970;213:1143–52.
4. Frolich E. In memoriam: Edward D. Freis, MD (1912–2005). Hypertension. 2005;45:825–7.
5. Vickers AJ. Clinical trials in crisis: four simple methodological fixes. Clin Trials. 2014;11 (6):615–21.
6. Institute of Medicine (US) Forum on Drug Discovery, Development, and Translation. Transforming Clinical Research in the United States: Challenges and Opportunities: Workshop Summary. Washington (DC): National Academies Press (US); 2010.
7. U.S.C. §1535.
8. U.S.C. § 3710a, et seq.
9. Weaver FM, Follett K, Stern M, Hur K, Harris C, Marks WJ Jr, Rothlind J, Sagher O, Reda D, Moy CS, Pahwa R, Burchiel K, Hogarth P, Lai EC, Duda JE, Holloway K, Samii A, Horn S, Bronstein J, Stoner G, Heemskerk J, Huang GD, CSP 468 Study Group. Bilateral deep brain stimulation vs best medical therapy for patients with advanced Parkinson disease: a randomized controlled trial. JAMA. 2009;301(1):63–73.
10. Follett KA, Weaver FM, Stern M, Hur K, Harris CL, Luo P, Marks WJ Jr, Rothlind J, Sagher O, Moy C, Pahwa R, Burchiel K, Hogarth P, Lai EC, Duda JE, Holloway K, Samii A, Horn S, Bronstein JM, Stoner G, Starr PA, Simpson R, Baltuch G, De Salles A, Huang GD, Reda DJ, CSP 468 Study Group. Pallidal versus subthalamic deep-brain stimulation for Parkinson's disease. N Engl J Med. 2010;362(22):2077–91.
11. Takaro T, Hultgren HN, Lipton MJ, Detre KM, et al. The VA cooperative randomized study of surgery for coronary arterial occlusive disease. II. Subgroup with significant left main lesions. Circulation 1976;54(Suppl 3):III-107–17.
12. Clarke JS, Condon RE, Bartlett JG, Gorbach SL, Nichols RL, Ochi S. Preoperative oral antibiotics reduce septic complications of colon operations: results of prospective, randomized, double-blind clinical study. Ann Surg. 1977;186(3):251–9.
13. Hammermeister K, Sethi GK, Henderson WG, Grover FL, Oprian C, Rahimtoola SH. Outcomes 15 years after valve replacement with a mechanical versus a bioprosthetic valve: final report of the veterans affairs randomized trial. J Am Coll Cardiol. 2000;36(4):1152–8.
14. Park WY, Thompson JS, Lee KK. Effect of epidural anesthesia and analgesia on perioperative outcome: a randomized, controlled veterans affairs cooperative study. Ann Surg. 2001;234 (4):560–9.
15. Spechler SJ, Lee E, Ahnen D, et al. Long-term outcome of medical and surgical therapies for gastroesophageal reflux disease—follow-up of a randomized controlled trial. JAMA. 2001;285(18):2331–8.

16. Lieberman DA, Weiss DG, Veterans Affairs Cooperative Study Group 380. One-time screening for colorectal cancer with combined fecal occult-blood testing and examination of the distal colon. N Engl J Med. 2001;345(8):555–60.
17. Lederle FA, Wilson SE, Johnson GR, Reinke DB, Littooy FN, Acher CW, Ballard DJ, Messina LM, Gordon IL, Chute EP, Krupski WC, Busuttil SJ, Barone GW, Sparks S, Graham LM, Rapp JH, Makaroun MS, Moneta GL, Cambria RA, Makhoul RG, Eton D, Ansel HJ, Freischlag JA, Bandyk D, Aneurysm Detection and Management Veterans Affairs Cooperative Study Group. Immediate repair compared with surveillance of small abdominal aortic aneurysms. N Engl J Med. 2002;346(19):1437–44.
18. Lederle FA, Johnson GR, Wilson SE, Ballard DJ, Jordan Jr WD, Blebea J, Littooy FN, Freischlag JA, Bandyk D, Rapp JH, Salam AA, Veterans Affairs Cooperative Study #417 Investigators. Rupture rate of large abdominal aortic aneurysms in patients refusing or unfit for elective repair. JAMA. 2002;287(22):2968–72.
19. Collins JF, Gaster RN, Krol WF, Colling CL, Kirk GF, Smith TJ, Department of Veterans Affairs Cooperative Cataract Study. Comparison of anterior chamber and posterior chamber intraocular lenses after vitreous presentation during cataract surgery: the department of veterans affairs cooperative cataract study. Am J Ophthalmol. 2003;136(1):1–9.
20. Goldman S, Zadina K, Moritz T, Ovitt T, Sethi G, Copeland JG, Thottapurathu L, Krasnicka B, Ellis N, Anderson RJ, Henderson W, VA Cooperative Study Group #207/297/364. Long-term patency of saphenous vein and left internal mammary artery grafts after coronary artery bypass surgery: results from a department of veterans affairs cooperative study. J Am Coll Cardiol. 2004;44(11):2149–56.
21. McFalls EO, Ward HB, Moritz TE, Goldman S, Krupski WC, Littooy F, Pierpont G, Santilli S, Rapp J, Hattler B, Shunk K, Jaenicke C, Thottapurathu L, Ellis N, Reda DJ, Henderson WG. Coronary-artery revascularization before elective major vascular surgery. N Engl J Med. 2004;351(27):2795–804.
22. Neumayer L, Giobbie-Hurder A, Jonasson O, Fitzgibbons R Jr, Dunlop D, Gibbs J, Reda D, Henderson W, Veterans Affairs Cooperative Studies Program 456 Investigators. Open mesh versus laparoscopic mesh repair of inguinal hernia. N Engl J Med. 2004;350(18):1819–27.
23. Zacharski LR, Chow BK, Howes PS, Shamayeva G, Baron JA, Dalman RL, Malenka DJ, Ozaki CK, Lavori PW. Reduction of iron stores and cardiovascular outcomes in patients with peripheral arterial disease: a randomized controlled trial. JAMA. 2007;297(6):603–10.
24. Boden WE, O'Rourke RA, Teo KK, Hartigan PM, Maron DJ, Kostuk WJ, Knudtson M, Dada M, Casperson P, Harris CL, Chaitman BR, Shaw L, Gosselin G, Nawaz S, Title LM, Gau G, Blaustein AS, Booth DC, Bates ER, Spertus JA, Berman DS, Mancini GB, Weintraub WS, COURAGE Trial Research Group. Optimal medical therapy with or without PCI for stable coronary disease. N Engl J Med. 2007;356(15):1503–16.
25. Montgomery B, Lavori P, Garzotto M, Lee K, Brophy M, Thaneemit-Chen S, Kelly W, Basler J, Ringer R, Yu W, Whittemore A, Lin DW. Veterans Affairs Cooperative Studies Program study 553: chemotherapy after prostatectomy, a phase III randomized study of prostatectomy versus prostatectomy with adjuvant docetaxel for patients with high-risk, localized prostate cancer. Urology. 2008;72(3):474–80.
26. Shroyer AL, Grover FL, Hattler B, Collins JF, McDonald GO, Kozora E, Lucke JC, Baltz JH, Novitzky D, Veterans Affairs Randomized On/Off Bypass (ROOBY) Study Group. On-pump versus off-pump coronary-artery bypass surgery. N Engl J Med. 2009;361(19):1827–37.
27. Lederle FA, Freischlag JA, Kyriakides TC, Padberg FT Jr, Matsumura JS, Kohler TR, Lin PH, Jean-Claude JM, Cikrit DF, Swanson KM, Peduzzi PN, Open Versus Endovascular Repair (OVER) Veterans Affairs Cooperative Study Group. Outcomes following endovascular vs open repair of abdominal aortic aneurysm: a randomized trial. JAMA. 2009;302 (14):1535–42.
28. Goldman S, Sethi GK, Holman W, Thai H, McFalls E, Ward HB, Kelly RF, Rhenman B, Tobler GH, Bakaeen FG, Huh J, Soltero E, Moursi M, Haime M, Crittenden M, Kasirajan V, Ratliff M, Pett S, Irimpen A, Gunnar W, Thomas D, Fremes S, Moritz T, Reda D, Harrison L, Wagner TH, Wang Y, Planting L, Miller M, Rodriguez Y, Juneman E, Morrison D,

Pierce MK, Kreamer S, Shih MC, Lee K. Radial artery grafts vs saphenous vein grafts in coronary artery bypass surgery: a randomized trial. JAMA. 2011;305(2):167–74.

29. Wilt TJ, Brawer MK, Jones KM, Barry MJ, Aronson WJ, Fox S, Gingrich JR, Wei JT, Gilhooly P, Grob BM, Nsouli I, Iyer P, Cartagena R, Snider G, Roehrborn C, Sharifi R, Blank W, Pandya P, Andriole GL, Culkin D, Wheeler T, Prostate Cancer Intervention versus Observation Trial (PIVOT) Study Group. Radical prostatectomy versus observation for localized prostate cancer. N Engl J Med. 2012;367(3):203–13.

30. Kamalesh M, Sharp TG, Tang XC, Shunk K, Ward HB, Walsh J, King S 3rd, Colling C, Moritz T, Stroupe K, Reda D, VA CARDS Investigators. Percutaneous coronary intervention versus coronary bypass surgery in United States veterans with diabetes. J Am Coll Cardiol. 2013;61(8):808–16.

31. Bhatt A. Quality of clinical trials: a moving target. Perspect Clin Res. 2011;2(4):124–8.

32. Meeker-O Connell A, Glessner C, Behm M, et al. Enhancing clinical evidence by proactively building quality into clinical trials. Clin Trials. 2016;3(4):439–44.

Part XI
Publication

Chapter 54
Publication

J. Michael Gaziano

Introduction

The goal of research is to address a gap in knowledge and to fill that gap with a research product, often the work of many years. Randomized trials fill an important niche in the spectrum of population studies that provide insights into health and disease. Population science has evolved in several phases and randomized trials are a relatively recent addition to the spectrum of study types. They provide the most reliable data on interventions of all types in health care.

Population science began with simple descriptive studies which were mere exercises in counting the cases or deaths. Next, in the preanalytic phase, associations were made by visual observation not involving any sophisticated analysis. For example, John Snow determined that the water supply in London was responsible for a cholera outbreak in the 1850s by mapping cases on a map that happened to have the water supply [1]. The association was made without any sophisticated analysis.

Two events occurred in 1948 that were pivotal in the development of the modern randomized controlled trial (RCT). The analytic phase of epidemiology began with case–control studies, but a shift in the disease paradigm occurred in 1948, when, in a small town in Massachusetts, a group of researchers founded the first large cohort study, the Framingham Heart Study (FHS). This study changed our perspective from thinking about diseases as having a single cause to diseases having multiple factors causing them. These early investigators gave us the term "risk factor" [2]. They were also the first to use logistic regression to address biologic processes

J.M. Gaziano (✉)
Medicine, VA Boston Healthcare System, Brigham and Women's Hospital,
Harvard Medical School, 150 S Huntington Ave, Boston, MA 02130, USA
e-mail: Michael.Gaziano@va.gov

© Springer International Publishing AG 2017
K.M.F. Itani and D.J. Reda (eds.), *Clinical Trials Design in Operative and Non Operative Invasive Procedures*, DOI 10.1007/978-3-319-53877-8_54

using a computer [3]. This concept was important in our understanding the power of randomization as essential for balancing the potentially causative factors that could possibly influence the outcomes of interest.

Another important event occurred in 1948, the first randomized controlled trial. It happened to be a trial funded by the Medical Research Council on the use of streptomycin for the treatment of tuberculosis [4]. A similar trial was conducted in the VA the same year. There had been other nonrandomized noncontrolled trials of other antibiotics, such as penicillin for pneumonia, but the big advance was control using random assignment to minimize selection bias, overt or even subconscious.

The process of developing standards for the conduct of trials evolved over the next decades. Systems for handling randomization and blinding and various quality controls over data collection evolved. The FDA played a key role in defining standards required for assessment of new drugs and devices [5]. Trials have been a mainstay of testing all manners of interventions in health care such as drugs, devices, quality improvement programs, and treatment strategies since those early beginnings.

As many other aspects of this book describe, trials have grown ever larger and more complex, but the conduct of trials has become standardized. A key element of the conduct of any trial is making the results accessible to others. The quality of the trial design and implementation is necessary to interpret the findings. The process by which trials are published has also become standardized [6–8]. In this chapter, I will describe the elements that go into the transparent reporting of trials.

Designing the Trial with Publication in Mind

The process of reporting the results of a trial begins with the design of the trial itself. There are clear design elements that will be required in order to have a trial published in a major peer-reviewed journal. There are key design features that a journal will look for when considering a manuscript for publication. The results of a trial must be judged in the context of the processes put in place at all steps of the conduct of the trial. These must all be included in the manuscript for a transparent assessment of the quality of the trial. These include a well-defined protocol, appropriate regulatory processes, clear trial oversight with appropriate monitoring, trial registration, a well-defined analysis plan, access to the data, as well as a clear plan for reporting the results.

Several journals published their own standard by which each journal would evaluate a manuscript reporting RCT results [9, 10]. There is a need for consistent transparent reporting of trial elements and processes when reporting trial results. In 1996, the first Consolidated Standards of Reporting Trials (CONSORT) document was published establishing guidance that many journals set as requirements for publication [6]. These were updated in 2001 [7] and again in 2010 [7]. These guidelines are a good starting point for understanding what will be required and should be read prior to embarking on the massive efforts of conducting a large-scale trial.

The CONSORT 2010 update contains a valuable checklist of the elements that should be in a trial manuscript [8] (see Fig. 54.1). While many of the guidelines refer to the manuscript, there are several items that refer to some elements of the design that must be considered prior to the conduct of the trial. Among these are the protocol with its analysis plan, trial registration, Institutional Review Board (IRB), and Data Safety Monitoring Board (DSMB) review and funding source.

CONSORT 2010 checklist of information to include when reporting a randomised trial*

Section/Topic	Item No	Checklist item	Reported on page No
Title and abstract			
	1a	Identification as a randomised trial in the title	
	1b	Structured summary of trial design, methods, results, and conclusions (for specific guidance see CONSORT for abstracts)	
Introduction			
Background and	2a	Scientific background and explanation of rationale	
objectives	2b	Specific objectives or hypotheses	
Methods			
Trial design	3a	Description of trial design (such as parallel, factorial) including allocation ratio	
	3b	Important changes to methods after trial commencement (such as eligibility criteria), with reasons	
Participants	4a	Eligibility criteria for participants	
	4b	Settings and locations where the data were collected	
Interventions	5	The interventions for each group with sufficient details to allow replication, including how and when they were actually administered	
Outcomes	6a	Completely defined pre-specified primary and secondary outcome measures, including how and when they were assessed	
	6b	Any changes to trial outcomes after the trial commenced, with reasons	
Sample size	7a	How sample size was determined	
	7b	When applicable, explanation of any interim analyses and stopping guidelines	
Randomisation:			
Sequence	8a	Method used to generate the random allocation sequence	
generation	8b	Type of randomisation; details of any restriction (such as blocking and block size)	
Allocation concealment mechanism	9	Mechanism used to implement the random allocation sequence (such as sequentially numbered containers), describing any steps taken to conceal the sequence until interventions were assigned	
Implementation	10	Who generated the random allocation sequence, who enrolled participants, and who assigned participants to interventions	
Blinding	11a	If done, who was blinded after assignment to interventions (for example, participants, care providers, those assessing outcomes) and how	
	11b	If relevant, description of the similarity of interventions	
Statistical methods	12a	Statistical methods used to compare groups for primary and secondary outcomes	
	12b	Methods for additional analyses, such as subgroup analyses and adjusted analyses	
Results			
Participant flow (a diagram is strongly recommended)	13a	For each group, the numbers of participants who were randomly assigned, received intended treatment, and were analysed for the primary outcome	
	13b	For each group, losses and exclusions after randomisation, together with reasons	
Recruitment	14a	Dates defining the periods of recruitment and follow-up	
	14b	Why the trial ended or was stopped	
Baseline data	15	A table showing baseline demographic and clinical characteristics for each group	
Numbers analysed	16	For each group, number of participants (denominator) included in each analysis and whether the analysis was by original assigned groups	
Outcomes and estimation	17a	For each primary and secondary outcome, results for each group, and the estimated effect size and its precision (such as 95% confidence interval)	
	17b	For binary outcomes, presentation of both absolute and relative effect sizes is recommended	
Ancillary analyses	18	Results of any other analyses performed, including subgroup analyses and adjusted analyses, distinguishing pre-specified from exploratory	
Harms	19	All important harms or unintended effects in each group (for specific guidance see CONSORT for harms)	
Discussion			
Limitations	20	Trial limitations, addressing sources of potential bias, imprecision, and, if relevant, multiplicity of analyses	
Generalisability	21	Generalisability (external validity, applicability) of the trial findings	
Interpretation	22	Interpretation consistent with results, balancing benefits and harms, and considering other relevant evidence	
Other information			
Registration	23	Registration number and name of trial registry	
Protocol	24	Where the full trial protocol can be accessed, if available	
Funding	25	Sources of funding and other support (such as supply of drugs), role of funders	

*We strongly recommend reading this statement in conjunction with the CONSORT 2010 Explanation and Elaboration for important clarifications on all the items. If relevant, we also recommend reading CONSORT extensions for cluster randomised trials, non-inferiority and equivalence trials, non-pharmacological treatments, herbal interventions, and pragmatic trials. Additional extensions are forthcoming: for those and for up to date references relevant to this checklist, see www.consort-statement.org.

Fig. 54.1 CONSORT check list provides information that should be included in the publication of a trial. [Reprinted with permission from Creative Commons Attribution CC BY 2.0]

The basic elements of the trial protocol should be available to the scientific community at the time of publication. Many journals require that it be submitted with the manuscript in order to allow the editors and peer reviewers the opportunity to refer to it during the review process. It may also be requested by scientists who want to refer to the details of the protocol or who may want to replicate the conditions in the trial for a follow-up trial or even use in clinical practice. The protocol lays out the key design elements that will need to be described in the methods. These elements include the study population and its assembly, sites, and their selection if applicable, intervention, outcomes, randomization scheme, analysis plan, power, and sample size. This means the protocol should be written in a format that can be easily read and referred to by others. It is inevitable that there will be changes to a protocol during the course of a large, complex longer term trial. These changes should be well-documented, and the appropriate approvals such as IRB review should also be documented.

The analysis plan is an essential part of the protocol that will be carefully scrutinized by peer reviewers, statistical reviewers, and editors. It will likely also be requested when you submit the manuscript alone or as part of the protocol. This is a part of the protocol that may need to be amended during the course of the trial. However, what an editor or peer reviewer will want to know is whether the analysis plan was finalized prior to any unblinding of the data. The analysis that is presented in the primary report of the RCT should conform to the analysis plan. This is a critical element of trial conduct because the interpretations of the results are predicated on analytic assumptions. Multiple looks at the data and multiple ways to analyze the outcome, for example, will impact the interpretation of the precision of the results. Therefore, well before the datasets are closed and analyses have begun, the analysis plan must be clearly specified so that it can be easily understood by others. The assumptions for power and sample size should be carefully thought out prior to the start of a study and well-documented. Any changes to the study design that impact power should prompt an update on power estimates.

Trial registration is another issue that can impact the publication of a trial such as in http://Clinicaltrials.gov [11]. Trial registration has been established for a number of reasons. It provides a cataloging of ongoing trials that can be queried by clinicians or patients who may want to enroll. It allows researchers in the field to know what trials are underway as new trials are designed. It also provides a resource for those who are pooling trial results to make them aware of trial data that have not yet been published. However, perhaps its main function is for investigators to register the main design elements prior to embarking on a trial. Some journals require that registration occur before recruitment begins, and there may need to be a clear explanation as to why the registration occurred later.

Funding sources must be reported with every manuscript and the role the funding entity played in the conduct of the trial must be clear. This requires clear delineation of these roles, and, thus, a discussion regarding these issues should occur early in the design phase of a trial. Each member of the research team should understand their role in all phases of the trial including the task of drafting the primary manuscript.

Another key element of a trial is all the regulatory requirements that must be met. As a manuscript is written, there will need to be a careful description of all regulatory and ethical issues. IRB approval will need to be described. Major changes that required IRB approval will also need to be addressed. Other ethical considerations such as vulnerable populations and children need to be carefully considered. The role of the DSMB should be spelled out in the protocol or in a DSMB charter. If an event such as early closure was recommended by the DSMB, the reason and justification such as prespecified stopping rules should be included.

Trial Implementation

Once the design considerations described above are in place, it is time to define the elements of the trial implementation that could impact the publication of the results of a trial. There will be inevitable changes to a large-scale, long-term trial. Those with complex aspects and with long duration are most subject to these types of troubleshooting. For example, recruitment might lag behind expected numbers, and adjustments to the inclusion or exclusion criteria may need to me made. Event rates may be less than anticipated thereby diminishing the original power. Loss to follow-up could impact expected person-years of follow-up time or event rates and could introduce bias if the loss to follow-up is nonrandom. Compliance rates may fall short of expectations.

All of these issues must be addressed in a thoughtful way so that there is a clear understanding of the full impact these problems might have on the original intended objectives. It should be noted that these types of issues are not uncommon. In fact, it is expected in large RCTs. The best advice is to clearly document any changes and the rationale behind them as well as the necessary discussions with the IRB and/or DSMB, funding agency, etc., so there is a clear trail of the decision-making process that can be clearly transmitted at the time of publication. It is best to do the documentation in real time rather than waiting until the end of a study when recollecting may be cloudy or when staff have turned over.

Presenting the Data to the World

As the trial is coming to a close, the study team will begin to lay out a thoughtful plan for reporting the results in a timely manner. The various formats where results can be presented include a poster or presentation at a national meeting. Generally, presentations as a poster or oral presentation at a national meeting will not jeopardize publication in a journal. Some journals will consider simultaneous publication either online or if feasible in print at the time of a presentation.

At times, there is a compelling reason to move results into the public realm as soon as possible. A press conference might be considered if a funding agency, such as the NIH, feels there is a justifiable reason to alert the public, patients, or clinicians as soon as possible. Bearing in mind that a press conference might jeopardize publication in a major journal, investigators should consider contacting the journal to inquire about the possibility of simultaneous publication. Many journals will consider this an opportunity for better exposure. It is important to contact the intended journal prior to the press conference. If the data are in a preliminary state, a "preliminary report" can be published with a full complete report to follow.

The next step is organizing the analysis so that it conforms to the analysis plan. The dataset must be completed and closed for analysis. Once this occurs, the investigators can begin analysis with the blinding removed, and envisioning the data tables and figures is an early step that provides the authors insight into the story that will be told.

Considering the right journal for your manuscript is a critical step. Trial results are important to move into publication in a timely manner because they often contribute high-quality data to the totality of evidence on an important topic. Many journals, which are eager to publish trial results, will work with authors to publish in a timely fashion and in conjunction with other presentations if warranted. Many editors will engage in a dialog about the feasibility of simultaneous publication and expedite the review process. However, advanced notice is often necessary to line up all the logistics of reviewing a paper and getting it ready for rapid publication.

Preparing the Manuscript

The CONSORT 2010 statement provides guidance on the key elements of the trial. These are provided in the reproduced statement for item numbers 1a through 25 [7]. The title should indicate that it was a randomized trial and should also include the intervention, outcome, and study population. The title page requirements are journal specific but generally include title, authors, and their affiliations, an address for correspondence, key words, and possibly a funding statement and a structured summary.

Introduction

The introduction should include the background and rationale as well as main objectives of the trial. Begin with the broad problem being addressed. This can be logically followed by the gap in knowledge that is to be addressed, and how the specific objectives and hypotheses being tested in the trial will fill in that gap. Finally, it is useful to describe the innovative aspects and potential clinical implications resulting from the trial. The introduction should be concise, however. Detailed discussions will happen later in the manuscript.

Design and Methods

Much of the design and methods section can be taken from the protocol and synthesized into a much more succinct description of the protocol as implemented. If needed, online documents can provide more detailed information. Start by providing a brief overview of the main design elements. Next define the study population and assembly of the trial cohort including a description of inclusion and exclusion criteria which could also be illustrated in a table. Site selection and management can be briefly described. Next, include a detailed description of the intervention as well as the primary and prespecified secondary end points, including any changes that were made to the main end points. The end point review process should be outlined. The randomization process is a critical element, so specifics are warranted. For instance, what type of blinding was used? Outline a careful discussion of follow-up methods and any challenges with maintaining high follow-up rates. Any changes in any of these components should be described and justified.

Sample size and power considerations give the reader a sense of how to interpret the results. Describe the main assumptions that were used to determine sample size estimation. Were there interim looks at the data or stopping rules that came into play? If the power was lower than expected due to a smaller sample size or fewer outcomes, it may be worth describing the power of the study as implemented.

Describe the analysis plan for the primary and prespecified secondary analyses. How were the groups compared? How was compliance data collected and used in the analysis? Was the primary analysis intention to treat? What sensitivity analyses were undertaken? What subgroup analyses were specified in the analysis plan?

Some studies choose to publish a design paper prior to publishing the main results paper. This can be done quite early in the conduct of the trial or it can be done shortly before the main paper is produced. If the design paper is produced early, it may make sense to wait until it is fully implemented so that early design changes can be included.

Results

The CONSORT recommendations suggest that a "CONSORT" flow diagram be included (Fig. 54.2) [8]. This diagram documents the flow of participants through the recruitment process, to randomization, and then to analysis. It should include loss to follow-up numbers and reasons. In the accompanying text, important dates of recruitment onset and study termination are useful.

Production of the result tables should begin early in the manuscript process. Choices about what tables to include in the final manuscript can come later. A baseline characteristics table divided by treatment group gives the reader an idea of how well randomization worked and describes the key characteristics of the population tested.

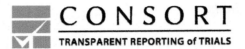

CONSORT 2010 Flow Diagram

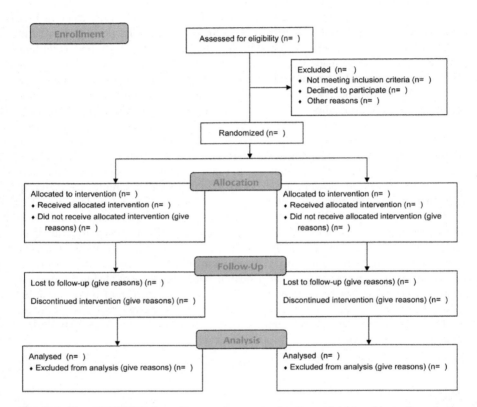

Fig. 54.2 The CONSORT flow diagram documents the flow of trial subjects through the recruitment and follow-up process so the reader can understand which participants are included in and excluded from the main analyses and why. [Reprinted with permission from Creative Commons Attribution CC BY 2.0]

The presentation of the main primary analysis and prespecified secondary analysis is dependent on the analysis plan. However, analyses presented should include specifically how many individuals are represented in a given analysis. Data should generally be presented by groups with main effects reported with the level of precision. About 95% confidence intervals are often used for this.

Data can be presented in a tabular form or as figures. The choice is at the discretion of the author, but figures should not merely duplicate what is in the tables. They should provide informative insights that a table cannot provide. In addition to the main primary and prespecified secondary analysis, information on compliance rates and side effects or harms are often included.

Additional analyses fall into several categories, and there are many ancillary categories that can be included. These include sensitivity analyses, compliance adjustment, subgroup analyses, effect modification, causal models, as well as analysis of secondary outcomes. It is important to make it clear to the reader which analyses were specified in the protocol's analysis plan and which are exploratory. Careful decisions should be made about what to include in the main manuscript, online materials, or for a future manuscript.

Discussion

Some journals provide a structure for the discussion, but most do not. I suggest beginning with a summary of the main findings of the paper. This should be more qualitative than quantitative since the numbers were just presented in the preceding section. It is often useful to follow this with a couple of paragraphs comparing and contrasting results of this trial with those of other similar trials or other relevant studies. Are there mechanistic studies or implications that are relevant? This does not need to be a completely comprehensive review of all the literature on a given topic.

The CONSORT recommendations suggest including a discussion of limitations of the present study, including a discussion of the potential impact that any limitations might have on the main findings [8]. I feel it is equally useful to include a summary of the strengths of your trial. A discussion of generalizability is also recommended. While considerations to insure feasibility and internal validity of the trial results may have led to necessary exclusions, these should be clearly discussed and transparent.

Finally, there should be a concluding section discussing how the results have been interpreted. What are the clinical implications? How do we balance the benefits with risk and harms? What are the cost implications? What are the next steps in terms of more research needed? It is best to let the data speak most loudly. Editors are cautious about over interpretation.

Other Sections

Information about funding and trial registration is generally required. The role of the sponsor should be well delineated. Acknowledgments can be included with degrees and affiliations of those mentioned. References should be formatted according to journal requirements. Journals often have specifications about how tables and figures should be formatted and uploaded. Copyright forms and conflict of interest forms are becoming more standardized [12] but there are still unique features that require careful attention to instructions.

Submission and Interaction with the Journal

All authors should have a meaningful opportunity to participate in the writing or review aspects of the manuscript. This requires coordination of the writing team which may be a subgroup of a large study team. The journals will require meeting the standard requirement for authorship [9].

Once the manuscript is in near final form, the team must begin the process of getting the submission completed. It is very important to read and follow all of the journal's specific requirements. Many submissions are electronic, and instructions are generally well laid out. If there are questions, many journals have staff that can be queried.

Once the paper is submitted, then preparations can be made for the next set of papers and for any public relations issues that should be addressed. Many journals have a public relations office. You may want to also notify the sponsor and your institution about an impending publication and discuss the potential need for contact with various media outlets.

Not all manuscripts are accepted for publication on the first submission, and resubmission of a manuscript is an exercise in diplomacy. There are usually excellent suggestions that will improve the manuscript. However, there also may be a peer review or editor recommendations with which you disagree. If you do not wish to accept a recommendation, a thoughtful explanation is required. Depending on the journal, a discussion with an editor might be possible and helpful.

Rejection should not be taken personally. The major journals publish only a small fraction of submitted papers. Some journals permit a thoughtful appeal while others do not. If you decide to submit to a new journal, the revision of a rejected paper can selectively include the improvements you received from reviewers of your initial submission and with which you agree. It is important to move the paper quickly to the next journal.

Summary

The conduct of trials is a mainstay of testing innovations in health care. They are costly and time-consuming and require extreme attention to detail but provide among the most reliable information about interventions. The publication of a clear, transparent manuscript describing the main design elements and reporting the results of a trial is the responsibility of every trialist. The CONSORT process provides a roadmap for how trials should be published. Discussions are now underway about making data from trials available to editors, reviewers, and possibly the readers. This will be a new consideration that trialists will have to contend with the future.

References

1. Snow J. Mode of communication of cholera. 2nd ed. London: John Churchill; 1855.
2. Kannel WB, Dawber TR, Kagan A, Revotskie N, Stokes JI. Factors of risk in the development of coronary heart disease—six year follow-up experience. The Framingham study. Ann Int Med. 1961;55:33–50.
3. Kahn HA. A method for analyzing longitudinal observations on individuals in the Framingham heart study. In: Goldfield ED, editor. American Statistical Association, Proceedings of the Social Statistics Section, 1961. American Statistical Association: Washington, DC; 1961.
4. Streptomycin in Tuberculosis Trials Committee. Streptomycin treatment of pulmonary tuberculosis. A medical research council investigation. Br Med J. 1948;2(4582):769–82.
5. Food and Drug Administration (FDA). FDA and clinical drug trials: a short history. April 2016. http://www.fda.gov/AboutFDA/WhatWeDo/History/Overviews/ucm304485.htm.
6. Begg C, Cho M, Eastwood S, Horton R, Moher D, Olkin I, et al. Improving the quality of reporting of randomized controlled trials. The CONSORT statement. JAMA. 1996;276:637–9.
7. Moher D, Schulz KF, Altman DG, CONSORT GROUP (Consolidated Standards of Reporting Trials). The CONSORT statement: revised recommendations for improving the quality of reports of parallel-group randomized trials. Ann Int Med. 2001;134:657–62.
8. Schultz KF, Altman DG, Moher D, for the CONSORT Group. CONSORT 2010 statement: updated guidelines for reporting parallel group randomized trials. Ann Intern Med. 2010;152 (11):1–8.
9. A proposal for structured reporting of randomized controlled trials. The Standards of Reporting Trials Group. JAMA. 1994;272:1926–31.
10. Call for comments on a proposal to improve reporting of clinical trials in the biomedical literature. Working group on recommendations for reporting of clinical trials in the biomedical literature. Ann Int Med. 1994;121:894–5.
11. ClinicalTrials.gov. A service of the U.S. National Institutes of Health. https://clinicaltrials.gov/.
12. International Committee of Medical Journal Editors (ICMJE). Defining the Role of Authors and Contributors. 2016. http://www.icmje.org/recommendations/browse/roles-and-responsibilities/defining-the-role-of-authors-and-contributors.html.

Index

Note: Page numbers followed by *f* and *t* indicate figures and tables respectively

A

Abdominal aortic aneurysm (AAA), 159, 160
Accreditation Council for Graduate Medical Education (ACGME), 88
Accuracy, 18
Action to Control Cardiovascular Risk in Diabetes (ACCORD), 46
Active control, 59
Adaptive randomization procedure, 134–135
Adaptive trial designs
  general considerations
    potential advantages, 100
    potential disadvantages, 100
  multi-arm adaptive designs
    adaptive randomization, 102–104
    enrichment designs, 104
    sample size re-estimation and internal pilot designs, 104–106
    sequential group designs, 101–102
Adjudication committee, 283
Advanced statistical methods
  multiple endpoints
    classic multiple testing correction methods, 165
    composite endpoints, 166–167
    Holm's step-down procedure, 164
    sequential testing procedures, 165–166
  site and operator heterogeneity, 170-173
  subgroup analysis
    biomarker-positive subgroup, 169–170
    Bonferroni correction, 169
    clinical/biological reasons, 169
    confirmatory, 168
    confirmatory phase III trials, 169
    exploratory subgroup analyses, 168
    false-negative conclusions, 168
    false-positive conclusions, 168
    parallel subgroup-specific design, 169

  statistical and methodological issues, 169
  types, 168
time-to-event endpoints
  clinical trial, 173
  Cox proportional hazard model, 176
  Kaplan–Meier survival curve, 174–175, 175*f*, 176*t*
  RMST, 176–177
  survival analysis, 174
  types, 174
Agency for Healthcare Research and Quality (AHRQ), 352
American College of Surgeons (ACS), 360
Analysis plan
  developing, 151–153
  operative procedures, studies evaluating effectiveness of
    carpal tunnel syndrome, example, 154
    ITT, 153
    long-term outcome, 154
    repeated measures over time, 154
    short-term outcomes, 154
  operative *vs.* nonoperative comparisons
    ADAM study, 159
    COURAGE study, 159–160
    AAA repair, 160
    TURP, 161
  secondary and supportive analyses
    cost-effectiveness analysis, 156
    interim analyses, 156
    REFLUX trial, 155–156
    safety, 154–155
    subgroups, 154
    supportive analyses, 155
  special considerations and cautions
    D1 *vs.* D2, 157
    learning curve, 157–158
    non-proportional hazards, 157
    PREVENT IV trial, 158–159

CPSIA information can be obtained
at www.ICGtesting.com
Printed in the USA
BVOW07*0244230517
484911BV00001B/10/P